Chemotherapy in Psychiatry

Chemotherapy in Psychiatry

Principles and Practice

REVISED AND ENLARGED EDITION

Ross J. Baldessarini, M.D.

Harvard University Press
Cambridge, Massachusetts, and London, England   1985

This book is printed on acid-free paper, and its binding
materials have been chosen for strength and durability.

Library of Congress Cataloging in Publication Data

Baldessarini, Ross J., 1937–
  Chemotherapy in psychiatry.

  Bibliography: p.
  Includes index.
  1. Mental illness—Chemotherapy.   2. Psychotropic
drugs.   I. Title. [DNLM: 1. Mental Disorders—drug
therapy.   2. Psychopharmacology.   QV 77 B176c]
RC483.B26 1985   616.89'18   85-7635
ISBN 0-674-11383-7 (alk. paper)

In memory of Buck, who lived to see the first edition

Preface

This updated survey of the various categories of psychotropic agents in current clinical use indicates that there are reasonably effective and safe medical treatments for most of the major psychiatric illnesses. Their usefulness is most apparent in the more acute and severe forms of psychiatric illness. Unfortunately, many persistent forms of psychosis, neurosis, and personality disorder respond less well to such medical treatments. Even in syndromes that do respond well to medications, the most efficient and humane use of medical therapies in psychiatry, as in general medicine, requires that applied medical technology be balanced with attention to the patient, family members, and clinician as individuals and as members of a social network. Effective application of psychiatric chemotherapy clearly requires more than recognition of a syndrome and selection of an appropriate agent and dose: personal sensitivity and effective application of more traditional psychological and social aspects of psychiatric care are still needed. The limited efficacy and occasionally serious toxicity of most of the available agents indicate the need to develop better drugs — a need that has existed for many years, since there have been very few fundamentally new agents since the 1950s.

In addition to its revolutionary impact on psychiatric practice, the development of effective chemotherapies has had an important impact on modern academic and theoretical psychiatry. Through the use and study of chemotherapy, psychiatry has come closer to the mainstream of scientific medicine. Biomedical research in psychiatry, though still disappointing in its practical contributions, has gained a new impetus, respect, and influence since the early 1950s. The careful description and critical differentiation of clinical syndromes have become increasingly important in the attempt to understand their biology as well as their psychology, and in matching the right treatment to the individual patient.

This book was developed over several years in seminars on psychopharmacology for students and psychiatric residents and in postgraduate seminars in psychiatry at the Massachusetts General and McLean hospitals. In recent years many reviews and monographs on various aspects of preclinical and clinical psychopharmacology have appeared, most of them technical or highly specialized. The interest expressed in this book by students and colleagues indicates the continuing need for a brief text to complement larger or more specialized monographs, to summarize a mass of information in this field, and particularly to make clinically useful information accessible to students and trainees as well as to clinicians attempting to keep up with this still rapidly developing field.

My aim in this book is to provide a brief but useful overview of principles and currently recommended practices for the clinical use of psychotropic agents in psychiatry and medicine. Some basic preclinical pharmacology is included, since it contributes to well-informed and rational use of medication. It is important to point out, especially for readers in other countries, that the agents and practices represented not only are biased toward those available in the United States, but also are modified in some instances by regional and local practices and personal experience. An attempt has been made to avoid controversial or idiosyncratic practices, and to indicate emerging ideas or usages that remain incompletely investigated or experimental. Occasionally, agents are mentioned because of their special interest or uniqueness, even if they are not currently available in American medicine. Indeed, a serious limitation for an American author in this field is the continued disparity between the much larger number of agents already in routine clinical use abroad and their investigational status or unavailability in the United States.

I should like to thank the following publishers for permission to use previously published material: data in Tables 11, 46, and 47 were derived from W. S. Appleton and J. M. Davis, *Practical Clinical Psychopharmacology* (copyright 1973 and 1980, The Williams & Wilkins Co., Baltimore); Table 28 was reprinted from Dunner et al., *Comprehensive Psychiatry* 18:561, 1977, by permission of Grune & Stratton; Table 57 was adapted from D. Burckhardt et al., *Journal of the American Medical Association* 239:213, 1978 (copyright 1978, American Medical Association); Table 61 was reprinted from M. Keller et al., *Journal of the American Medical Association* 248:1851, 1982 (copyright 1982, American Medical Association); Table 74 was reprinted from N. Klein et al., *Jour-

nal of Clinical Psychopharmacology 2:434, 1982 (copyright 1982, The Williams & Wilkins Co., Baltimore).

This work was partially supported by a Career Research Scientist award from the National Institute of Mental Health (MH-47370). The book was made possible by the research, teaching, and clinical programs of the Mailman Laboratories for Psychiatric Research at McLean Hospital, as well as the clinical and training programs of the McLean and Massachusetts General hospitals and the Department of Psychiatry of Harvard Medical School and the Neuroscience Program of the School. Portions of the material are based on reviews, chapters, and other monographs I have prepared since the appearance of the first edition. The artwork for the figures and chemical formulas in the book was provided by Mrs. Edith Lipinski. Assistance in preparing the manuscript was provided by Mrs. Mila Cason and Mrs. Bea Bradley.

Boston, Massachusetts
March 1985

Contents

Macbeth: How does your patient, doctor?

Doctor: Not so sick, my lord, as she is troubled with thick-coming fantasies, that keep her from her rest.

Macbeth: Cure her of that: Canst thou not minister to a mind diseas'd; pluck from the memory a rooted sorrow; raze out the written troubles of the brain; and with some sweet oblivious antidote cleanse the stuff'd bosom of that perilous stuff which weighs upon the heart?

Doctor: Therein the patient must minister to himself.

—William Shakespeare, *Macbeth*

1

Modern Psychopharmacology and Psychiatric Treatment

Throughout the recorded history of medicine, attempts have been made to utilize chemical or medicinal means to modify abnormal behavior and emotional pain. Alcohol and opiates have been used for centuries not only by physicians and healers but also spontaneously for their soothing or mind-altering effects. Stimulant and hallucinogenic plant products have also been a part of folk practices for centuries. More recently, man has applied modern technology, first to "rediscovering" and purifying many natural products, later to synthesizing and manufacturing their active principles or structural variants with desired effects. Throughout the discussion that follows, the classes of chemicals used for their *psychotropic* effects (altering feelings, thinking, and behavior) will be referred to by the somewhat awkward terms *antipsychotic, antidepressant,* and *antianxiety* agents. This system of terminology grows out of the *allopathic* tradition of modern scientific medicine, which treats with drugs producing effects opposite or antagonistic to those of a given illness.

The modern era of psychopharmacology has been dated from 1949, when the antimanic effects of the lithium ion were discovered, or 1952, when reserpine was isolated and the special properties of chlorpromazine were recognized. The antidepressant monoamine oxidase (MAO) inhibitor iproniazid was also introduced in the early 1950s, and soon thereafter the "tricyclic" antidepressant imipramine. Use of meprobamate began in 1954, and chlordiazepoxide was being developed before 1960 as an antianxiety agent. Thus, by the end of the 1950s, medicine and psychiatry had available therapeutic agents for the major psychoses—including schizophrenia, mania, and severe depression—and the neurotic or anxiety disorders. Remarkably few new kinds of psychiatrically therapeutic agents have come along since that time. The past thirty years have been marked by an accumulation of structural analogues of the earlier agents, with very similar effects, and by considerable gains in understanding the biological and clinical actions of the drugs and their appropriate use.

The impact of modern psychopharmaceuticals on the practice of psychiatry in the 1950s and 1960s has been compared to the impact of the antibiotics on medicine. Quantitatively, the utilization of chlorpromazine compares well with that of penicillin: in the first decade of its availability this antipsychotic drug was given to approximately 50 million patients throughout the world, and some 10,000 scientific papers were written about it. In the 1980s tens of millions of prescriptions for psychoactive agents in the United States account for about 20% of all prescriptions, and are used by about 10% of the entire population. These facts underscore the revolutionary impact of these drugs on clinical as well as theoretical psychiatry.

Prior to the 1950s most severely disturbed psychiatric patients were managed in relatively secluded private or public institutions, usually with locked doors, barred windows, and other physical restraints. The few medical means of managing them included the use of barbiturates, bromides, narcotics, and anticholinergic drugs such as scopolamine for sedation; other treatments were soothing baths and wet packs, "shock" therapies with insulin, atropine, or convulsant drugs, and later electrically induced convulsions, and neurosurgical techniques including prefrontal leucotomy. Since then most of those forms of treatment, except for electroconvulsive treatment (ECT), have virtually disappeared; most locked doors have opened; patients and psychiatric facilities themselves have been returned to "the community," to general hospitals, to open day-hospitals, and to hospital-based or local outpatient clinics. To conclude that modern drugs have been solely responsible for these changes would be a gross exaggeration. In the same period, partly independent changes in the management of psychiatric patients were also beginning; these included the use of group and milieu techniques, an appreciation of the untoward regressive effects of institutions on behavior, and a strongly increased social consciousness throughout medicine, particularly in community psychiatry. A fair conclusion would be that these social and administrative changes and the new drugs had mutually facilitating and enabling effects, which resulted in a melioristic trend toward progress and change.

Statistics emphasizing the important impact of the antipsychotic and antidepressant drugs on hospital practice include the observation that in the United States the number of hospitalized psychiatric patients in public psychiatric facilities reached a peak of close to 0.60 million in 1955, with an initially rapid and now slower downward trend (to about 0.15

million currently), despite an increase in the total population. This change has resulted not only from beneficial effects of the modern drugs but also from policy decisions to alter the pattern of health care delivery, including decisions to reduce the number of available beds in many public institutions. Rates of new admissions and of readmissions have declined less than the potentially misleading decline in prevalence of psychiatric hospitalization; in certain categories, especially among the very young and the very old, new admission rates have remained high or increased since the 1950s, and there continues to be a high turnover rate of hospitalized patients in all categories. Many patients who might formerly have been hospitalized are now kept in "the community," sometimes under conditions of marginal or inadequate adjustment that cause considerable distress to patients and their families. Nevertheless, a large proportion of patients formerly kept in hospitals for many months are now capable of returning to useful and productive lives in weeks or even days thanks to the current philosophy of care combined with the effects of modern chemotherapy.

A number of serious problems remain despite the striking improvements in the management of patients with psychoses. Whereas many acute episodes of psychosis can be interrupted or shortened with modern therapies, and highly disturbed or disorganized behavior is now relatively infrequent even in public mental institutions, the available chemotherapies have severe shortcomings, including limitations of efficacy and problems of toxicity. Many chronic and difficult schizophrenic patients do not respond well to antipsychotic drugs, and the temptation to "do something" by continuing to use these medications indefinitely runs the risk of potentially irreversible neurological toxicity. The antidepressant drugs are not only relatively toxic, potentially lethal, and used in a population at high suicidal risk, but are also slow and clinically unsatisfactory drugs; their efficacy in comparison to placebo has not always been obvious.

An additional complication in the medical treatment of psychiatric disorders is the uncertainty of diagnosis that is characteristic of psychiatry. Diagnosis is more important than ever, especially in order to optimize the chances of a beneficial response to treatment. The advent of modern psychopharmacologic treatments has, perhaps more than any other single factor, contributed to a vigorous renewal of interest in nosology and its ally, psychiatric epidemiology. Since etiology (biological or psychological) in most psychiatric disorders remains unknown, nosology rests on the description of clinical features of syndromes, their course or natural history, their familial associations, their outcome, and their responses to treatment. Despite the fundamentally unsatisfactory basis of psychiatric nosology, and the inescapable contributions of individuality to even the most classic syndromes, diagnosis continues to gain objectivity, coherence, and reliability. Associations between specific clinical syndromes and predictable responses to psychotropic agents continue to support efforts to improve psychiatric classifications. The current standard for psychiatric diagnosis in the United States and in some other countries is the *Diagnostic and Statistical Manual* of the American Psychiatric Association. The World Health Organization has sponsored development of a psychiatric component in its *International Classification of Diseases,* which is commonly followed in Europe and elsewhere. Additional systems of diagnosis and the gathering of clinical information have been developed for specialized research purposes. However, even the best of available systems for research or clinical use require gathering and interpretation of data by and from individual persons, so that subjective and idiosyncratic elements in their application are hard to avoid.

The Development of New Agents

Most of the available psychopharmaceuticals have been developed in one of three basic ways: rediscovering and exploiting a folk usage of a natural product, often with the synthesis of similar molecules with comparable effects (for example, reserpine, opioids, and centrally active sympathomimetics); serendipitous or accidental observation that an agent developed for another purpose has a desirable but unexpected clinical effect (chlorpromazine, the butyrophenones, iproniazid, imipramine, meprobamate, trazodone); or synthesizing and screening structural analogues of known agents or entirely novel compounds (piperazine, phenothiazines, thioxanthenes, butyrophenones, diphenylbutylpiperidines). One important guiding principle that underlies the process of drug development in the psychopharmaceutical industry is the profit motive: psychoactive compounds represent tens of millions of prescriptions and hundreds of millions of dollars annually in this country alone. There is a tendency to rediscover only slightly altered old drugs, owing partly to a desire to break into a highly profitable market and partly to the limited possibility of predicting structure-activity relationships in new molecules. There is also a fundamental limitation to developing novel agents on a fully rational, scientific basis because of the lack of knowledge of biological bases of most major mental illnesses, which remain idiopathic.

The current procedure for developing new agents in the United States is established by tradition and by the regulations of the U.S. Food and Drug Administration (FDA); similar procedures are followed in many other countries. Once the potential clinical usefulness of a new molecule is suspected, initial animal experimentation is conducted to establish its spectrum of activities and, more important, to evaluate its toxicity and gain a preliminary estimate of the *therapeutic index* (ratio of lethal or toxic dose to dose producing a desired effect). Next, the evaluation of the new agent proceeds along several paths: basic pharmacology is studied in pharmaceutical research institutes or in universities, and human studies are initiated, usually by a pharmaceutical company. The first phase of human experimentation (phase I) involves toxicologic studies in healthy human volunteers. If these are successful, preliminary clinical trials are begun in selected patients under rigorously supervised conditions (phase II). If the initial trials suggest that an agent has desirable effects and little toxicity, broader trials are permitted under more realistic clinical conditions by a number of cooperating investigators, usually located in public institutions or teaching hospitals (phase III). If all of these phases are successful, the drug can be licensed for general use. An important additional phase of development ("after-marketing" or "phase IV") is the refinement of clinical usage based on accumulated experience. In this phase, dosage schedules may be modified and indications are often broadened; increasing knowledge of the actions, distribution and metabolism, and toxicology of the new agent modify clinical practice.

The preclinical phase of drug development, which involves screening of whole-animal or isolated tissue or biochemical responses as predictors of clinical activities, has become something of a scientific subspecialty within psychopharmacology. The simplest animal tests entail measurement of vital signs and rating of behavioral or neurological signs (such as activity, sleep, coordination, grooming, reflexes, muscle tone, posture, defecation, simple social interactions, or aggression). More precise tests include objective measurement of selected aspects of behavior (such as electrical or mechanical measurements of locomotion, coordination tests based on the ability to remain on a rod or screen placed at various angles, the occurrence of catalepsy, or the ability to survive various stresses). A number of indirect tests involve potentiating or antagonizing effects of relatively familiar, standard test substances (such as classical sedatives, stimulants, or neurotoxins); changes in seizure threshold; antagonism of vomiting, stereotyped gnawing, or other movements induced by apomorphine, the dopamine agonist; ability to reverse the syndrome of sedation, hypothermia, hypotension, miosis, and ptosis induced by reserpine, or to potentiate drugs known to reverse this syndrome, such as L-dopa, which may be stimulant or mood-elevating. In addition, conditioning paradigms are commonly applied to the evaluation of potential psychotropic agents: passive or active avoidance or escape behavior, classically conditioned escape behaviors or autonomic responses, operant or instrumental conditioning with positive or negative reinforcement, "experimental neurosis" induced by conflicted or ambiguous contingencies, and the orienting or startle response to a novel stimulus. With the striking progress in biochemical psychopharmacology in the past decade have come many in vitro laboratory methods to assess interactions of new agents with neurotransmitter metabolism, enzymes, and receptors or binding sites. Although such tests have usually been developed on the basis of rather obvious, or at least theoretical, relationships between the behavior measured and the clinical effect desired (*modeling*), in fact they are useful to the extent that drugs with known clinical effects produce consistent changes in the tests (*isomorphism*).

Once a new agent is found to have behavioral efficacy in animal screening tests and minimal toxicity in animals or human volunteers, clinical trials must demonstrate or deny the predicted efficacy of the drug. Again, a subdiscipline within psychopharmacology has emerged in the past three decades to manage the design, conduct, and evaluation of drug trials. The rigorous application of certain accepted scientific principles in phase II trials is essential to provide a convincing and objective demonstration of the efficacy of a new drug, and this is also desirable, though not always possible, in phase III. A general appreciation of these principles is necessary for a critical appraisal of this aspect of the literature of clinical psychopharmacology, which is frankly uneven in quality.

The most obvious requirement is that a study have clearly defined and diagnostically homogeneous subjects in sufficient number (N) to permit confidence in the results. Sometimes a large N can work against the investigator if the group under study is very heterogeneous or the condition under study is highly variable over time; the result may be a tendency for the data to regress to the mean, with a false-negative (type II, or beta-error) interpretation of the results: no specific benefit of a truly effective drug compared with placebo or another drug. (This same phenomenon can also complicate the design and interpretation of metabolic experiments that seek to define unique biological characteristics of a particular diagnostic category of patients. It is just as much a problem in psychotherapy research as in psychopharmacology.) One way to manage the problem is to utilize a large N with respect to events rather than subjects, that is, to seek an effect more than once in a given subject as by alternating periods of treatment with placebo and active drug when the time course of the changes makes this approach practical. The task of obtaining a sufficient number of patients of a clearly defined diagnostic type is often difficult in psychiatry. One practical, though statistically awkward, approach has been the development of large multicenter collaborative projects such as those coordinated by the National Institute of Mental Health (NIMH) and the Veterans Administration (VA) for the evaluation of antipsychotic and antidepressant drugs. Another important consideration is the natural history of the illness being studied: for example, many acute psychiatric illnesses, especially affective disorders, remit spontaneously within a few months, and beneficial drug effects must be distinguished from spontaneous remissions.

The experimental regimen chosen for a clinical trial should conform to previously established facts concerning the pharmacokinetics, duration, and latency of action of the drug under study. For example, it may not be fair, or safe, to compare chlorpromazine and a lithium salt administered in single daily doses. Also, it would not be reasonable to compare imipramine and ECT after a week, because of the slow onset of effect of the tricyclic antidepressant. In chronically ill populations who may be recruited repeatedly into drug trials, it is important to consider the washout time of a previous agent before a new treatment is started (at least several weeks for most antipsychotic agents). Comparison of equivalent doses of different agents may not be possible until considerable experience with a newer agent has accumulated. For example, early trials of chlorpromazine that used less than 300 mg/day in schizophrenics gave results that were inferior to those of more recent trials employing higher doses. It is also clear that it would not be reasonable to test 300 mg of chlorpromazine against 300 mg of trifluoperazine or against 300 mg of thiothixene (see Table 1). A similar consideration is that the dose-response curves of many agents tend to be biphasic, with benefit increasing to a maximum followed by diminishing gains or even clinical worsening and toxicity with increasing doses. This problem is particularly evident with the tricyclic antidepressants.

Perhaps the most important development in clinical psychopharmacology has been the attempt to exclude or control bias. Bias can enter a clinical drug trial at several levels. There may be bias in the selection and assignment of patients: "sicker" patients may be overly represented in a group predicted to have a "more effective" treatment, and even subtler differences may occur in comparisons of a chemotherapy and a psychosocial therapy. There may also be bias in the taking of drugs: an agent with an unpleasant side effect may appear to be ineffective if patients omit doses. Chemical assay of the concentration, or at least the presence, of a drug in blood or urine represents the only certain means of controlling this artifact. In most careful studies an inert dummy or placebo, identical in appearance to the active drug, is included for comparison in order to control for beneficial effects ("placebo effects") not related to the actions of a drug. Unfortunately, even this strategy may not be adequate if side effects of the drug make the difference obvious to the patients and the observers. In some cases it is possible to design more elaborate placebos, for example, a benzodiazepine to produce sedation and a small amount of atropine to produce anticholinergic effects. It is also a good idea to include in each study of a new agent a drug of proven efficacy for comparison. In most clinical trials it is now routine to arrange the situation so that the patients and the evaluators of their responses are uninformed as to the type or dose of medication (a *double-blind* design); sometimes only the patient is kept unaware (a *single-blind* design), although it is at least as critical that the observers remain objective. The evaluation should be done with one or more standardized "objective instruments," which usually are rating scales extensively tested to establish their reliability. It is not enough to assume reliability, even of a well-standardized scale, and it must be demonstrated repeatedly in each study and with each set of observers.

Despite all these attempts to control bias and other spurious variables, the power of the placebo effect and the closely related observer bias (patients want to get better and doctors want to cure them) may dominate a study and contribute to either the success or the failure of a drug being tested. These effects are so pervasive that the availability of a new treatment may even affect differential diagnosis. For example, there is evidence that the introduction of the phenothiazines was associated with increased diagnosis of schizophrenia relative to affective psychoses, and the advent of lithium salts was associated with a reversal of this trend. It is also clear that enthusiasm for any drug is greatest soon after its introduction. Since it is difficult in practice to conduct a scientifically impeccable clinical trial, and since even an extremely careful single trial cannot provide compelling evidence of the efficacy of a new agent, the accumulation of consistently replicated results in a large number of independent studies is needed.

In the testing of new medications, subtle but crucial ethical problems may arise. Effective treatments now exist for most of the major psychiatric illnesses, and withholding them for purely scientific or academic reasons is not easily justified. To deal with the ethical problem of adequate treatment, an investigator may forgo the scientific luxury of a placebo control group and make comparisons only between a treatment known to be effective and a newer one of probable, but not proven, efficacy. It is increasingly common to compare a standard and a new agent without a placebo condition. The resulting data may permit the conclusion that the two treatments yielded similar results; they do not necessarily prove that the new treatment is effective. Such a design retains the risk of false-positive results if the standard drug does not perform as well as expected. That is, "not different from" is not equivalent to "as good as." Theoretically, too, omission of a placebo group can increase the number of patients and duration of risk of morbidity due to inferior treatment as statistically sufficient data are gathered. It is possible to start an effective treatment as soon as it is clear that a new treatment is either less effective or slower than a previously established treatment. Also available is the "crossover" technique of assigning a patient to more than one treatment, including a placebo in sequence, with perhaps several changes made to increase the number of measurable events. This strategy is generally limited in practice to illnesses that remit and relapse rapidly in a matter of days or weeks. Crossover designs are also open to contamination by residual effects of the preceding treatment. A related problem, which is becoming increasingly evident, is that because of the considerable success of medical treatment of common and typical psychiatric syndromes, many patients who are enlisted as research subjects in academic or research centers present atypical, complex, or treatment-refractory conditions.

The increased difficulty and cost imposed by current standards to prove efficacy and disprove toxicity of new drugs has markedly slowed their rate of development, especially in this country. The difficulties and expense of developing new drugs call for increased cooperation among the pharmaceutical industry, federal regulatory agencies, and academic psychopharmacologists, not only because the rate of development of new and significantly better agents has slowed in the past two decades but also because the shortcomings of existing agents (the toxicity of antipsychotic agents and the ineffectiveness and toxicity of antidepressants) have become increasingly evident.

Biological Hypotheses in Psychiatry

The introduction of relatively effective and selective agents for the treatment of schizophrenic and manic-depressive patients in the 1950s and 1960s encouraged formulation of biological hypotheses of the pathogenesis of these and other major mental illnesses. These were further stimulated by increased knowledge of the actions of the new drugs and of agents that induced or mimicked some features of psychiatric syndromes. For example, an association between depressed mood in some vulnerable persons and the use of reserpine or other antiadrenergic compounds for the treatment of hypertension, as well as between stimulant or mood-elevating effects and sympathomimetic actions of many agents (such as amphetamine, cocaine, L-dopa, or imipramine) led to speculations concerning a possible deficiency of adrenergic synaptic neurotransmission in the brains of patients with major mood disorders. Further, the stimulation of mood or the induction of acute psychosis by stimulant drugs with dopamine-potentiating effects, and the antipsychotic and antimanic actions of the antidopaminergic neuroleptics, encouraged speculation that the function of dopamine as a neurotransmitter in the brain may be excessive in psychotic or manic patients. Alternatives considered included searches for endogenous toxins which, by analogy to natural or synthetic agents with hallucinogenic or psychotoxic actions, might contribute to the cause of some psychoses. Such lines of reasoning led to a "pharmacocentric" approach to the construction of hypotheses in a field that has come to be known as biological psychiatry.

The approach is strongly appealing in its seeming rationality, and it has gained apparent support by studies of the actions of most available antipsychotic or mood-altering agents. Nevertheless, despite extensive efforts for many years, attempts in clinical investigations to document metabolic changes predicted by the new biological hypotheses have not, on balance, provided consistent or compelling corroboration. Simultaneously, genetic studies have suggested that inherited factors contribute only to a portion of risk, but specific genetic defects have not been revealed, and there is much room for environmental or psychological hypotheses as well. The hopes of the 1950s and 1960s for the discovery of clearly defined, genetically determined inborn errors of metabolism to explain major psychiatric disorders have not been realized. On the other hand, such efforts have contributed to a greatly enriched *description* of biological features of acute psychiatric syndromes, as well as encouraging research and adding biological factors to aid in defining clinical entities.

It may be that the lack of solid clinical metabolic findings to support biological hypotheses based on the actions of drugs arises not from the technical shortcomings of modern medical biology but from oversimplifications and false expectations arising from pharmacology. It was commonly hoped that improved understanding of the actions of psychotropic agents would lead, more or less directly, to the discovery of fundamental pathophysiologic or even etiologic abnormalities in psychiatric patients. Furthermore, it was expected that such changes would be, in some way, opposite to the effects of the drugs that ameliorated symptoms of conditions such as schizophrenia or major affective disorders. This speculation has not proved to be the case. One difficulty is that the actions of psychotropic agents remain elusive. Typically, their immediate effects, many of which have been appreciated for twenty years, are dissimilar or even opposite to later effects, which may be more pertinent to the clinical situation. However, more fundamental limitations may be at work.

The antipsychotic, antimanic, and antidepressant drugs have effects on brain mechanisms that underlie the regulation of consciousness, arousal, activity, mood, and autonomic functions. It is not unreasonable to suppose that modification of such mechanisms by drugs might have important behavioral consequences and useful clinical effects regardless of the nature or cause of the mental disorder so treated. There are many examples in general medicine of agents with powerful clinical benefits whose pharmacology is not likely to have led directly to the etiology of the illness treated (examples include the effects of antipyretics in infections, and the effects of diuretics in congestive heart failure). A related issue is that the seeming similarity of actions of agents within a given class of psychotropic drugs is not necessarily a clue to effects that are either necessary or sufficient to improve the conditions for which they are used clinically. Such similarity is more likely a feature of the highly conservative and repetitive nature of drug development, in which new agents are found largely by imitation of molecular structures or actions of earlier agents of a similar type. Moreover, it is important to realize that most psychotropic agents are not highly syndrome-specific. Antipsychotic agents, for example, are effective in schizophrenia, but also at least as effective in mania and many organic mental disorders. Additional problems for biological studies arising from psychopharmacology include the almost certain biological heterogeneity of even the most carefully diagnosed groups of patients, and technical difficulties in conducting metabolic studies in conditions that may change profoundly over short periods of time. Ironically, one of the most common technical problems arises from the fact that the prevalent use of psychotropic drugs may induce complex artifactual changes in tissue metabolism that are not easily reversed.

Despite the conceptual and technical limitations of a pharmacocentric biological psychiatry, there have been many advances and gains in the past generation. A fundamental gain has been strong general encouragement of all forms of research in psychiatry, the development of a cadre of well-trained scientific investigators, and support for objective and critical appraisal of information and an experimental philosophy. Pharmacological and allied biological investigations have strongly supported a worldwide renaissance of interest in psychiatric nosology, epidemiology, genetics, and experimental therapeutics. These efforts have led to sophisticated research techniques and improved methods of classification and assessment. In short, psychiatry has drawn closer to the mainstream of modern medicine. At present, the available information does not permit a conclusion as to whether discrete biological lesions are a crucial basis of the major, idiopathic psychiatric disorders not associated with coarse brain lesions or intoxications. Indeed, it is not necessary to presume that such a biological basis is at work in order to provide effective medical treatment of psychiatric patients. Moreover, it would be clinical folly to underestimate the importance of psychological and social factors in the manifestations of mental illnesses or to overlook individualized, psychological aspects of the conduct of medical treatments and the overall care of psychiatric patients.

Summary

The development of modern psychopharmacology has had a striking impact on psychiatry in the second half of the twentieth century. Effective and relatively safe medical treatments are now available for most of the major psychiatric disorders. These treatments have had beneficial interactions with changes in the philosophy and administration of health care delivery programs and have contributed to a decreasing importance of prolonged hospitalization. In addition, the development of psychopharmacology has contributed to a heightened awareness of the medical and scientific traditions of psychiatry and encouraged a greater reliance on preclinical and clinical experimental studies of diagnosis, epidemiology, pathophysiology, and treatment, especially of the psychoses and severe mood disorders. The scientific design and conduct of objective controlled clinical trials of new drugs in psychiatry have become increasingly sophisticated and serve as a model for other medical specialties. An important limitation to the discovery of new agents is that many of the preclinical methods for screening compounds with potentially useful effects have led to the discovery of more compounds with previously known effects and toxic actions. Drug development remains highly empirical and remarkably conservative. Progress is hampered by a lack of knowledge of biological causes or of precise pathophysiologic bases of the major mental disorders, most of which remain idiopathic. The partial success of older treatments contributes further to the problem of testing new agents, in part because of ethically based compromises in the design of drug trials, and partly because of an apparently increasing proportion of atypical patients available for study.

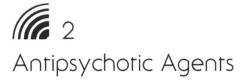 2

Antipsychotic Agents

Antipsychotic agents include a large number of compounds proven effective in the management of a broad range of psychotic symptoms and found to be particularly useful in the treatment of schizophrenia and mania. Nearly all of the currently available agents produce a variety of neurological effects in animals and in patients, and there has been considerable speculation that the extrapyramidal effects of these drugs may be necessary and even desirable. Psychopharmacologists have been so struck by the regular association between antipsychotic effects and extrapyramidal effects that they have suggested the term *neuroleptic* ("affecting the nervous system," but, essentially, producing signs of neurological disorder) for this class of drugs. The preclinical screening of new agents in this class has depended almost entirely on the observation of altered posture and movement in animals. Although this manner of developing new agents has had practical advantages, it may have retarded the search for agents that have antipsychotic effects without neurological side effects. The description of at least one agent (clozapine) that may have such desirable properties supports the conclusion that the more general and hopeful term *antipsychotic* is to be preferred while the search for drugs lacking neurological toxicity is pursued.

The earliest antipsychotic drugs were the phenothiazines and the *Rauwolfia* alkaloids, notably reserpine (1952–1953), although the usefulness of lithium salts for the management of excited or manic patients had been described earlier (1949). The first antipsychotic phenothiazine, chlorpromazine, was developed by the Rhône-Poulenc Laboratories in France. The phenothiazine nucleus had been synthesized late in the nineteenth century with the development of such aniline dyes as methylene blue (1876). The history of the study of these dyestuffs is intimately related to the early development by Paul Ehrlich and others of the theory of specific drug-tissue interactions — a cornerstone of general pharmacology. Like several of the thionine dyes, phenothiazine itself was for a time used clinically as an antimicrobial agent. In the late 1930s a phenothiazine derivative, promethazine (Phenergan), was noted to have antihistaminic and sedative properties by Paul Charpentier at the Rhône-Poulenc Laboratories, and it was in the hope of finding molecules with similar properties that chlorpromazine was developed. Antihistaminic sedative agents had been given to agitated psychotic patients in the 1940s with little benefit, so the eventual success of chlorpromazine was unexpected. Chlorpromazine was first tried clinically in 1951 as a preanesthetic sedative by the French surgeon Henri Laborit, who described some of its peculiar effects on behavior ("artificial hibernation"); these included retention of consciousness associated with striking indifference to the surroundings. In 1951–1952 in Paris, several psychiatrists noted the ability of the new agent to increase the efficacy with which barbiturates sedated manic and other psychotic patients. In 1952–1953 Jean Delay and Pierre Deniker reported further experience with the new agent used alone in psychiatric patients in Paris. The drug was given as early as 1954 in the United States, where at first its unique usefulness in psychosis was not appreciated, although it was used as an antiemetic, sedative, and hypothermic agent. Many pharmaceutical companies then rapidly developed chemically analogous compounds, and by the 1960s, prototypes of most of the classes of antipsychotic agents currently in use were known.

Pharmacology

Types of Molecules with Antipsychotic Effects

Nearly 20 phenothiazines have reached the state of clinical application since the introduction of chlorpromazine (Figure 1; see Table 1). The term *phenothiazine* should not be used loosely as a synonym for *antipsychotic agent;* it refers only to those compounds containing a tricyclic nucleus of two benzene rings (*pheno*), joined through a central ring containing a sulfur atom (*thio*) and a nitrogen atom (*azo*), to which is attached a carbon side chain terminating in either a tertiary amine or a cyclic structural analogue of a tertiary amine. The several types of phenothiazines differ in the nature of the side chain. The terminal amine moiety may have methyl or other alkyl substituents with a straight chain of carbon atoms (*aliphatic* or *aminoalkyl* phenothiazines, such as chlorpro-

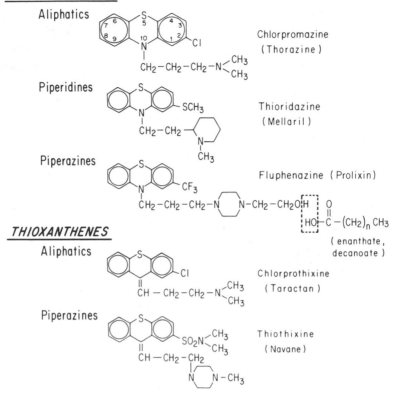

Figure 1 Chemical structures of tricyclic antipsychotic agents.

BUTYROPHENONES (PHENYLBUTYLPIPERIDINES)

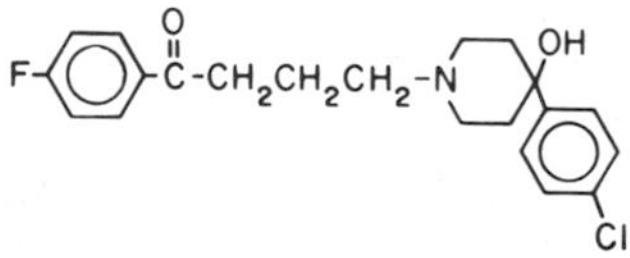

Haloperidol (Haldol)

DIPHENYLBUTYLPIPERIDINES

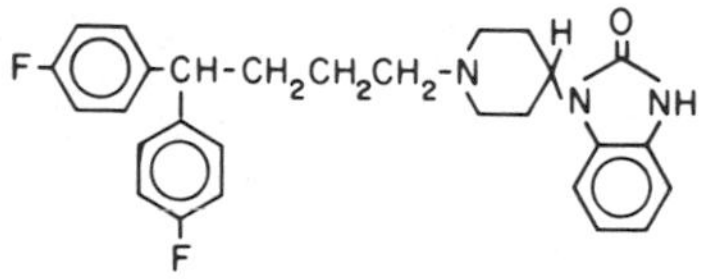

Pimozide (Orap)

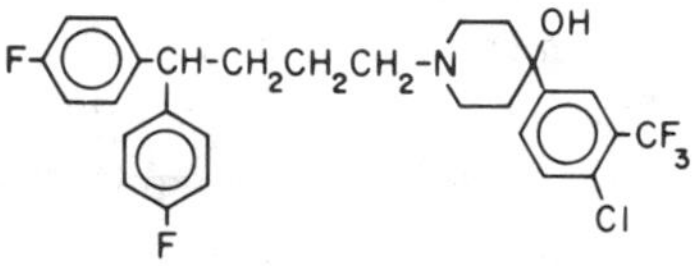

Penfluridol

INDOLIC COMPOUNDS

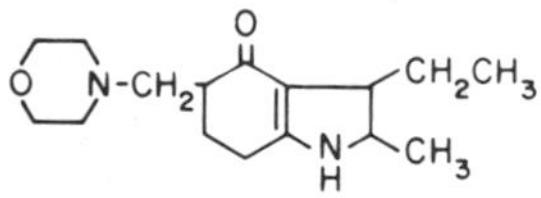

Molindone (Moban)

BENZAMIDES

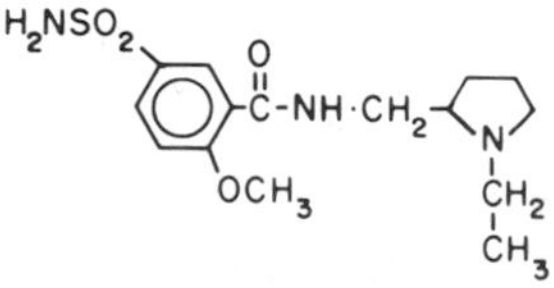

Sulpiride (Dogmatil)

AMINE-DEPLETING AGENTS

Rauwolfia Alkaloids

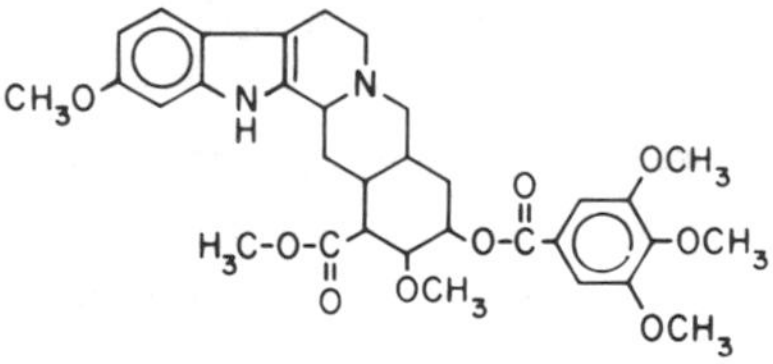

Reserpine (Serpasil)

Benzoquinolizines

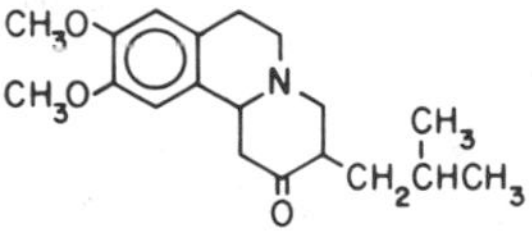

Tetrabenazine (Nitoman)

Figure 2 Chemical structures of other antipsychotic drugs.

mazine, triflupromazine, and promazine); or it may incorporate the amino nitrogen atom into a cyclic structure, as in the *piperidine* derivatives (such as thioridazine and mesoridazine) and the potent *piperazine* derivatives (such as trifluoperazine, perphenazine, and fluphenazine). The tricyclic core of the molecules was also altered, without loss of antipsychotic effects, first by replacing the nitrogen atom of the central ring with a carbon atom but leaving the sulfur atom. Since this type of molecule was a sulfur-containing (*thio*) structural analogue of xanthene, which contains an oxygen atom in the central ring (not to be confused with the *xanthine* alkaloids, including caffeine and theophylline), the drugs were designated *thioxanthenes* and became the first nonphenothiazine antipsychotic agents. The thioxanthenes also include molecules with side chains of the aliphatic type (for example, chlorprothixene) and several potent piperazines (for example, thiothixene). Further experimentation with the tricyclic structure has resulted in other variants of the phenothiazines, notably the still-experimental *acridanes,* which are similar to the acridine dyes and have a nitrogen atom in the central ring but no sulfur atom.

The general rules of structure-activity relationships among these tricyclic antipsychotic agents include the requirement for a side chain of three carbon atoms (at position 10) separating the amino nitrogen atom from the central ring. The addition of an electronegative substituent in position 2 (such as Cl, CF_3, or SCH_3) generally increases the efficacy of the molecule, possibly by contributing a stereochemical bias to the three-dimensional configuration of the molecule. Substitution of a piperazine group for an aliphatic or piperidine moiety on the side chain generally imparts only markedly increased potency (*not* greater clinical efficacy). Higher potency is generally associated with somewhat less tendency to produce sedation and hypotension but an increased incidence of extrapyramidal reactions.

In 1959 Paul Janssen, in Belgium, while experimenting with derivatives of meperidine (Demerol) in search of a new analgesic, developed the *butyrophenones,* which can also be called *phenylbutylpiperidines* (Figure 2). The only butyrophenone routinely used in the United States as an antipsychotic agent is haloperidol (Haldol). Droperidol (Inapsine) is antipsychotic but also very sedating and short-acting, and is recommended only as an anesthetic agent (although it is sometimes also used in psychiatric emergencies). The butyrophenones share with the piperazine phenothiazines high potency and a strong tendency to affect the extrapyramidal motor system, but haloperidol has much less tendency to produce sedation, hypotension, and anticholinergic effects at ordinarily employed doses.

Several new compounds that are structurally related to the butyro-phenones are undergoing clinical study at the present time. These compounds include the *diphenylbutylpiperidines,* such as pimozide, penfluridol, and fluspiriline (Figure 2). Pimozide is a potent neuroleptic with relatively selective actions at dopamine receptors in the brain. Penfluridol and fluspiriline have relatively prolonged actions for about one week, and penfluridol is long-acting even after oral administration. Except for pimozide (recently released as Orap), these agents remain investigational in the United States even though they have been in long use abroad.

The only other long-acting neuroleptic agents are long-chain aliphatic, fatty-acid esters of standard antipsychotic compounds (Figure 1), notably fluphenazine esters (including the 7-carbon enanthate ester and the somewhat longer-acting 12-carbon decanoate ester, which is currently the most commonly used agent of this type in the United States). These compounds are believed to act as precursors or *prodrugs* of the free, and presumably active, neuroleptic by the action of esterases in plasma and many tissues after slow, secondary release from sites of storage of the ester in body fat and other tissues. At least ten other agents exist as fatty acid esters as well, including other phenothiazines (for example, perphenazine enanthate), thioxanthenes (for example, clopenthixol decanoate), and butyrophenones (for example, haloperidol decanoate). They remain investigational in the United States, although haloperidol decanoate may soon be available. These compounds are useful in the management of chronically psychotic outpatients who are unreliable in taking oral medication, since their effects last from one to four weeks after depot injection in an oily vehicle.

Another class of antipsychotic agents of potentially great importance are the piperazine derivatives of *dibenzazepine* tricyclic molecules (Figure 1). Those with two nitrogen atoms in the central ring are dibenzo*diaz*epines (for example, clozapine and fluperlapine). Loxapine, a dibenz*ox*azepine, has an oxygen atom instead of a second nitrogen atom in the central ring. Metiapine and clothiapine are dibenzo*thia*zepines, with a sulfur atom replacing the same nitrogen atom. Loxapine, metiapine, and clothiapine are typical neuroleptic agents with strong antidopaminergic and extrapyramidal neurological effects, but clozapine and its congeners are *atypical* antipsychotic agents with considerable theoretical and practical importance; they have little extrapyramidal activity and are only weakly antidopaminergic. Clozapine has an uncertain clinical status because of its occasional association with severe depression of bone marrow function. Nevertheless, the discovery of atypical agents of this type supports the hope that other drugs can be developed that will retain desired antipsychotic properties without extrapyramidal reaction.

Another group of experimental agents, the substituted *benzamides* (notably, sulpiride; see Figure 2) are somewhat less likely to induce extrapyramidal side effects, at least at low doses, and may exert clinically useful antipsychotic actions at high doses. Sulpiride is a relatively water-soluble agent that seems to penetrate the blood-brain diffusion barrier with difficulty; high doses are required for clear effects on the brain, while small doses elevate prolactin levels to reflect the fact that the anterior pituitary is outside the blood-brain barrier. On a worldwide basis, it is one of the most commonly prescribed antipsychotic agents, even though it remains experimental in the United States. Another agent of this class, metoclopramide (Reglan), is used in gastroenterology; it has been associated with extrapyramidal toxicity but is not known to be antipsychotic.

Other types of molecules with demonstrated antipsychotic effects include indole derivatives (such as oxypertine and molindone; see Figure 2). A large number of other agents have been evaluated partially but are not yet commercially available. One interesting agent undergoing clinical trials, a tricyclic agent with some structural similarity to phenothiazines but without typical neuroleptic actions, is currently designated BW-234U (*cis*–9–[3–(3,5–dimethyl–1–piperazinyl) propyl] carbazole · 2HCl).

Several alkaloids derived originally from the Indian snakeroot plant *Rauwolfia serpentina* and later synthesized, notably reserpine, rescinnamine, and deserpidine, are known to have antipsychotic actions, and for a short while in the early 1950s there was considerable interest in their clinical effects. Several synthetic polycyclic compounds, such as *tetrabenazine* (Figure 2) and benzquinamide, share with *Rauwolfia* alkaloids an ability to deplete amine stores from cells containing catecholamines and indoleamines, particularly in the brain. Oxypertine also shares with this group some amine-depleting activity. The actions of tetrabenazine are complex and may include some direct, antiadrenergic receptor effects. Although all of these amine-depleting agents have some antipsychotic efficacy, they have not held up well in controlled comparisons with the phenothiazines and other neuroleptics. Their limited efficacy, side effects (especially sedation, hypotension, and marked cholinergic dominance in the gut, with diarrhea) and tendency to induce depression have led to their virtual abandonment for the treatment of psychosis. Although reserpine had been implicated as a possible contributor to risk of breast cancer, this effect seems unlikely in light of more recent epidemiological studies.

Despite its many limitations, reserpine, in much higher doses (5–10 mg/day, or more) than are customary for the treatment of hypertension, can be utilized if side effects or allergic reactions preclude the use of other antipsychotic drugs.

Dose-Effect Relationships

Despite the clinical availability of antipsychotic drugs for more than three decades, there is a striking dearth of quantitative pharmacologic information based on human studies, although a few general principles can be derived from studies in laboratory animals and from the available clinical literature. An adequate dose-response relationship has not been worked out for any antipsychotic drug in man. Some of the best available information is derived from reanalysis of published "success rates" (meaning that a drug is superior to a placebo in overall group response) in studies comparing the antipsychotic effects of chlorpromazine with a placebo. These results suggest that the chance of a study's reporting success was about 60% when less than 300 mg of chlorpromazine was given per day, 80–90% at doses of 300–500 mg, and virtually 100% at doses of 500–800 mg or more. Doses as low as 100 mg/day may be effective in many acutely psychotic or elderly patients, however. The dose-response relationship in man must be very broad since it is usually possible to obtain clinical estimates only of approximately minimum effective doses, whereas maximally effective doses are not known. What can be offered are approximately equivalent doses of antipsychotic agents (Table 1), based on clinical trials and clinical experience over many years. In comparisons of standard recommended doses of potent antipsychotic agents, such as fluphenazine and haloperidol, with doses more than ten times higher, it has not been possible to demonstrate consistently appreciable increases in group success rates, particularly when the comparison was extended for two to three months. Recommended doses are thus usually set above minimum effective doses but low enough to avoid toxicity. There are two important clinical problems in the attempt to establish an ideal dose: the available methods have not provided quantitative evaluation of partial responses, and antipsychotic effects seem to have steep dose-effect curves, or to be virtually all-or-none phenomena and not clearly dose-related, except in the region of a "threshold" dose.

In many early clinical studies of antipsychotic agents, serious problems obscured clinical dose-effect relationships, including the application of broad diagnostic criteria as well as inadequate control of doses and short follow-up periods. In most studies patients were called "schizophrenic,"

Table 1 Approximately equivalent doses of commonly used antipsychotic agents by chemical type

Generic name	Commercial name[a]	Approximate equivalent dose (mg)[b]	Relative potency
Phenothiazines			
Aliphatic			
Chlorpromazine	Thorazine, etc. (generic)	100	Low
Triflupromazine	Vesprin	30	Low
Piperidines			
Mesoridazine	Serentil	50	Low
Thioridazine	Mellaril	90–100	Low
Piperazines			
Acetophenazine	Tindal	15	Intermediate
Perphenazine	Trilafon	10	Intermediate
Trifluoperazine	Stelazine	5	High
Fluphenazine[c]	Prolixin, Permitil	2	High
Thioxanthenes			
Aliphatic			
Chlorprothixene	Taractan	75	Low
Piperazine			
Thiothixene	Navane	3–5	High
Dibenzazepines			
Clozapine	(Leponex, experimental)	150	Low
Loxapine	Loxitane, Daxolin	10–15	Intermediate
Butyrophenones			
Haloperidol[c]	Haldol	2–3	High
Droperidol	Inapsine (for injection)	1–2	High
Diphenylbutylpiperidines			
Penfluridol	(Semap, experimental)	2 (1 week dose)[c]	High
Pimozide[c]	Orap	1–2	High
Indoles			
Molindone	Moban, Lidone	8–10	Intermediate
Rauwolfia			
Reserpine	Serpasil, etc. (generic)	3–5	High

a. Trade names in parentheses are not yet licensed in the United States. Many other agents used elsewhere are not available in the United States. The commercial preparations are available as soluble salts (most are hydrochlorides; Loxitane or Daxolin is a succinate; Tindal is a maleate; Serentil is a benzylate: see Table 2). Other agents that are not commonly but often mixed populations were evaluated. Recent controlled studies of fixed, moderate doses of neuroleptics suggest that an effective dose in acute idiopathic psychoses may be as low as 100–200 mg of chlorpromazine per day or the equivalent. The dose-effect relationship in prolonged treatment aimed at reducing risk of exacerbations of chronic psychotic disorders is even less well studied. Doses below the equivalent of 100 mg/day of chlorpromazine may suffice for many chronically psychotic patients. An evaluation of published reports of the results of treating schizophrenic patients with controlled doses of fluphenazine decanoate for one year indicates that the half-maximally effective dose (ED_{50}) may be only 5 mg/2 weeks, while doses of about 10–25 mg/2 weeks yield apparently optimal results, and higher doses may be associated with an excessive risk of neurological toxicity and inferior clinical outcome (Teicher and Baldessarini, 1985). The poorer results with higher doses may be due in part to nonrandom assignment of sicker patients to the higher doses, but may also reflect the increased risk of extrapyramidal and other neurotoxic effects. Currently recommended doses (Table 2) are set above estimated

---

used now or are less effective in the treatment of psychoses are not included, for example, butaperazine (Repoise), carphenazine (Proketazine), mepazine (Pacatal), promazine (Sparine), piperacetazine (Quide), and thiopropazate (Dartal). Droperidol (Inapsine) is an extremely potent, short-acting neuroleptic, now used mainly as a preanesthetic or coanesthetic agent intramuscularly or intravenously, although it has powerful antipsychotic-sedative effects that might also be useful in psychiatric emergencies. Pimozide (Orap) is a potent diphenylbutylpiperidine currently recommended only for the Itard-Tourette syndrome. In addition, prochlorperazine (Compazine) and thiethylperazine (Torecan), while having typical neuroleptic (and some antipsychotic) effects, are mainly used as antiemetic agents. Reserpine and other amine-depleting agents are inferior antipsychotic drugs but are sometimes used in the management of tardive dyskinesia. While the other tabulated drugs vary by more than 100-fold in *potency,* they are very similar in their clinical *efficacy.*

b. Data are summarized as averages from several sources, some of which vary greatly. These numbers are only an approximate guide, and dosage for each patient must be established by clinical response. In switching from high doses of one agent to a dissimilar one, it is well to proceed gradually over several days to decrease the risk of side effects from the newly introduced drug. It is also important to realize that these equivalent doses are *not therapeutic doses* (which are typically several times higher).

c. Injectable fluphenazine esters are commonly used in doses of 12.5–50 mg intramuscularly every one to four weeks. The enanthate (derived from a 7-carbon fatty acid) typically acts for two weeks, and the currently more popular decanoate (ester of a 12-carbon carboxylic acid) for about three weeks. As an approximate equivalence, 25 mg (2 ml) of intramuscular fluphenazine decanoate every two to three weeks resembles in effectiveness about 10 mg of fluphenazine HCl (orally) per day (or 500 mg of chlorpromazine). The decanoate ester of haloperidol is also available and is given every 3 or 4 weeks in intramuscular doses of 20 times the daily oral dose. Some long-lasting diphenylbutylpiperidines (experimental in the United States) can be used once weekly; penfluridol can be used at about 2% of a *weekly* dose of chlorpromazine (that is, 40 mg/week can replace 2,100 mg/week of chlorpromazine). Pimozide (Orap) has recently been released in the United States for the treatment of Gilles de la Tourette's syndrome, but is also an effective antipsychotic agent.

Table 2 *Selected antipsychotic drugs: Chemical structures, doses, side effects, and dosage forms*

Phenothiazines — Main Structure

Ring positions 1, 2, 3, 4, 5, 6, 7, 8, 9, 10; N–R_1; R_2 at position 2.

Dosage form key:

Oral: T = tablet (mg), C = capsule (mg), S = syrup, E = elixer, C = concentrate, CS = concentrated suspension

Injection: A = ampule, V = vial, S = syringe

R_1	R_2	Antipsychotic daily dosage — Usual[b] (mg)	Extreme[b] (mg)	Single IM dose[a] (mg)	Sedative	Extrapyramidal	Hypotensive	Oral	Injection
Chlorpromazine HCl (Thorazine)[d] $-(CH_2)_3-N(CH_3)_2$	$-Cl$	300–800	25–2000	25–50	+++	++	IM+++ Oral++	(T) 10, 25, 50, 100, 200; (C) sustained release, 30, 75, 150, 200, 300; (S) 10 mg/5ml; (C) 30 mg/ml, 100 mg/ml[c]	(A) 25 mg/ml, 50 mg/2ml; (V) 25 mg/ml in 10 ml
Triflupromazine HCl (Vesprin) $-(CH_2)_3-N(CH_3)_2$	$-CF_3$	100–150	25–300	20–50	++	+++	++	(T) 10, 25, 50; (CS) 50 mg/5ml[c]	(V) 10 mg/ml in 10 ml; 20 mg/ml; (S) 10 mg/ml
Mesoridazine besylate (Serentil) $-(CH_2)_2-$ [piperidine] $N-CH_3$	$-SCH_3$ =O	75–300	25–400	25	+++	+	++	(T) 10, 25, 50, 100; (C) 25 mg/ml	(A) 25 mg/ml

Drug	R							Dosage forms
Piperacetazine (Quide) -(CH₂)₃-N⟨⟩(CH₂)₂OH	-COCH₃	20-160	5-200	—	++	++	+	(T) 10, 25
Thioridazine HCl[d] (Mellaril) -(CH₂)₂ ⟨⟩ N-CH₃	-SCH₃	200-600	50-800	—	+++	+	++	(T) 10, 15, 25, 50 100, 150, 200; (C) 30 mg/ml 100 mg/ml (CS; 25 and 100 mg/5 ml[c])
Acetophenazine maleate (Tindal) -(CH₂)₃-N⟨⟩N-(CH₂)₂-OH	-COCH₃	60-120	20-600	—	++	++	+	(T) 20
Fluphenazine HCl enanthate, decancate[a] (Permitil, Prolixin) -(CH₂)₃-N⟨⟩N-(CH₂)₂-OH	-CF₃	25-20	1-30	1.25-2.5 (HCl); 25-50, decanoate or enanthate q. 1-3 wks	+	+++	+++	(T) 0.25, 1, 2.5, 5, 10; (T) sustained release, 1; (C) 5 mg/ml; (E) 2.5 mg/5 ml; (V) 2.5 mg/ml in 10 ml (HCl); (S) 25 mg/ml (esters); (V) 25 mg/ml (esters) in 5 ml
Perphenazine (Trilafon) -(CH₂)₃-N⟨⟩N-(CH₂)₂-OH	-Cl	8-32	4-64	5-10	++	++	+	(T) 2, 4, 8, 16; (T) sustained release, 8; (C) 15 mg/5 ml; (A) 5 mg/ml
Trifluoperazine HCl[d] (Stelazine) -(CH₂)₃-N⟨⟩N-(CH₂)₂-OH	-CF₃	6-20	2-60	1-2	+	+++	+	(T) 1, 2, 5, 10; (C) 10 mg/ml; (V) 2 mg/ml in 10 ml

Table 2 (continued)

Chemical structure		Dose			Side Effects			Dosage forms	
R₁	R₂	Antipsychotic daily dosage		Single IM dose[a] (mg)	Sedative	Extra-pyramidal	Hypo-tensive	Oral	Injection
		Usual[b] (mg)	Extreme[b] (mg)						
Thioxanthenes Main Structure									
Chlorprothixene (Taractan) $CH-(CH_2)_2-N(CH_3)_2$	$-Cl$	50–400	30–600	25–50	+++	++	++	(T) 10, 25, 50, 100 (C) 100 mg/5 ml	(A) 25 mg/2 ml
Thiothixene HCl (Navane) $CH(CH_2)_2-N$⟨piperazine⟩$N-CH_3$	$-SO_2-N\genfrac{}{}{0pt}{}{CH_3}{CH_3}$	6–30	6–60	2–6	+	+++	+	(C) 1, 2, 5, 10, 20[c] (C) 5 mg/ml	(A) 4 mg/2 ml
Other Heterocyclic Compounds Haloperidol (and decanoate)[a] (Haldol)		6–20	2–100	2.5–5	+	+++	+	(T) 0.5, 1.2, 5, 10 (C) 2 mg/ml as the lactate	(A) 5 mg/ml, as the lactate (V) 5 mg/ml, as the lactate, in 10 ml (A) 50 and 100 mg/ml as 70.5 and 141 mg of the decanoate

Drug							
Pimozide[e] (Orap)	2–10	0.5–20	—	+	+++	±	(T)2
Loxapine succinate (Daxolin, Loxitane)	60–100	20–250	12.5–25	++	++	+	(C) 5, 10, 25, 50; (C) 25 mg/ml, as the HCl; (A) 50 mg/ml as the HCl; (V) 50 mg/ml in 10 ml as the HCl
Molindone HCl (Lidone, Moban)	50–225	15–400	—	++	+	0	(T) 5, 10, 25; (C) 5, 10, 25; (C) 20 mg/ml

Note: Side effects are rated as follows: 0, rarely encountered; ±, equivocal but small risk; +, mild; ++, moderate; +++, severe.

a. Except for the ester forms of fluphenazine and haloperidol, dosage can be given intramuscularly up to every 6 hours for agitated patients; haloperidol has also been used cautiously intravenously.

b. Extreme dosage ranges are occasionally exceeded cautiously and only when other appropriate measures have failed. Doses for elderly patients are typically one-half to one-third the usual daily adult oral dose.

c. Chlorpromazine is available as the free base in rectal suppositories in 25- and 100-mg sizes; the hydrochloride is also available in nonproprietary preparations. Thiothixene is available as the free base in 1-, 2-, 5-, and 10-mg capsules. Trifluopromazine is available as the free base in oral suspension, *equivalent to* 50 mg of the hydrochloride per 5 ml; thioridazine base is also available as an oral suspension (equivalent to 25 and 100 mg of the HCl per 5 ml).

d. Also available as generic drugs; trade names are in parentheses.

e. Pimozide is recommended only for the treatment of the Itard–Gilles de la Tourette syndrome (severe tics and vocalization) above age 12, but has been used in schizophrenia as well; it should be discontinued if ECG changes indicate depressed conduction (QT > 500 msec).

minimum effective doses. The maximum recommended doses are based on more limited research data and on clinical experience.

An undetermined percentage of patients respond inadequately even to doses equivalent to more than 2,000 mg of chlorpromazine a day. An occasional unresponsive patient may improve with a higher dose than usual, with injected medication, or after several months of continued treatment, but such individuals are not easily identified clinically, short of an empirical trial of such treatment when ordinary dosing proves ineffective and not toxic. Unique but as yet ill-documented metabolic characteristics of some unresponsive patients might account for their failure to respond to antipsychotic medications. Moreover, many clinicians believe that a major reason for poor response is failure to take medication as prescribed. Compliance can be increased by the use of injected medication or liquid oral preparations of antipsychotic drugs to avoid surreptitious disposal of pills.

Guidelines to approximately clinically equivalent doses of commonly prescribed neuroleptic agents are summarized in Table 1. When these doses are used to guide changes between agents, the changes should be made gradually and cautiously. Thus, while 500 mg of chlorpromazine and 25 mg of trifluoperazine may be approximately equivalent in antipsychotic efficacy, a sudden switch from high doses of one to the other may result in severe reactions. These include dystonia on changing to a more potent agent or sedation and hypotension on changing to a less potent drug.

Studies of laboratory animals provide quantitative determinations of dose-response relationships but do not meaningfully predict clinical responses. Nevertheless, they do reflect what is also known clinically, namely that the *therapeutic index* (the ratio of a severely toxic or lethal dose to a dose that produces noticeable behavior effects) for most of the antipsychotic agents is extremely high. Lethal clinical doses cannot be ascertained. It is almost impossible for a patient to commit suicide with these agents unless medical assistance is unavailable, secondary complications of severe medical illness arise, other toxins have also been ingested, or there is preexisting serious medical illness. More than 10 g of chlorpromazine has been ingested acutely by patients who survived.

The generalization that most neuroleptic agents have an unusually high therapeutic index requires some clarification, however, in that doses regularly associated with unwanted acute extrapyramidal effects overlap those which are effectively antipsychotic. In practice, it is virtually impossible to avoid some extrapyramidal effects, even at low doses of typical antipsychotic agents. Dosage forms and usual adult doses are summarized in Table 2. Effective agents and doses for use in children under 16 years of age are only slightly more limited than for late adolescent or adult patients. Current recommendations for children are discussed later in the chapter and summarized in Table 3.

Pharmacokinetics and Metabolism

The pharmacokinetics and metabolism of the antipsychotic drugs are being investigated actively. At present, however, only a few clinically relevant conclusions can be drawn, partly because of limitations of the laboratory techniques involved, the low plasma levels of most antipsychotic drugs (on the order of nanograms, or 10^{-6} mg, per milliliter), the complex metabolism of some antipsychotic agents, and the many problems inherent in diagnosis and objective evaluation of clinical change in psychotic patients. Other problems have included the study of patients unlikely to respond clearly or rapidly to medication, as well as doses that have often been inadequately controlled or so high as to minimize the range of clinical outcomes.

Nevertheless, a few generalizations can be made. Many antipsychotics have somewhat erratic and unpredictable patterns of absorption among individuals, particularly after oral administration, and blood concentrations of a drug vary widely among individual patients. Neuroleptics are highly lipophilic and highly membrane-bound or protein-bound; they accumulate in the brain, lung, and other tissues with a high blood supply. Accumulation may be particularly striking after repeated exposure to high doses of the less potent agents. The main routes of metabolism of the antipsychotic drugs are oxidative, mediated largely by hepatic microsomal drug-metabolizing enzymes. Conjugation with glucuronic acid is an important route of metabolism. Water-soluble, or hydrophilic, metabolites of neuroleptic agents are excreted in the urine and, to some extent, in the bile. Most oxidized metabolites of antipsychotic drugs are biologically inactive, but some are not (for example, mesoridazine, 7-hydroxychlorpromazine, 7-hydroxynorloxapine) and may contribute to the biological activity of the parent drug substances. Active metabolites that form unpredictably in individual patients also complicate attempts to correlate chemical assays of drug molecules in blood with clinical effects. The less potent antipsychotic drugs may weakly induce their own hepatic metabolism or conjugation, since concentrations of chlorpromazine and other phenothiazines in blood are often lower after several weeks of treat-

Table 3   Antipsychotic agents recommended for children

Agent (route)	Single dose (mg/kg)	Typical daily dose (mg)	Daily maximum (mg) <6 yr	6–12 yr
Chlorpromazine HCl				
Oral	0.50	10–50	—	—
Intramuscular	0.50	—	40	75
Rectal	1.0	—	—	—
Triflupromazine HCl				
Oral	0.50	10–50	—	—
Intramuscular	0.2–0.25	—	10(>2½ yrs)	10
Thioridazine HCl				
Oral	0.25–0.50	5–50	—	—
Fluphenazine HCl				
Oral	0.05–0.10	0.75–5	0(<5 yrs)	10(≥5 yrs)
Perphenazine HCl				
Oral	0.05–0.10	1–5	4(>1 yr)	6
Prochlorperazine maleate				
Oral	0.10	5–10	—	—
Intramuscular	0.05	1–2	—	—
Trifluoperazine HCl				
Oral	0.50	1–10	0	15
Intramuscular	0.05–0.10	1–2	0	2
Chlorprothixene				
Oral	0.5–1.0	30–100	0	100
Pimozide				
Oral	0.05–0.10	2–10	0	20

At the lower limit of age, there is little reported experience in infants or the preschool age from 1 or 2, to 5 or 6 years. For adolescents aged 12 to 16 years, the lower range of adult doses can be used for most neuroleptic agents. For all children, *divided* daily doses are recommended (typically, three times a day). For late adolescents over 16, adult doses are used as required individually. Note that only eight agents are recommended by their manufacturers for oral use, and only four for parenteral (intramuscular) use; Thorazine can also be administered by rectal suppository; the liquid Compazine edisylate is not recommended for children. Agents not included are not recommended for use in children by their manufacturers. Haloperidol has been used safely and effectively in children with Gilles de la Tourette's syndrome (Itard-Tourette syndrome). Pimozide (Orap) has also been used for this purpose, especially when haloperidol or other neuroleptics fail, but there is little experience with its use in children below age 12; it should be discontinued if the Q-T interval on the ECG exceeds 470 msec in a child. It should be noted that these recommendations are based on FDA-approved guidelines provided by their manufacturers. However, clinical practice with severely disturbed, psychotic children indicates that doses in the range required for acutely psychotic adults are often required, and are well tolerated. Thus, total daily doses of 500 mg of chlorpromazine for a 50-kg child (10 mg/kg), or its equivalent, are not rare in institutional practice.

ment with the same dosage. Alterations of gastrointestinal motility might be partly responsible for such changes.

In practice, attempts to correlate chemically measured plasma concentrations of neuroleptic agents or their metabolites with clinical response have not been especially successful, since plasma concentrations vary widely among individual patients. These variations may range from 10-fold to 100-fold and are not eliminated by controlling the dose, timing, or prior exposure to a drug; this variability suggests the involvement of genetic or other individual factors. Chemical assays of clinical plasma concentrations of chlorpromazine and of haloperidol, for example, have been reported to be typically on the order of tens of nanograms per milliliter, while levels of hundreds of nanograms per milliliter may be toxic. To complement chemical assays, a biological assay has been introduced which detects a drug and its pharmacologically active metabolites in blood. This method depends on competition for binding of a radioactively labeled standard neuroleptic to "receptors" (binding sites that may represent sites of action) in animal brain tissue and so is known as *radioreceptor assay*. Attempts to relate the levels of neuroleptic activity detected by such radioreceptor assays to clinical actions have met some success under controlled experimental conditions, including studies in which fixed moderate doses of a neuroleptic were given to acutely ill patients with a favorable short-term prognosis. Nevertheless, in general, assays of blood concentration of neuroleptics by any technique are not sufficiently well developed for routine use in guiding clinical practice, and plasma concentrations that best predict optimal clinical responses cannot yet be stated.

Age is an important determinant of the rate of metabolism and excretion of antipsychotic drugs. The fetus, the infant, and the elderly have diminished capacity to metabolize and eliminate these agents and are more sensitive to them, while children eliminate them *more* rapidly than adults. Accordingly, relatively smaller doses are used for elderly patients, but effective daily doses of antipsychotic drugs in children are not much lower than adult doses.

Detailed comments on pharmacokinetics can be offered for only a few agents that have been well studied, such as chlorpromazine, thioridazine, and haloperidol (see Table 4). The low-potency phenothiazines are sometimes favored for such evaluations because they are used in large doses, and relatively high concentrations of drug and metabolites are present for chemical assay. However, complex metabolism makes their evaluation more difficult.

The absorption of tablets of chlorpromazine is particularly erratic; perhaps two-thirds may be metabolized on the "first pass" through the gut and liver en route to the systemic circulation. The loss of haloperidol after oral administration is reportedly somewhat less marked and variable than that of chlorpromazine. The relatively strong anticholinergic effects of thioridazine can modify its intestinal absorption. The bioavailability of antipsychotic agents is increased somewhat by using liquid concentrates, but these preparations are relatively expensive and inconvenient to use. Peak concentrations of the phenothiazines and of haloperidol are attained in plasma about 2 to 4 hours after an oral dose. Intramuscular injection of neuroleptics avoids much of the first-pass metabolism in the gut and liver that occurs after oral administration and provides measurable concentrations in plasma within 15 to 30 minutes. Peak plasma levels may be increased up to tenfold by injection, but a clinical guideline is to expect about a threefold or fourfold increase in potency of injected over orally administered antipsychotic agents. The gastrointestinal absorption of chlorpromazine is modified unpredictably by food and is reported to be decreased by orally administered colloidal antacids. Early reports also suggested that anticholinergic drugs, such as antiparkinsonism agents, may decrease the gastrointestinal absorption of phenothiazines, but this impression has not been supported by more recent, well-controlled studies.

Plasma concentrations of antipsychotic agents, as they are commonly assayed, are not equivalent to brain levels for all neuroleptics. Most neuroleptics are highly lipid-soluble, pass the blood-brain diffusion barrier easily, and may be retained in brain tissue. Concentrations of some neuroleptics in brain (for example, haloperidol) are more than ten times those in blood. Total plasma levels of neuroleptic molecules by chemical assay or of neuroleptic activity by radioreceptor assay correlate closely with levels in brain tissue and with behavioral effects of the drugs in animals under laboratory conditions.

Neuroleptic drugs bind significantly and tightly in tissue membranes or to lipids and to plasma albumin; most are more than 90% bound in plasma. It follows that it is virtually impossible (and usually not necessary) to remove these agents by dialysis after an overdose. Technical difficulties have precluded meaningful attempts to evaluate the relationship between unbound or free levels of neuroleptics in plasma with corresponding brain levels in animals or with clinical effects in patients.

Thioridazine and its important active metabolite, mesoridazine, are exceptional agents. Total plasma levels of thioridazine are typically 10 to 100 times higher than those of many other antipsychotic agents. They are relatively polar or water-soluble molecules, and are much less extensively or firmly bound to plasma proteins than are other neuroleptics. Such properties of thioridazine as well as of the benzamides (such as sulpiride) contribute to their lesser ability to pass the blood-brain barrier than other neuroleptics.

A correlate of the ability of neuroleptic drugs to enter and accumulate in the central nervous system (CNS) is their ability to enter the fetal circulation easily. It is not known whether those agents that enter the CNS with relative difficulty also have more limited access through the maternal blood-placental barrier.

The pharmacokinetics of all antipsychotic drugs follow a multiphasic pattern. The disappearance of neuroleptics from plasma typically includes a rapid, distribution, alpha phase (half-life, $t_{1/2}$, about 2 hours) and a slower, average elimination, beta phase ($t_{1/2}$, about 20 or 30 hours), as well as a terminal elimination phase with a prolonged $t_{1/2}$ of perhaps 60 hours. Elimination from the plasma may be more rapid than from sites of high lipid content and binding, notably in the CNS. Markedly variable values of plasma elimination half-life have been reported among agents and among individual patients, but these rates are typically 10 to 40 hours (Table 4). Nevertheless, the biological effects of a single dose of a neuroleptic may persist for many days. The large margin of safety of even relatively high peak tissue levels of neuroleptics, along with their slow elimination, supports the feasibility of taking the entire daily dose at one time. This practice is common once a patient has accommodated to the initial side effects of the drug. Similar dosing schedules are safe for antidepressants under some circumstances, but not with the lithium salts, mainly because of their low margin of safety (therapeutic index; Table 5).

The more prolonged, depot-like characteristics of fatty acid esters of neuroleptics are illustrated by the approximate half-lives of elimination of preparations of fluphenazine. While the orally administered hydrochloride is half-eliminated in 10 to 20 hours, the enanthate requires three to four days and the decanoate seven to ten days. On injection of the esters, however, sufficient free fluphenazine is commonly liberated to induce neurological side effects. Characteristics of most of the long-acting antipsychotic agents are summarized in Table 6.

It is important to realize that the antiparkinsonism agents sometimes given with a neuroleptic are eliminated much more rapidly than the latter

Table 4 Clinical pharmacokinetic characteristics of antipsychotic agents

Drug	Bioavailability (%)	Plasma binding (%)	Distribution volume (L/kg)	Plasma half-life[a] (hr)	Active metabolites	Typical plasma levels (ng/ml)[b]
Chlorpromazine	ca. 30	95	7–20	5–16	7-OH	100–600
Thioridazine	ca. 30	98	?	7–42	2-SOCH$_3$	100–800
Fluphenazine	?	?	10	16–24	?	?
Perphenazine	low	?	10–35	8–21	?	?
Thiothixene	?	?	?	34	?	10–150
Haloperidol	65	92	17–30	13–36	none[c]	2–260
Pimozide	50	?	?	55	none known	?

Source: Adapted from Morselli (1977) and Hollister (1978); these values are highly tentative, and there are some marked differences among studies using different methods.

a. Refers to the slow elimination (beta) phase as an estimated, average value.

b. These are typical values encountered in psychotic patients receiving various, but clinically reasonable, doses and for various periods of time; at present it is not possible to state reliable data for highly standardized conditions, much less to suggest guidelines for clinically optimal levels.

c. A reduced (keto group → OH) form of haloperidol, of uncertain biological significance, occurs in human plasma.

Table 5   Pharmacologic characteristics of major psychotropic agents and dosing regimens

Agent	Elimination half-life (hr)	Therapeutic index (TD:ED)	Maintenance dosing (per day)
Neuroleptics	20–30	ca. 100[a]	1
Tricyclic antidepressants	20–30	ca. 10	1–2
Lithium salts	10–20	ca. 3	2–3

Note: The balance of relatively slow elimination and a high margin of safety encourages common once-daily dosing regimens with most usual doses of antipsychotic agents, with moderate doses of most antidepressants in healthy young adults, but not with lithium salts.

   a. It should be noted that this high degree of relative safety of the neuroleptic drugs refers to severe, potentially life-threatening toxicity, whereas extrapyramidal neurologic effects occur at clinically effective doses.

and have a low margin of safety. Accordingly, they are prescribed in divided daily doses and are continued for several days after discontinuing a neuroleptic agent.

The half-life of elimination of neuroleptic molecules from the human brain is unknown. In animal studies, behavioral effects of neuroleptics persist after brain levels are no longer detectable by the most sensitive assays. A single small dose of haloperidol can exert neuroleptic activity in the rat for more than a month, for example (Campbell and Baldessarini, 1985). Such effects suggest a slow dissociation of a small, critical pool of drug, possibly including specific receptor sites. Even slower phases of elimination probably occur, especially after repeated dosing; and neuroleptic molecules can accumulate in human lipid and connective tissues, including the eye, skin, and probably the brain. Metabolites of some agents have been detected in human urine for as long as several months after the drug has been discontinued. Slow removal of drug may contribute to the typically slow exacerbation of psychosis after drug treatment is discontinued.

The most important site of metabolic alteration of antipsychotic agents is the liver, in which microsomal oxidation and conjugation mechanisms operate. The phenothiazines and thioxanthenes yield large numbers of metabolic products with various, largely unknown, pharmacologic activities. An example of a neuropharmacologically active metabolite is mesoridazine, which accounts for some of the neuroleptic activity of its precursor, thioridazine, and is itself marketed as the antipsychotic drug Serentil. Haloperidol and other butyrophenones are metabolically split into two inactive products but may also yield active hydroxy-derivatives. Many

Table 6 Long-acting neuroleptics

Agent	Route[a]	Approximate equivalent dose (mg)	Approximate duration (weeks)
Fatty acid ester prodrugs			
Clopenthixol decanoate[b]	IM	100	2–3
Haloperidol decanoate	IM	100	3–4
Flupenthixol decanoate[b]	IM	100	2–3
Fluphenazine enanthate	IM	100	2–3
Fluphenazine decanoate	IM	100	3–4
Oxyprothepine decanoate[b]	IM	—	2–3
Perphenazine enanthate[b]	IM	5	2–3
Pipothiazine palmitate[b]	IM	150	3–4
Pipothiazine undecylenate[b]	IM	200	2–3
Lipophilic free agents			
Fluspirilene[b]	IM	25	1
Penfluridol[b]	PO	100	1

Source: Data adapted from D. Johnson (ed), *Therapeutics Today,* vol. 2 (Adis Press, New York, 1982).

Note: Only approximate guidelines can be provided for estimating dosage requirements in changing between oral and long-acting injected forms of such agents. One approach that has been used with fluphenazine decanoate is to rely on extensive experience that indicates the approximate equivalence of 25 mg (1.0 ml) every two weeks, with 10–15 mg of the oral hydrochloride daily. Another simple and more general approach is to equate the milligrams of the free base or parent molecule in the long-acting form, divided by the dosing interval in days, with the approximately daily requirement of oral medication. A refinement of the latter approach is to correct for the approximate oral bioavailability (see Table 4). For example, a monthly injection of haloperidol decanoate equal to 150 mg of free haloperidol would be equivalent to (200 mg × 0.65 availability)/28 days = 4.6 mg/day of oral medication. Assays of haloperidol also indicate that plasma levels obtained near the end of a month of such a dose are similar to those obtained the day following an oral dose of 5–10 mg.

a. Routes of administration: oral (PO), intramuscular (IM) in an oily vehicle.

b. Not available in the United States; oldest is fluphenazine enanthate (1962).

products of hepatic metabolism of neuroleptic agents are pharmacologically inactive. Most are also more water-soluble and thus more easily excreted by the kidneys than are the parent substances.

Mechanisms of Action

The mechanisms of action of the antipsychotic drugs are only partially known. Moreover, the hope that such knowledge would provide important clues to the rational development of safer or more effective antipsychotic agents, let alone the pathophysiology of idiopathic psychotic illnesses, has not been realized. However, observations of the effects of most antipsychotic agents strongly suggest pathophysiological mechanisms that underlie their neurological side effects.

Although the antipsychotic drugs represent a wide variety of chemical structures (see Figures 1 and 2), their pharmacology and clinical activities are remarkably similar. The antipsychotic agents in current use in this country all regularly produce a variety of disorders of the control of posture, muscle tone, and movement, presumably as a result of dysfunction of the extrapyramidal nervous system. A crucial question is whether the almost routinely encountered neurologic ("neuroleptic") effects of the antipsychotic drugs are essential to their beneficial actions. The fact that several apparently effective, atypical antipsychotic drugs only rarely induce acute neurologic reactions (dystonias, parkinsonism, and restlessness) challenges the inevitability of an association of neurologic and antipsychotic effects and encourages the hope that more selective antipsychotic agents, with lesser neurologic side effects, can be developed.

Since the pharmacologic basis of the selectivity of the so-called atypical antipsychotic agents remains obscure, the activity of an agent such as clozapine is not adequately predicted by current theory or preclinical laboratory techniques. Some atypical antipsychotic agents, such as clozapine and thioridazine, are strongly anticholinergic, but molindone and sulpiride are not. Most of the atypical agents have weak activity in typical laboratory tests of antidopamine actions. They also have little ability to induce supersensitivity to dopamine agonists (such as apomorphine) in laboratory animals given clinically relevant doses — a putative predictive test of risk of tardive dyskinesia. Despite this partial understanding, there is no effective means of predicting the activity of atypical antipsychotic agents short of empirical clinical trials. The methods of screening new substances for potential antipsychotic activity which have led to most of the existing typical antipsychotic agents have essentially involved seeking neurological reactions in laboratory animals because of the lack of satisfactory animal tests for psychosis. This impasse has contributed to repeated "rediscovery" over the past three decades of agents with similar actions and limitations.

The antipsychotic drugs differ from most other CNS depressants in several ways. Charpentier and Laborit in Paris first noted chlorpromazine's ability to reduce emotional reactivity without inducing somnolence or anesthesia as part of their description of the "neuroleptic syndrome," or "artificial hibernation," in the early 1950s. In general, neuroleptic agents have limited ability to induce the sedative or hypnotic effects that are common to sedatives and other CNS depressants, especially the more potent agents. Coma or respiratory depression is uncommon even after large overdoses. Dependence or addiction is unknown, and tolerance to the main (antipsychotic) clinical effects of these agents is not prominent. The antipsychotic drugs have a remarkably low potential for lethality on acute overdose. In laboratory animals the therapeutic index (ratio of lethal to pharmacologically effective doses, or $LD_{50}:ED_{50}$) ranges from about 25–200 for low-potency phenothiazines to more than 1,000 for high-potency piperazines and butyrophenones.

Antipsychotic agents have a low potential for abuse and dependence: Patients experience no craving for them, and they do not produce euphoria. Rebound excitation has been reported in animals after the abrupt discontinuation of high, prolonged doses of phenothiazines. A possibly analogous reaction can also occur in humans; thus, abrupt discontinuation of ultra-high doses (hundreds of milligrams per day) of powerful neuroleptic agents, such as fluphenazine, can lead to severe, acute dyskinesias. Milder acute dyskinesias are sometimes also encountered after rapid discontinuation of more ordinary doses. Rapid discontinuation of moderate doses of neuroleptic agents following their prolonged use sometimes leads to symptoms of an apparent withdrawal syndrome, such as malaise and gastrointestinal dysfunction. There are also suggestive case reports of sharp, but typically transient, exacerbation of psychotic symptoms on rapid discontinuation of neuroleptics in some patients. Accordingly, withdrawal is ordinarily slowly graded by lowering the dose not more than 10% a day, accompanied by even slower removal of a more rapidly cleared antiparkinsonism agent if one is used.

Routine or early tolerance to the main effects of the antipsychotic drugs is not evident, whereas tolerance is found with many side effects of neuroleptics, including sedation, hypotension, anticholinergic effects, acute dystonic reactions, and possibly parkinsonism. Some tolerance to antipsychotic effects may also be possible, most likely after more than two years of continuous treatment. One recent study noted such adaptation in fewer than 3% of patients maintained on depot injections of an ester of fluphenazine (Chouinard and Jones, 1980).

In further contrast to sedatives, neuroleptics are more capable of diminishing conditioned behavioral responses than of depressing unconditioned responses. They selectively dampen neurophysiologic effects of peripheral stimuli in the forebrain while inhibiting to a much lesser extent the effects of direct stimulation of the brainstem. This difference may lie in actions of the antipsychotic agents at the level of the brainstem reticular activating system, which has a crucial regulatory action on forebrain activity and behavioral arousal. Antipsychotic drugs also have striking inhibitory effects on autonomic and motoric expressions of arousal and strong affect in animals, presumably mediated by actions in the limbic forebrain and hypothalamus. The cellular and biochemical events underlying these behavioral and physiologic actions, however, have remained obscure until recently.

In the early 1960s European pharmacologists proposed that the neurologic, and possibly also the antipsychotic, effects of neuroleptic drugs may reflect their ability to interfere with synaptic transmission mediated by dopamine. This suggestion arose largely from the observation that one of the biochemical properties of neuroleptic drugs was that levels of the metabolites of dopamine consistently and selectively increased, drawing attention to the possibility of unique drug interactions with this monoamine neurotransmitter. Dopamine is prominent in the hypothalamus and in the nigroneostriatal tract, which links the midbrain and basal ganglia. In addition, there are dopamine-containing projections from midbrain nuclei to forebrain regions associated with the limbic system as well as temporal and medial prefrontal cerebral cortical areas closely interlinked with the limbic system (Figure 3). In these regions, dopamine serves as a catecholamine synaptic neurotransmitter at nerve terminals that contain the metabolic apparatus found in sympathetic, adrenergic nerve terminals, except the enzyme dopamine-beta-hydroxylase which converts dopamine to norepinephrine (Figure 4). A somewhat simplistic, but attractive, concept has been that many extrapyramidal neurologic effects of the antipsychotic drugs may be mediated by antidopamine effects in the basal ganglia and that some of their antipsychotic effects may be mediated by the antagonism of dopaminergic neurotransmission in the limbic system, hypothalamus, and cortex.

In recent years much information has accumulated to support the theory that the antagonism of dopamine-mediated synaptic neurotransmission is an important action of these drugs (Table 7). Thus, antipsychotic agents, but not their nonantipsychotic congeners, increase the rate of production of dopamine metabolites in animal and human brain, as well as increasing both the rate of conversion of precursor amino acids to dopamine and its metabolites and the firing rate of dopamine-containing neurons in the CNS of animals. These effects have been interpreted as compensatory responses aimed at maintaining homeostasis in the face of an interruption of synaptic transmission at dopamine terminals in the forebrain.

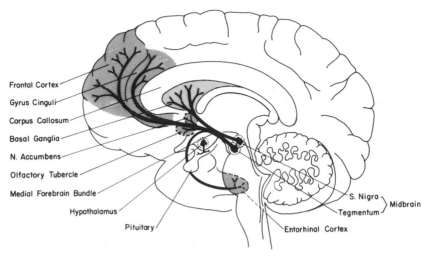

Frontal Cortex
Gyrus Cinguli
Corpus Callosum
Basal Ganglia
N. Accumbens
Olfactory Tubercle
Medial Forebrain Bundle
Hypothalamus
Pituitary
S. Nigra
Tegmentum
Midbrain
Entorhinal Cortex

Figure 3 Dopamine-containing neurons in the human brain. The major systems involving dopamine are the nigrostriatal *pathway from the zona compacta of the midbrain substantia nigra to the neostriatum (caudate-putamen);* mesolimbic *projections from midbrain tegmentum through the lateral hypothalamus to limbic structures, including the septal nuclei (for example, nucleus accumbens septi) and olfactory tubercle; and related* mesocortical *projections, also arising in the midbrain, and projecting particularly to mesial-prefrontal and temporal areas of the cerebral cortex. There is also a* tubero-infundibular *dopamine-containing (TIDA) system within the hypothalamus which provides dopamine, by secretion, to the pituitary gland by way of the hypophysioportal circulation.*

Evidence that a crucial primary event may be the blockade of postsynaptic dopamine receptor sites includes the ability of small doses of antipsychotic agents to block behavioral or neuroendocrine effects of dopamine agonists. Examples are stereotyped behaviors in rodents induced by the dopamine agonist apomorphine, the locomotor excitement induced by the injection of dopamine into limbic sites, or the prolactin-decreasing response of dopamine agonists believed to be mediated by pituitary dopamine receptors. Such tests have been used as screening methods to detect even more agents of the kinds already available.

More direct evidence of a receptor blockade has been provided by the antagonism of dopamine-sensitive adenylate cyclase activity in forebrain tissue and the interference with electrophysiological reponses to dopamine locally applied to receptive forebrain cells in animal brains. A more recent development is the application of experimental radioligand binding assays using homogenates of caudate nucleus or other forebrain tissues and low (nanomolar) concentrations of intensely radioactive, tritium-labeled butyrophenones or other neuroleptic drugs. Such binding is proposed to represent an interaction with dopamine receptor sites. Correlations between the clinical potency of most types of antipsychotic drugs and their ability to interfere with the binding of a butyrophenone are impressive. Clinically inactive analogues or isomers of the antipsychotic drugs compete only weakly for the binding sites. Neuroleptics generally

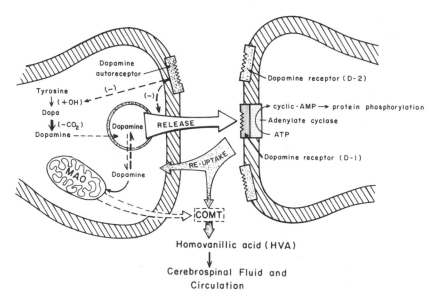

Figure 4 Metabolism at dopamine synapse in the brain. Dopamine is formed from L-tyrosine by hydroxylation (the rate-limiting step) to L-dihydroxyphenylalanine (dopa), which is rapidly decarboxylated. Dopamine is stored in presynaptic vesicles (shaded circle), *from which release occurs into the synaptic cleft by neuronal depolarization in the presence of calcium ion. The released amine has a postsynaptic effect, possibly mediated by a recognition molecule (receptor, type D-1) associated with adenylate cyclase that converts adenosine triphosphate (ATP) to adenosine 3',5'-(cyclic) monophosphate (cyclic AMP), which may, in turn, exert biochemical effects leading to altered neurophysiological sensitivity in the receptive cell. Other receptors, with a high affinity for neuroleptics, are termed type D-2. The neurotransmitter is inactivated largely by efficient high-affinity uptake into the presynaptic terminals; excess dopamine that is not stored can be metabolized by monoamine oxidase (MAO) in the mitochondria and catechol-O-methyltransferase (COMT), largely extraneuronal, to produce homovanillic acid (HVA) from dihydroxy-phenylacetic acid, an intermediary metabolite; the metabolites are removed in the cerebrospinal fluid and venous circulation by a probenecid-sensitive uptake process, largely at the choroid plexus.*

Table 7 Effects of neuroleptic drugs on dopamine (DA) neurons in the brain

Secondary or indirect effects

- DA metabolism increased acutely (increased tyrosine hydroxylation and metabolite production)
- Midbrain DA cell firing increased acutely

Primary or direct effects

- Plasma prolactin increased in rat and man in proportion to behavioral or clinical potency of neuroleptic
- Behavioral actions of systemically administered DA agonists blocked (e.g., L-dopa, apomorphine, amphetamine)
- Self-stimulation through electrodes in DA-rich forebrain regions blocked in rat
- Arousal in response to local injections of DA agonists in forebrain DA target areas blocked in rat
- Iontophoretic effects of DA (but not of cyclic-AMP) blocked in caudatoputamen (striatum) of rat
- DA-sensitive adenylate cyclase in forebrain homogenates blocked by most neuroleptics (butyrophenones are atypically weak)
- Binding of tritiated neuroleptics to membranes in forebrain homogenates antagonized with potency corresponding closely to behavioral and clinical effects

interact with dopamine *agonist* receptor sites in poor correspondence with clinical potency, in contrast to binding sites defined by antagonists such as labeled butyrophenones (see Table 8).

These findings, taken together, strongly support the theory that antipsychotic agents interfere with the actions of dopamine as a synaptic neurotransmitter in the brain. They do not prove, however, that antidopamine effects are either necessary or sufficient for antipsychotic efficacy. They do strongly suggest that some of the extrapyramidal neurologic effects and neuroendocrine actions (prolactin elevation) of this class of agents may be produced by antagonism of dopamine receptors in the basal ganglia and pituitary, respectively. This theory, as it regards extrapyramidal effects, is based largely on analogy to Parkinson's disease, with its demonstrated loss of dopamine in the caudate nucleus and putamen and its beneficial responses to L-dopa, the immediate precursor of dopamine, as well as to other dopamine agonists (for example, apomorphine, bromocriptine). Although it is plausible to assume that the antidopamine actions of neuroleptics play a role in mediating some of their neurological and neuroendocrine effects, there is no fully satisfactory way to account for the antipsychotic effects of these agents.

Table 8 *Effects of antipsychotic agents at dopamine receptors in mammalian brain*

Agent	Anti-apomorphine ED_{50}[a] (mg/kg)	Anti-adenylate cyclase IC_{50}[b] (μM)	^{3}H-Spiroperidol binding IC_{50} or K_i[c] (nM)	Prolactin elevation ED_{200}[a] (mg/kg)	Limbic DA synthesis stimulation ED_{50}[a] (mg/kg)
Fluphenazine	0.05	0.1	0.8	—	—
Haloperidol	0.05	2.0	1.1	4.5	0.07
cis-Flupenthixol[d]	—	0.02	1.2	10	—
Chlorpromazine[d]	0.3	0.6	18	8.5	0.6
Norchlorpromazine[d]	—	—	40	—	—
7-OH-chlorpromazine[d]	—	—	56	—	—
Chlorpromazine-SO_2[d]	(weak)	—	>10,000	—	—
Thioridazine[d]	6.0	0.5	12	8.5	2.5
Mesoridazine[d]	—	—	5	—	—
Sulforidazine[d]	—	—	17	—	—
Thioridazine-SO_2[d]	(weak)	—	4,500	—	—
Molindone	—	—	7.5	7.0	—
Sulpiride	20	700	—	0.01	20
Clozapine	10	0.6	20	20	13

Note: Clinical potency and potency vs. apomorphine effects and to increase DA-turnover correlate well; haloperidol (and other butyrophenones and diphenylbutylpiperidines) are atypically weak vs. DA-sensitive adenylate cyclase in all brain regions (so-called D-1 receptor sites); the thioxanthene cis-flupenthixol and the experimental agent SCH-23390 are selective at such sites; sulpiride has access and high potency at D-2 sites of pituitary mammotrophic cells to increase prolactin levels, but is weak at D-1 sites; competition vs. spiroperidol binding (D-2 sites) correlates well with in vivo and clinical potency for most antipsychotic agents.

a. Data adapted from Carlsson, in *Psychopharmacology: A Generation of Progress*, ed. M. A. Lipton, A. DiMascio, and K. F. Killam (Raven Press, New York, 1978), p. 1057, re rat, as half-maximally effective dose (ED_{50}) or dose to double plasma prolactin level (ED_{200}).

b. Data adapted from Sulser and Robinson, ibid., p. 943, re D-1 receptors in rat.

c. Data from B. M. Cohen (personal communication, 1983) and review by Baldessarini, *N. Engl. J. Med.*, 297:988, 1978 re D-2 receptors in beef and rat brain; half-maximally effective inhibitor concentration (IC_{50}) or inhibitor affinity (K_i).

d. Potencies for phenothiazine metabolites accord well with their neuroleptic pharmacologic activities.

It is reasonable to suppose that limbic and cortical mechanisms are involved in the manifestations of psychosis and their suppression by neuroleptic drugs; yet progress beyond such a generalization has been difficult. Moreover, the selective effects of the atypical antipsychotic agents cannot be explained adequately by antidopamine actions. They are, generally, weak dopamine antagonists and do not exert impressive regionally selective actions, for example at limbic or cerebral cortical dopamine sites as opposed to the basal ganglia of the extrapyramidal system or the anterior pituitary. Thus, no coherent pharmacologic theory is available to guide future development of selective antipsychotic drugs free of neurological or neuroendocrine side effects.

The dopamine receptor–antagonism theory may account for some of the neurological side effects of neuroleptic agents, such as signs of parkinsonism. It probably also contributes to their useful antidyskinetic actions, as in Huntington's disease and Gilles de la Tourette's syndrome. It almost certainly explains why most antipsychotic agents elevate levels of prolactin, whose release is tonically inhibited by actions of dopamine at receptors of the anterior pituitary. Antidopamine effects in the brainstem "chemoreactive trigger zone" or emesis center may also contribute to the antinausea and antiemetic actions of most typical neuroleptics. The dopamine theory does not, however, account for all effects of these drugs. Generally the less potent neuroleptics are less selective in blocking dopamine receptors and interact with many other systems as well. Some side effects, including sedation, hypotension, sexual dysfunction, and other autonomic effects, which are commonly associated with the less potent compounds may reflect their ability to block adrenergic (especially alpha-adrenergic) and histamine receptors (Table 9). Since even potent neuroleptics exert central anti-alpha-adrenergic effects, these may contribute to the antipsychotic or antimanic actions of this class of drugs. Many apparent antiparasympathetic actions of the antipsychotic drugs on cardiac, ophthalmic, gastrointestinal, bladder, and genital tissues have been ascribed to anticholinergic effects at muscarinic receptors. Antimuscarinic actions are more common with the less potent agents and are especially characteristic of clozapine and thioridazine (Table 10). There is also strong evidence that dopamine exerts an important inhibitory action on cholinergic interneurons in the basal ganglia, so that in addition to direct antimuscarinic effects of the less potent neuroleptics, there can be indirect facilitation of cholinergic transmission in some brain areas, especially by potent neuroleptics. This acetylcholine-facilitating effect seems to be short-lived, however. Finally, recent evidence suggests that some neuro-

Table 9   Correlations of clinical potency versus receptor affinity of antipsychotic agents

Receptor type	Method of assay	r
Dopamine		
D-1	DA-sensitive adenylate cyclase	+0.41
	(excluding butyrophenones)	(+0.85)
D-2	^{3}H-neuroleptic binding (caudate-putamen)	+0.94
D-agonist[a]	^{3}H-DA-agonist binding	+0.10
Noradrenergic		
Alpha$_1$	^{3}H-α-antagonist binding (WB-4101)	+0.24
Acetylcholine		
Muscarinic	^{3}H-muscarinic antagonist binding (QNB)	−0.74
	(phenothiazines only)	(−0.84)
Histamine		
H-1	^{3}H-antihistamine binding (mepyramine)	−0.44
Serotonin		
5HT-2	^{3}H-spiroperidol binding (cortex)	+0.32

Sources: Data were taken for analysis from Peroutka and Snyder, *Science* 210:88, 1980; Seeman, *Pharmacol. Rev.* 32:229, 1980; Arana et al., *Biochem. Pharmacol.* 32:2873, 1984.

Note: Butyrophenones and diphenylbutylpiperidines are atypically weak vs. D-1 dopamine receptors, and the inverse correlation between potency and antimuscarinic activity is very high among the phenothiazines (see Table 10).

a. DA agonist binding is not well defined physiologically, but probably includes sites defined as type D-2 receptors (not associated with stimulation of adenylate cyclase, and found for example in anterior pituitary mammotropic cells), but possibly also type D-1 receptors (defined by association with stimulation of the formation of cyclic AMP, and found for example in parathyroid cells and some components of the intermediate and posterior pituitary); the physiological characterization of DA receptors in forebrain remains incomplete and uncertain.

leptic agents interact with sites thought to mediate actions of serotonin, particularly in forebrain regions other than the extrapyramidal motor system. Interaction with such so-called serotonin type 2 receptors is characteristic of butyrophenones, but the physiological significance of this interaction is unknown.

In summary, effects of the antipsychotic drugs at the level of the limbic system, cerebral cortex, and reticular formation appear to correlate well with their observed behavioral and clinical effects, while other effects on the hypothalamus, pituitary, and basal ganglia seem to account for many of the autonomic, neuroendocrine, and neurological side effects of these

Table 10 Antimuscarinic potency of antipsychotic and other agents

Agent	Effective concentration (nM)
Atropine	0.4
Trihexyphenidyl (Artane)	0.6
Benztropine (Cogentin)	0.8
Amitriptyline (Elavil, etc.)	16
Imipramine (Tofranil, etc.)	89
Desipramine (Norpramin, etc.)	116
Clozapine (Leponex)	15
Thioridazine (Mellaril, etc.)	105
Triflupromazine (Vesprin)	1,000
Chlorpromazine (Thorazine, etc.)	1,500
Acetophenazine (Tindal)	7,000
Fluphenazine (Prolixin, etc.)	7,000
Perphenazine (Trilafon)	7,500
Trifluoperazine (Stelazine)	16,500
Haloperidol (Haldol)	27,500

Data are averages of measurements of EC_{50} or affinity for competition with the labeled muscarinic antagonist, quinuclinidyl benzilate (^{3}H-QNB) in rat brain (adapted from Snyder and Yamamura, *Arch. Gen. Psychiatry* 34:236, 1977) or the stimulation of synthesis of $3',5'$(cyclic)-guanosine-monophosphate (cyclic-GMP) by carbamylcholine (a stable acetylcholine analogue) in cultured neuroblastoma cells (adapted from Richelson and Divinetz-Romero, *Biol. Psychiatry* 12:711, 1977). Note that smaller numbers indicate *higher* affinity.

agents. Many of these local actions are probably mediated by the effects of these drugs at the surface of neuronal membranes—including sites of action of dopamine as a neurotransmitter in the CNS—but the precise local chemical changes and their neurophysiological consequences remain obscure. The basis of the apparently selective antipsychotic effects of the atypical agents such as clozapine is not known.

Clinical Use

Drug Selection

It can be difficult to choose among the large variety of antipsychotic compounds now available. An important generalization that simplifies the problem, however, is that most antipsychotic drugs are remarkably similar in their main actions and overall antipsychotic efficacy. A survey of thousands of patients in the Veterans Administration (VA) medical system in the late 1970s indicates that the most commonly prescribed antipsychotics were chlorpromazine, thioridazine, haloperidol, fluphenazine, trifluoperazine, thiothixene, and perphenazine (Baldessarini et al., 1984).

A practical consideration, especially with prolonged use of neuroleptic agents, is their cost. In a recent unpublished survey of costs of a typical month's supply of antipsychotic drugs (equivalent to 400 mg/day of chlorpromazine), prices ranged from about $10 to $30 a month (Baldessarini, 1983). Since prices may vary in different regions, one should check with local suppliers for the best values. It is worth noting that chlorpromazine and thioridazine have already outlived their patent protection and that they are now available as generic agents; haloperidol and other older drugs will soon follow, presumably with more competitive pricing. Finally, one can realize significant savings (more than fivefold) by the use of unit doses of larger size (more milligrams per tablet).

Available data from controlled clinical trials of many drugs do not support rational selection of a class of agents, much less a particular drug, for a specific type of illness. Nonetheless, antipsychotic drugs may not all be equally effective for an individual patient. It is reasonable to try several dissimilar agents serially in adequate and increasing doses, even by injection, and to persist with these trials for several months, so that a patient who at first responds poorly may have the benefit of any doubt. Nevertheless, given adequate doses and duration of treatment, the chances of added success by a change in agent are probably small. The success rate of treatment with an antipsychotic drug, defined in terms of clinical improvement of psychosis or ability to leave a hospital, has averaged 75% or more. For example, in a large National Institute of Mental Health cooperative study, 75% of patients diagnosed as schizophrenic and given a phenothiazine improved within six weeks and only 5% became clinically worse, while of those given a placebo, only 25% improved and 50% were unchanged or worse (NIMH, 1968).

The *potency* (effect per milligram) of antipsychotic agents varies by more than a hundredfold (see Tables 1 and 2), but the overall clinical *efficacy* of most agents is remarkably similar, provided adequate doses are used. This conclusion arises from controlled comparisons of agents given to many patients called "schizophrenics" prior to the early 1970s. Based on current diagnostic standards, many of these studies may have included several types of psychotic patients, although most patients were evidently severely and chronically ill. Studies done in the 1960s and early 1970s indicated that daily doses of an antipsychotic drug equivalent to 300 to 800 mg of chlorpromazine were needed for consistent benefit in such populations. For example, in a review of 65 placebo-controlled studies of the short-term efficacy of chlorpromazine in such patients, all studies found statistically significant results favoring the active agent if the daily dose exceeded 500 mg (Appleton and Davis, 1980). Only two-thirds of the studies employing daily doses below 300 mg found significant effects, and intermediate doses gave intermediate chances of success of chlorpromazine. In a survey of more than 17,000 psychiatric patients in the U.S. Veterans Administration facilities in the late 1970s, the average daily *chlorpromazine-equivalent* dose (see Table 1) for hospitalized patients was 600 mg (ranging from 300 mg for thioridazine to 1,000 mg for haloperidol and fluphenazine). For outpatients, the average daily dose was about 300 mg (Baldessarini et al., 1984). Relatively high chlorpromazine-equivalent doses of the high-potency agents are easily attained but carry a higher risk of neurotoxic effects.

Although figures such as these may reflect average, common clinical practices, there have been very few systematic investigations of dose-effect relationships, or comparisons of specific types of agents, in large numbers of psychotic patients diagnosed by reliable methods. Such studies are notably lacking among patients with acute or intermittent psychoses. A few recent studies suggest that some acutely psychotic or manic patients may do well with daily doses as low as the equivalent of 100 to 300 mg of chlorpromazine, and that many chronic schizophrenics can be maintained adequately on even lower doses, possibly as low as 50 to 100 mg per day.

There are a few exceptions to the rule that most neuroleptics are approximately equally effective. For example, in about 60% of controlled studies, promazine (Sparine) and mepazine (Pacatal) were no better than a placebo, and reserpine failed to produce results better than placebo in about a third of its trials. Furthermore, prochlorperazine (Compazine) failed in about 22% of comparisons with a placebo and is associated with a high risk of acute dystonic reactions. It cannot be recommended for routine use as an antipsychotic agent and currently is more commonly used for treating nausea and vomiting. Loxapine, in a relatively small number of trials, has not been consistently as effective as other antipsychotic drugs; yet its chemical dissimilarity to the phenothiazines may provide a useful alternative, for example in cases of dangerous toxic reactions. The same advantage is offered by haloperidol, molindone, and possibly reserpine. To date, molindone has been associated with late dyskinesias less often than most other neuroleptics, although its efficacy and long-term utility are not as securely established as for many older and more extensively evaluated agents. Nearly every other antipsychotic agent currently in common use produced better results than a placebo in at least 80% to 90% of comparisons (Table 11).

It may seem remarkable that chlorpromazine failed to be more effective than a placebo in 17% of 66 controlled studies. However, these results cannot be taken as important evidence against the efficacy of chlorpromazine because they include some very early studies of the 1950s with drug doses that were probably inadequate for some patients; moreover, in more than 100 studies that have made direct comparisons of antipsychotic agents in schizophrenia, no agent has been found to be more effective than chlorpromazine.

Sedatives such as phenobarbital, as well as normal or even high doses of diazepam (Valium), have nearly always failed to produce better results than an inactive placebo in the treatment of chronically psychotic patients. Nevertheless, sedative agents may have a specialized role in the management of acutely disturbed patients. For example, the early management of highly agitated, assaultive, or manic patients can be enhanced by administration of a benzodiazepine (for example, diazepam in 5–10 mg doses or lorazepam in 1–2 mg doses) in frequently repeated (half-hourly or hourly) doses until sedation develops. Droperidol (Inapsine), a potent, short-acting, sedating butyrophenone neuroleptic, can also be used to sedate acutely agitated psychotic patients. Barbiturates and other sedatives are rarely used in this way now, because their depression of respiration and enhancement of metabolism of other agents, including neuroleptics, complicate their use. A direct comparison of the short-term efficacy of rapidly repeated intravenous haloperidol or diazepam (2.5 to 10 mg every 30 to 60 minutes) showed similar benefits with both agents given to acutely psychotic patients after several hours or the next day (Lerner et al., 1979). Selectivity of either type of agent in producing antipsychotic, as opposed to sedative, effects in such short-term, high-dose treatment has not been shown. This apparent short-term similarity of sedative and antipsychotic agents does not, however, contradict the conclusion that the former have not been proved effective in the treatment of chronic psychoses.

Sedative and antianxiety agents, particularly the benzodiazepines, are currently considered somewhat safer than neuroleptics in the management of psychotic and excited states associated with certain cerebral toxins, including phencyclidine (PCP), lysergic acid diethylamide (LSD),

Table 11 Frequency with which drugs proved more effective than placebos or equal to chlorpromazine as a standard comparison agent in schizophrenia

Agent	Percentage of trials superior to placebo	Percentage of trials equal to chlorpromazine
Phenothiazines		
Butaperazine (Repoise)	100	100
Carphenazine (Proketazine)	100	100
Fluphenazine (Prolixin, etc.)	100	100
Mesoridazine (Serentil)	100	100
Perphenazine (Trilafon)	100	100
Thioridazine (Mellaril, etc.)	100	100
Triflupromazine (Vesprin)	90	100
Trifluoperazine (Stelazine)	89	100
Chlorpromazine (Thorazine, etc.)	83	—
Prochlorperazine (Compazine)	78	100
Promazine (Sparine)	43	33
Mepazine (Pacatal)	40	0
Non-phenothiazines		
Chlorprothixene (Taractan)	100	100
Haloperidol (Haldol)	100	100
Molindone (Moban)	100	100
Loxapine (Loxitane, etc.)	83	93
Reserpine (Serpasil, etc.)	69	—
Phenobarbital	0	0
Diazepam (Valium; high doses)	0	—

Data are adapted from Appleton and Davis, *Practical Clinical Psychopharmacology* (Williams and Wilkins, Baltimore, 1980), who reviewed 206 placebo-controlled studies of antipsychotic agents (mean = 10 studies per agent; range = 1–66) and 119 comparisons with chlorpromazine (mean = 7 studies per agent; range = 2–15). Although the data are tentative for some agents in which few studies were available for review, it appears that most agents except mepazine, promazine, reserpine, and possibly loxapine and prochlorperazine were consistently effective. Phenobarbital has been consistently ineffective, and diazepam appears to be ineffective (though infrequently studied in schizophrenia), although sedative and antianxiety agents may have useful short-term effects in acutely psychotic patients. The imperfect record for chlorpromazine probably reflects inclusion of early studies in which relatively low doses were employed.

and strongly anticholinergic agents. Long-acting benzodiazepines, such as diazepam, are also agents of choice in the management of withdrawal from alcohol. Neuroleptic agents, particularly low-potency phenothiazines, can increase the risk of grand mal seizures and may induce unpredictable changes in blood pressure and temperature in patients with delirium tremens. Neuroleptics may, however, have a place in the management of paranoid illnesses or hallucinosis occasionally encountered in alcoholics following detoxification.

It is questionable practice to use antipsychotic agents for the routine treatment of anxiety or neuroses. Neuroleptics are not particularly effective antianxiety agents, and their extrapyramidal side effects may even worsen anxiety as well as creating neurological risks that can usually be avoided by alternative forms of treatment. The selectivity of action of the neuroleptic agents in psychosis refutes the idea that they are simply stronger ("major") "tranquilizers" than older sedatives. Neuroleptics are occasionally considered for anxious patients previously dependent on alcohol, sedatives, or anxiolytic agents.

Clinical folklore based on anecdotal experiences and perhaps on a misinterpretation of the significance of certain side effects has led to a common but probably erroneous impression that certain high-potency agents (particularly the piperazine phenothiazines and thioxanthenes, as well as the butyrophenones and diphenylbutylpiperidines) are somehow more "incisive" in their ability to interrupt florid psychotic symptoms, or that the same agents are uniquely beneficial for more withdrawn and apathetic schizophrenics because of putative "activating" effects. Few firm data derived from controlled clinical trials support these concepts. Although there is no significant basis for these views, there is also no reason *not* to select the more potent antipsychotic agents either for floridly psychotic or withdrawn patients.

Attempts to tailor treatment to the individual patient's requirements are reasonable. One approach is to select a specific agent on the basis of avoiding specific side effects that are likely to be encountered. For example, hypotensive or potential mild cardiac depressant effects of some low-potency agents (such as the piperidine phenothiazines and aliphatic phenothiazines or thioxanthenes) might wisely be avoided in elderly, infirm, or cardiac patients. On the other hand, the early sedative effects of such low-potency agents may be desirable for a severely agitated, assaultive, manic, or sleepless patient. Such sedative effects would be undesirable in a school-aged child or an adult engaged in potentially hazardous work. High-potency agents may be especially poorly tolerated by young adult, male paranoid patients who may resent and misinterpret their neurological side effects. Such patients may also be disturbed by altered libido or orgasmic and ejaculatory function sometimes associated with low-potency antipsychotic agents. The risk of an acute dystonic reaction in an outpatient whose trust is still to be gained may also encourage caution in the use of a high-potency neuroleptic. In most cases the avoidance of long-acting depot preparations or of excessive doses of any neuroleptic *early* in treatment, as well as avoiding routine use of single daily doses, are sound practices. The usefulness of blood level assays to assure optimal doses of an antipsychotic agent or to monitor compliance with prolonged treatment has not been established.

In some instances it may seem reasonable to consider combinations of agents during antipsychotic drug treatment, but there is rarely a rational basis for the use of more than one neuroleptic at a time. The short-term addition of a sedative agent to manage a dangerous, acutely agitated patient has already been mentioned. On the other hand, the routine addition of a nighttime sedative-hypnotic agent for sleep is almost always unnecessary. Sustained use of sedatives or hypnotics, especially of the barbiturate or other non-benzodiazepine classes, can complicate the determination of dosage requirements for an antipsychotic agent by inducing its increased hepatic metabolism and inactivation. The provision of an extra amount of a neuroleptic of any type at bedtime is often an adequate treatment of insomnia in psychosis. Sometimes it may seem desirable to conteract the sedative effects of a neuroleptic or to minimize the apathy of many schizophrenic patients by adding a stimulant or antidepressant; however, this tactic is rarely helpful, adds unnecessary complexity to treatment, and may increase psychotic agitation or the risk of cerebral intoxication.

Short-Term Use of Antipsychotic Agents

The antipsychotic drugs reduce and can even interrupt specific acute features of psychotic illnesses. Such symptom-relief includes relatively early modification of delusions and hallucinations, followed by a gradual disappearance of thought disorder. The antipsychotic drugs are not specifically "antischizophrenic" agents, since their effects are not limited to schizophrenia and indeed have their least striking benefits in chronically psychotic patients. Rather, they exert beneficial actions in a number of severe psychiatric illnesses including schizophrenia, mania, melancholia, psychotic reactions to stimulants, and even some aspects of dementia and acute brain syndromes. This class of agents is generally palliative rather than curative, and their antipsychotic effects are most readily observed in acute and florid psychotic excitement with considerable anxiety and agi-

Table 12 Indications for short-term use of neuroleptics

- Acute psychotic episodes, regardless of type
- Exacerbations of schizophrenia
- Acute manic excitement while deferring use of lithium or awaiting onset of its effects
- Adjunctive therapy for major depression with prominent psychotic symptoms, or when an antidepressant or ECT alone is not successful
- For agitation in delirium, dementia, or severe mental retardation while seeking to identify and treat the primary basis of the problem
- In certain chronic, degenerative, or idiopathic neuropsychiatric disorders with dyskinesias, such as Huntington's disease or Gilles de la Tourette's syndrome; or for ballism or hemiballism
- Childhood psychoses or apparently allied conditions marked by severe agitation or aggressive behavior
- Miscellaneous medical indications, notably nausea and vomiting, or intractable hiccups

tation. Currently accepted short-term indications for antipsychotic agents are summarized in Table 12.

Target symptoms that consistently benefit from treatment with antipsychotic drugs include combativeness, hyperactivity, hostility, negativism, hallucinations, acute delusions, insomnia, poor self-care, anorexia, and sometimes seclusiveness. Improvement in insight, judgment, memory, and orientation is also likely in cases of acute psychosis or phases of acute exacerbation in recurrent psychoses, such as bipolar illness. In contrast, responses of the latter features in (chronic) schizophrenia and dementias are more variable and often unsatisfactory.

In addition to acuteness and excitation, other clinical factors also suggest that a patient will have a favorable response to antipsychotic drugs and a good prognosis. They include lack of insidious, prolonged onset or chronicity; history of a relatively healthy premorbid adjustment and of social, educational, and occupational accomplishment; current psychotic episode being the first; remissions between episodes; and previous favorable responses to similar medications or other medical treatments.

In an effort to maximize clinical benefit in the minimum time and to limit the total dose of antipsychotic agents, several uncontrolled trials and a few partially controlled trials of unusually high or rapidly increasing doses of antipsychotic agents have been conducted early in acute psychoses or acute exacerbations of schizophrenia. Because of the excessive sedation and hypotension associated with high parenteral doses of low-potency neuroleptics such as chlorpromazine, these trials have usually used a butyrophenone or a potent piperazine phenothiazine or thioxanthene. Such approaches can reduce some psychotic symptoms early, sometimes within a few hours. However, the hope that aggressive early intervention might shorten or even prevent hospitalization has not been fulfilled, and outcome at one week or after several weeks did not differ when very intensive and more standard neuroleptic regimens were compared. A few studies failed to show consistent differences between high, rapid dosing versus more ordinary treatment even within the first day. Whether the apparent benefits reported are due to the rapid induction of antipsychotic effects or to sedation is not clear. As mentioned above, at least one comparison of rapidly repeated intravenous injections of diazepam or haloperidol failed to find a significant difference in efficacy within the first day (Lerner et al., 1979), suggesting that sedative or other nonspecific central depressant effects may have contributed to the outcome. Indeed, a clinical distinction between "sedation" and antipsychotic effect is often difficult in acutely disturbed and agitated patients; a prevalent impression that "real" antipsychotic effects (on disturbed, irrational thinking, delusions, hallucinations, and the like) may require several weeks to be manifest is based mainly on experience with less acutely disturbed chronic schizophrenic patients, although rapid calming effects followed by slower recovery in acute, as well as chronic, psychosis are usual (Figure 5). One final note concerning the use of "rapid neuroleptization" regimens is that they require close medical and nursing supervision because of the risk of inducing excessive sedation, occasionally with hypotension or compromised respiration. Rare fatalities have occurred.

There has also been a tendency to increase dosages of antipsychotic medications for more prolonged use in the hope that a greater percentage of favorable responses would be obtained. Controlled studies indicate that the use of hundreds of milligrams of potent antipsychotic agents such as fluphenazine, trifluoperazine, or haloperidol probably does not increase the overall rate of favorable responses. Although a few patients may respond somewhat better, the overall effects of doses more than ten times greater than those usually recommended are similar to ordinary doses at the end of several weeks, based on studies which, for the most part, have involved schizophrenic patients. The success of antipsychotic drug treatment may have raised expectations of rapid and dramatic responses in every case, even though this prospect is not realistic. Many psychotic patients, especially schizophrenics, respond gradually over many weeks,

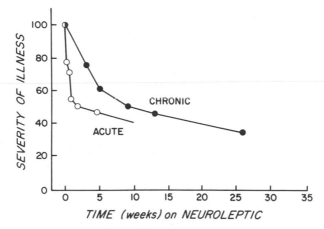

Figure 5 Time course of improvement during neuroleptic treatment. Data in open circles represent mean trends reported in four studies of early use of a neuroleptic (haloperidol) in acutely psychotic patients (some were schizophrenic). Comparisons between high and ordinary dose regimens were included (total of seven treatment cohorts) and, since there were no differences, were pooled. Data are adapted from Lerner et al., Am. J. Psychiatry *136:195, 1979; Appleton and Davis:* Practical Clinical Psychopharmacology *(Williams and Wilkins, Baltimore, 1980); and Neborsky et al.,* Arch. Gen. Psychiatry *38:195, 1981. Data in filled circles represent mean trends reported in three NIMH-sponsored studies of phenothiazines in chronic schizophrenia, adapted from NIMH Study Group,* Am. J. Psychiatry *124:900, 1968. In both curves, 100 is equated to the most disturbed initial clinical scores (usually by the Brief Psychiatric Rating Scale, BPRS). For both groups there were at least two apparent phases of response: rapid improvement over the first week (acute cases) or month (chronic cases), followed by slower improvement thereafter. It is likely that early effects include calming of acute agitation and florid symptoms, while more complete recovery of rationality and function evidently requires a longer time.*

as shown in Figure 5, and it has not been demonstrated that the rate of improvement is increased by use of unusually high doses of neuroleptics. Early use of extraordinarily high doses is almost always unnecessary and increases the risk of toxicity as well as the expense of treatment.

Early uncontrolled studies also suggested that acute neurological side effects of high doses of antipsychotic drugs were no greater than were encountered with ordinary doses, and perhaps even less than usual (the "side effect breakthrough" hypothesis). However, the higher doses are not innocuous. There is an increased incidence of acute dystonic reactions with higher doses as well as other undesirable effects on the CNS, including impressive akinetic and sedative effects that contribute to an apparent worsening of mental status in some cases. There may also be an increased risk of hepatic and autonomic toxicity. The safety of *prolonged* exposure to high doses of these drugs is not established, and there is a suspicion that increases of the total dose and length of exposure may increase the risk of late neurological toxicity. Thus, caution in the use of unusually high doses of antipsychotic agents is appropriate.

To summarize, unusually high doses of antipsychotic medication can be tried temporarily when responses to vigorous treatment with more ordinary daily doses, say up to 1,200 mg of chlorpromazine or 30 mg of fluphenazine or haloperidol or their equivalent, are unsatisfactory after several weeks. If higher doses do not bring about appreciable benefit within two or three months, they should be reduced or abandoned. Prolonged use of extreme doses has not been established as safe and should be avoided unless a clearly demonstrable effect in an individual patient can be obtained in no other way. The unique value of very rapid increases to high doses within a matter of hours in the first few days of an acute psychotic illness has not been established.

In the early exposure of a psychotic patient to a neuroleptic agent, it is best to rely on *divided* doses for safety and to assure sustained availability of the drug throughout the day. Cautious addition of "as needed" supplemental doses of an antipsychotic agent may be useful in the first hours or days of initiating treatment in order to guide selection of an optimal daily dose. However, the burden for close medical supervision and dosing remains with the treating physician, and the routine delegation of this responsibility to nurses or other clinical colleagues is not recommended. Gradually, many patients can tolerate most or all of a day's medication in a single dose. The simplicity of this practice is especially attractive for treatment that extends for more than a few weeks. Most of the day's dose is given typically at bedtime to minimize the risk of sedative and extrapyramidal side effects during the waking hours. Nevertheless, a reduction in the amount of drug required may be possible by dosing only in the morning or by relying on a schedule of two or three times per day, with relatively small doses selected to minimize side effects.

Sometimes, following initial improvement early in the use of an antipsychotic agent, the mental status of a patient may worsen. Although the adequacy of dosage and of compliance should be reviewed, one should also consider other explanations such as worsening of the primary disorder under treatment or misinterpretation of worsening extrapyramidal or other CNS side effects. The latter neurotoxic reactions, which may include akathisia, the neuroleptic "malignant syndrome," delirium, or other manifestations of cerebral intoxication, are especially likely if large doses of a neuroleptic or multiple centrally active medications are used.

In conclusion, evidence is abundant that currently available antipsychotic drugs are effective in treating relatively acute cases of psychosis, regardless of the cause or specific diagnostic type, at least in reducing symptom severity, facilitating clinical management, and supporting early rehabilitation (see Table 12). Controlled short-term studies using more than 300 mg per day of chlorpromazine or the equivalent of other drugs have consistently shown efficacy—for the most part in patients diagnosed as schizophrenic. Recent studies suggest that even lower doses may be adequate for many acutely psychotic patients. These results have led to the impression that it would be irresponsible not to treat acute psychosis or relatively acute exacerbations of schizophrenia with adequate doses of antipsychotic medication. The next question is whether and how long to pursue the treatment.

Long-Term Treatment

There is good evidence that sustained use of an antipsychotic agent prevents or delays exacerbations of psychotic illness in patients diagnosed as schizophrenic. (The term *exacerbation* is consistent with the current concept of schizophrenia as a chronic illness with sustained disability, with the possibility of acute worsening, but not as a pattern of relapses and full remissions as may occur in manic-depressive, schizophreniform, or atypical psychotic conditions.) Most of this evidence has been obtained in controlled prospective studies in which patients who benefited from neuroleptic treatment in the short term were then treated with active medication or a placebo. Thus, patients who responded poorly to initial treatment would not even be candidates for such a study. The representation of such treatment-unresponsive patients among a general population of psychotic patients is not known, but an estimate would be perhaps 20 to 30% or more if only chronically psychotic schizophrenic or demented patients are considered. The available data indicate predictable risks of relapse or exacerbation following recovery from an acute psychotic illness or an acute phase of a chronic illness, especially after abrupt discontinuation of medication on discharge from the hospital. Neuroleptic agents can reduce this risk substantially, but many questions remain.

In nearly 30 studies, patients diagnosed as "schizophrenic" were followed for various periods, typically for three to six months after initial

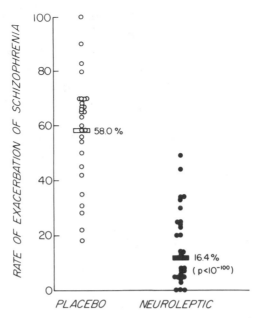

Figure 6 Rate of exacerbation in schizophrenia. The 28 studies evaluated involved controlled prospective assignment to a neuroleptic, usually a phenothiazine (filled circles), or a placebo (open circles) and clinical follow-up (typically for three to six months). Exacerbation was defined typically as gross psychotic decompensation or rehospitalization. The mean difference is highly significant. Based on studies reviewed by Baldessarini and Davis, Psychiatry Res. 3:115, 1980.

improvement, during after-care with either active neuroleptic medication or an inactive placebo, presumably assigned randomly. The overall results of an analysis of most of these studies (Figure 6) indicate a mean rate of clinical exacerbation (obvious worsening of psychosis or rehospitalization) of only 16.4% of patients on active medication versus 58% of those on placebo. This difference, indicating a 42% sparing of exacerbation as a result of active medication, is highly significant statistically ($p < 10^{-100}$). Nevertheless, there has been striking variability in outcome across studies. Among cohorts of patients assigned to a placebo (Figure 6), the rate of exacerbation ranged from 100% to less than 20%. Some of this variability among studies may reflect varying definitions of relapse as well as differences in the duration of follow-up or the average dose of medication. An additional, and possibly more important, source of variance almost certainly has been the broad application of the term *schizophrenia* in the period when most of these studies were carried out (mainly in the 1960s and early 1970s). It is probable that many cases would not meet current research criteria for schizophrenia or the standards of the American Psychiatric Association's *Diagnostic and Statistical Manual of Mental Disorders,* and that cases of acute psychosis, mania, psychotic depression, severe "neuroses" or character disorders, as well as dementia, retardation, or pervasive developmental disorder (autism) might well have been included. Long-term outcome studies with different treatments among separate disorders formerly included among "schizophrenias" remain to be made. Such long-term trials based on currently accepted diagnoses might clarify the indications for prolonged, uninterrupted neuroleptic therapy. Moreover, long-term studies of agents other than phenothiazines (mainly chlorpromazine, thioridazine, or fluphenazine) are few.

At present one can point to several conclusions that are supported by adequate research or clinical experience. Risk of exacerbation is clearly high among schizophrenics who have recently improved in response to short-term treatment with a neuroleptic drug. Those maintained on a placebo, on the average, underwent exacerbation ("relapse") at the rate of about 5 to 10% per month over the first six to twelve months of follow-up; about 50% relapsed within six months. This risk was reduced by a factor of two or three by continued medication (Figure 7). There is little information about the risk of relapse after more than a year of follow-up in controlled studies, and the available results are almost certainly contaminated by the statistical problem of bias in drop-out rates with increasing time as well as by the inclusion of patients with differing degrees of illness. An additional limitation of such studies of maintenance treatment is that they demonstrate effects soon after initial response to treatment, and thus may reflect prevention of early relapse of an index episode of acute illness rather than true prophylaxis against future acute episodes. A further theoretical possibility is that the results of such studies of neuroleptic discontinuation may include effects of relatively rapid removal of medication, particularly if neuropharmacologic effects disappear only gradually over weeks or even months. Thus it should not be assumed that indefinite and continuous maintenance treatment is required for all patients, or that alternative methods of treatment should not be considered. For example, some chronically psychotic patients may do well with temporary neuroleptic treatment followed by slow reduction of dosage or even discontinuation, perhaps with rapid and aggressive additional medication if signs of exacerbation or periods of additional stress are encountered.

Clinical experience indicates that the long-term benefits of indefinitely prolonged antipsychotic therapy become increasingly difficult to demon-

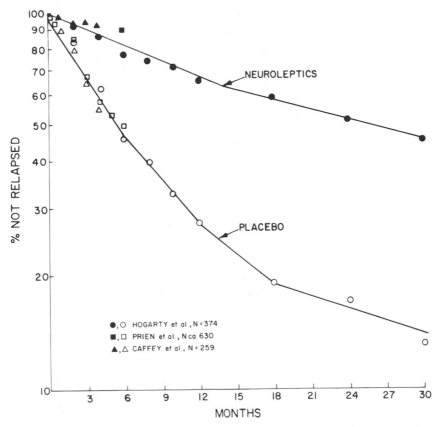

Figure 7 Rate of non-relapse of schizophrenics treated with a neuroleptic or placebo versus time. Data are adapted from Caffey et al., J. Chron. Dis. 17:347, 1964; Prien et al., Brit. J. Psychiatry 115:679, 1969; and Hogarty et al., Arch. Gen. Psychiatry 28:54, 1977, and indicate rates of non-exacerbation ("survival") during follow-up after improvement of schizophrenia and assignment to continued neuroleptic (phenothiazine) treatment or a placebo. The rate of exacerbation ("relapse") is remarkably similar in all studies for the placebo groups over at least six months (about 5 to 10% per month).

strate in truly chronic "poor-prognosis" schizophrenia, especially as the duration of illness and of treatment increases. Long-term use of an antipsychotic agent thus requires repeated attention to an objective justification in each case. Such justification is required in view of the risks involved, particularly the potentially irreversible neurological sequelae, including tardive dyskinesia and subtle impairment of some higher cortical functions and psychomotor skills. These issues are matters of concern not only among psychiatrists and other medical professionals, but also for the general public. Mutual agreements are required between clinician and patient or family based on judgments that weigh the possible benefits and risks of neuroleptic treatment continued longer than six months. There is wide agreement that patients with sustained psychotic symptoms and functional impairment are candidates for indefinitely prolonged treatment if reevaluation indicates that the signs and symptoms are not only still present but also responsive to medication to a degree that justifies the risk of late toxic effects of the neuroleptics.

At present there is almost no scientific support for sustained use of neuroleptics in intermittent psychotic conditions such as bipolar (manic-depressive) illness; however, the long-term benefits of lithium salts in bipolar illness are indisputable, and the safety and efficacy of sustained treatment with lithium or an antidepressant for rapidly recurring, severe, nonpolar major depressions are gaining growing support. A summary of possible indications for prolonged use (more than six months) of an antipsychotic medication is provided in Table 13.

Attempts to specify dosage requirements in prolonged maintenance treatment of chronically psychotic patients are difficult, since most of the available studies have been inadequate and poorly controlled. In a recent analysis of nearly 30 studies (see Figure 6) that gave sufficient data to permit computations of mean daily antipsychotic drug doses in terms of the approximately equivalent amount of chlorpromazine, doses ranged from 125 to 2,000 mg daily. The rate of presumed drug effect (difference between the rate of exacerbation on placebo minus that of the drug-treated cohort) ranged from about 10% to 75%. The correlation between these two measures ($r = 0.07$) was almost nil. One possible explanation for this apparent lack of dose-effect relationship is that most of the studies only partially controlled the dose of medication and allowed some degree of dosage adjustment to meet clinical indications, thus obscuring any relationship. Another interpretation is that even the lower range of doses (daily equivalent of 125 to 300 mg of chlorpromazine) may exceed the requirements for many patients. In a recent review of 11 controlled studies involving more than 700 schizophrenic patients, the patients were randomly continued at high but usual doses of a neuroleptic, equivalent to 600 mg of chlorpromazine daily, or given a very high dose, averaging approximately 15 times more (9.2 grams of chlorpromazine daily). There was little improvement in psychosis, but a 64% increase in the prevalence of extrapyramidal toxicity (Aubree and Lader, 1980). Several recent pro-

Table 13 Possible indications for continuous long-term use of neuroleptics (for more than six months)

Primary indications
• Schizophrenia
• Paranoia[a,b]
• Childhood psychoses[a,b]
• Some degenerative or idiopathic neuropsychiatric disorders (notably, Huntington's disease and Gilles de la Tourette's syndrome)[b]

Secondary indications
• Extremely unstable manic-depressive or other episodic psychoses (unusual)[b]
• Otherwise unmanageable behavior symptoms in dementia, amentia, or other brain syndromes[a,b]

Questionable indications
• Chronic characterological disorders with schizoid, "borderline," or neurotic characteristics; substance abuse; or antisocial behavior[a,b]
• Recurrent mood disorders[a,b]

Note: It is important to clarify that there may be times when a neuroleptic drug is used in the short-term management of exacerbations and crises of chronic or recurrent conditions such as those outlined above. Moreover, there may be justification for even more prolonged uses based on clinical judgment in individual cases and objective demonstration of important benefits. It is also important to state that clinical research has not yet provided compelling support for long-term uses in cases other than chronic schizophrenia, nor has it provided evidence that such uses are contraindicated. Clinicians are left to rely on their evaluations of individual patients and on their clinical experience as additional research data continue to be gathered and assessed. Thus, the recommendations provided above can only be viewed as tentative and are based on an attempt to balance the available research literature and clinical experience.
    a. Efficacy has not been adequately demonstrated in controlled studies.
    b. Long-term neurological safety has not been demonstrated.

spective studies indicate that a critical portion of a hypothesized dose-effect relationship in long-term treatment may occur at daily doses well below 300 mg of chlorpromazine or its equivalent in other agents. Several recent reports indicate that a majority of patients were adequately maintained at doses equivalent to 50–100 mg of chlorpromazine per day (see Baldessarini et al., 1984). The results of several such studies, in which doses were known with certainty by the use of injected fluphenazine decanoate, are summarized in Table 14. They suggest not only that small doses are often adequate, but also that large doses may give inferior results, presumably due to toxic or other effects and not merely to the artifactual assignment of the sickest patients to the highest doses.

Table 14 Dose-effect relationship for fluphenazine decanoate in the treatment of schizophrenic patients for one year

Study	Year	N	Mean dose[a] (mg/2 weeks)	Relapse rate[b] (%)
Hogarty et al.	1979	55	41	35.1
Marder et al.	1984	22	36	20.2
Rifkin et al.	1977	19	31	5.3
Kane et al.	1983/4	64	31	7.0
Marder et al.	1984	28	7	22.4
Kane et al.	1984	36	6	20.0
Kane et al.	1983/4	62	3	56.0
Hogarty et al.	1976	41	0	67.4
Rifkin et al.	1977	19	0	68.4

Source: Teicher and Baldessarini, *Arch. Gen. Psychiatry,* 1985 (in press) and references cited therein concerning six studies that involved a total of 346 chronically ill schizophrenic patients given a controlled dose of fluphenazine ester by injection every two weeks, and followed clinically for a year. A computer-assisted analysis of the dose-effect data suggest a half-maximally effective dose of only 5 mg/2 weeks, as well as an antitherapeutic effect at higher doses, at $ED_{50} = 45$ mg/2 weeks (apparent therapeutic index = 9). These doses may be equivalent to daily doses of chlorpromazine of about 50 and 500 mg, respectively. There is no evidence that less responsive patients were nonrandomly assigned to higher doses.

a. Represents best estimate of weighted mean, based on information provided in each report.

b. Proportion of patients experiencing clinical relapse within one year of follow-up, excluding subjects dropped because of severe toxicity or for administrative reasons.

Studies such as these, as well as clinical experience with chronically psychotic patients, strongly encourage attempts to seek the lowest effective dose of antipsychotic medication with each patient. Usually such low doses are best attained gradually, and with added nonpharmacologic support and encouragement. It is also likely that requirements for neuroleptic medication will change over time with fluctuations in clinical status, responses to stressful changes in life events, or other uncertain factors in individual patients.

Injected long-acting preparations of antipsychotic agents (see Table 6) are sometimes used for convenience, efficiency, or to overcome unreasonable reluctance to cooperate with oral medication regimens. Some studies indicate that rates of exacerbation can be reduced significantly by use of injected medication in prospective comparisons with oral regimens; others find that similar benefits are obtained with either form of treatment. Results of representative studies are shown in Table 15. It is

Table 15 *Oral versus injected neuroleptic in treatment of schizophrenic patients*

Study	Year	Total N	Relapse rates (%)					
			0–12 months			0–24 months		
			Oral	Intramuscular		Oral	Intramuscular	
Johnson	1979	260	43.0	12.0		59.0	34.0	
Hogarty et al.	1979	105	39.5	35.1		64.7	40.3	
Schooler et al.	1980	214	32.8	24.3		—	—	
Total/weighted mean	—	579	38.6	20.7		60.6	35.8	
Sparing by IM over PO				17.9%/year			24.8%/2 years	

Sources: Data are adapted from the following reports: Johnson, *Brit. J. Psychiatry* 135:524, 1979; Hogarty et al., *Arch. Gen. Psychiatry* 36:128, 1979; and Schooler et al.: *Arch. Gen. Psychiatry* 37:16, 1980; the latter two studies compared fluphenazine hydrochloride (PO, orally) and fluphenazine decanoate (IM, intramuscularly), whereas Johnson studied patients given various oral and intramuscular agents. The results suggest a moderate overall advantage of injected agents for the first year, with an increase of that advantage by the end of two years of follow-up.

Table 16 Possible tolerance to antipsychotic effects of fluphenazine esters

Year of treatment	Dose (mg/2 weeks)	Annual dose increase (%)
1	50 ± 14	—
2	59 ± 10	18
3	157 ± 33	166
4	234 ± 69	49

Ten patients of mean age 34 years were drawn from an outpatient clinic population of 300 schizophrenics treated for at least three years with fluphenazine decanoate or enanthate injections (doses are means ± S.E.M.). Serum prolactin was elevated in all cases (70 ± 11 ng/mL), and 80% had mild or moderate tardive dyskinesia, the severity of which corresponded only weakly with the increasing dosage requirements. The data are adapted from Chouinard and Jones, *Am. J. Psychiatry* 137:16, 1980. The findings suggest that tolerance may occur to the antipsychotic effects of some neuroleptics in a minority of patients after several years of continuous treatment; they do not prove that new, iatrogenic dysfunction was added.

possible that differences in patients or in the level of enthusiasm or vigor of the treating staff contribute to such differences between clinics. One potentially important recent observation arising from the prolonged use of injected esters of fluphenazine is that the amount of medication required to maintain antipsychotic effects rose sharply in a significant minority of patients after two or three years of continuous treatment (Table 16). While such findings have led to speculations concerning the possibility that psychosis may eventually worsen under such conditions, possibly by altered function of dopamine in the limbic system, there is no evidence that the psychosis encountered is different from previous manifestations of the primary illness. These observations do, however, raise the possibility that *tolerance* to the main antipsychotic effects of certain neuroleptics may eventually occur in some patients.

In conclusion, dosage guidelines for long-term use of neuroleptics are hard to establish from research studies. Many patients are maintained by doses that are less than half of those used for management of acute psychosis. The selection of a low but effective dose for maintenance treatment is best worked out empirically and is a matter of clinical judgment. Good practice includes objective and repeated assessments of benefits and side effects and repeated attempts to reduce doses gradually or to try periods of time without medication. In this way patients with acute psychoses who no longer require medication can be found, and those with relentless and unyielding chronic illnesses will also be better recognized. For both, the risks of long-term side effects and toxicity will be minimized.

Influence of Age on the Use of Antipsychotic Agents

The use of antipsychotic agents in patients at the extremes of the age spectrum raises some special considerations. Many elderly patients have psychotic illnesses, including dementias, psychotic depression, paranoia (delusional disorder), or exacerbations of previously present schizophrenia or bipolar disorder. While the antipsychotic agents are useful in treating these conditions, it is common to prescribe doses about one-half or one-third those commonly used for younger adults. Nevertheless, a small number of controlled trials suggest that daily doses below 200 to 300 mg of chlorpromazine or the equivalent of another agent are not effectively antipsychotic for some patients. There is, however, a marked increase in the incidence of side effects and toxicity in the elderly which often limits the doses that can be tolerated. Thus, doses initially should be small, divided, and increased slowly in small increments.

The low-potency antipsychotic agents tend to induce toxic CNS reactions in the elderly, including confusion, disorientation, and lethargy or restlessness and agitation. Thioridazine has been popular for older patients, partly because of its lower incidence of extrapyramidal reactions and its possible antidepressant effects. Nevertheless, because of its strong anticholinergic and other actions on the autonomic systems, it is particularly likely to induce serious parasympatholytic side effects, toxic delirium, and possibly cardiac arrhythmia. Thioridazine and other low-potency agents are also associated with a high risk of postural hypotension, which is potentially dangerous in the elderly. More potent agents in *moderate, divided* doses may be preferable for older patients with psychotic illnesses marked by agitation, delusions, hallucinations, and hostility. Alternatively, agents of moderate potency, such as perphenazine or acetophenazine, in moderate doses, may offer a compromise between the risk of anticholinergic autonomic and sedative effects of low-potency agents and the extrapyramidal effects of high-potency agents. More benign states of agitation that are not associated with psychoses or organic mental syndromes can often be managed by cautious use of short-acting benzodiazepines, but these have a high risk of inducing cerebral intoxication in the elderly. Other sedatives, especially barbiturates and long-acting benzodiazepines, should be used cautiously, if at all, because of their tendency to induce ataxia and confusion and thus to worsen agitation.

Paranoid delusional disorders in the elderly are particularly difficult to manage with any medication, but moderate doses of the more potent antipsychotic agents can be tried.

At the other end of the age range, the efficacy and safety of the antipsychotic agents have been demonstrated consistently in the management of children with psychoses and allied conditions marked by severe agitation and aggressive behavior, or with severe behavioral disturbances associated with brain damage. These drugs are not used for neurotic or mild behavior disorders or for hyperactivity, however, because of their potential to impair cognition and the risk of extrapyramidal reactions. They *are* used in the management of Gilles de la Tourette's syndrome (particularly haloperidol) and are sometimes included in the treatment of autistic children (with pervasive developmental disorder), with variable success. The most extensive experience has been in the management of adolescent patients diagnosed as schizophrenic, in whom these drugs relieve psychotic thinking and disturbed (and disturbing) behavior, as they do in adults. Doses effective against psychosis in school-age children are not much lower than those given to adults and thus may be even higher than adult dosages on the basis of weight (milligrams per kilogram). The recent acceptance of relatively high doses of neuroleptic and other psychotropic agents for children, particularly for hospital treatment, reflects experimental evidence that rates of metabolism and clearance of these agents in children may be perhaps twice those in adults. The dosage in young children is usually lower than for those above age 12; this is determined partly by smaller body size but also reflects a greater awareness of side effects that may impair intellectual and other functions in school-age patients, and possibly an increased sensitivity to some extrapyramidal effects in children. When antipsychotic agents are used for prolonged periods in young children, the patients are monitored closely for signs of impairment of their physical and scholastic development, as well as the side effects typical of adult patients. Low-potency agents are usually avoided, and moderate doses of the less sedating agents, such as trifluoperazine, fluphenazine, thiothixene, and haloperidol, have been preferred. Apart from the question of side effects, most antipsychotic agents in common use are probably as effective in childhood psychoses as they are in the adult illnesses. Nevertheless, current manufacturers' recommendations remain conservative regarding the agents, doses, and routes of administration suggested for children under age 12, as shown in Table 3 earlier in the chapter. Based on accumulating research and clinical experience, such guidelines appear to be excessively restrictive and cannot be recommended as standards for the treatment of severely ill, psychotic children.

Toxicology

The most important point to clarify about the toxicity and side effects of the antipsychotic agents is that they are among the safest drugs available in medicine. This safety, in no small measure, accounts for their widespread use. The overall incidence of important problems, other than extrapyramidal reactions, is only a few percent; and some regularly occurring effects are more annoying than dangerous. The latter include feelings of heaviness, sluggishness, weakness, or faintness and a variety of mild effects presumed to be anticholinergic, including dry mouth and blurred vision. Postural hypotension can be a problem, especially early in treatment with low-potency agents and in elderly patients. Among the most common side effects characteristic of neuroleptic agents are those involving posture and movements, which are evidently mediated by effects on the extrapyramidal motor system.

Neurological Effects of Neuroleptic Drugs

The common and sometimes troublesome neurological side effects of most antipsychotic drugs represent a unique constellation of syndromes not associated with other psychotropic agents. These reactions can be divided into six categories, as outlined in Table 17. Other classes of psychotropic drugs, including sedatives (such as barbiturates), tranquilizer-antianxiety agents (such as benzodiazepines), and even antidepressants and lithium salts, are more likely to induce toxic delirium and, at higher doses, coma and death. In contrast, CNS toxicity of the antipsychotic agents is manifested in several characteristic motor syndromes. Except for parkinsonism, the pathophysiology of these reactions is still poorly understood, although it is suspected that effects on dopamine-mediated systems in the basal ganglia are involved. These syndromes are discussed in the following paragraphs.

Acute dystonias typically occur within the first few hours or days of treatment and are most likely to be associated with the more potent neuroleptics. They involve sustained hyperkinesias of the muscles of the neck, jaw, and tongue, as well as the eyes and trunk. Signs may include trismus, opisthotonos, or tonic oculogyric movements or deviations of the eyes ("oculogyric crisis"). Facial grimacing, perioral spasms, protrusions or torsion of the tongue, and dysphagia are common. Laryngeal or pharyngeal spasm with dyspnea or life-threatening respiratory distress may develop, and a few fatalities have occurred. The reaction may be accompanied by sweating or pallor and fever. Severe anxiety is the rule. Such reactions seem to be especially common in adolescent and young adult male patients. The pathophysiology of the condition remains obscure, partly because of the wide and inconsistent variety of agents reported to be of benefit. It has been found that the period of maximum risk for neuroleptic-induced dystonias is during the phase of rapid decrease of blood levels of a neuroleptic drug. If dystonic reactions recur frequently, hypocalcemia may be present. Typically, tolerance to dystonias develops following days or weeks of treatment; possible exceptions include the sudden change from a neuroleptic of low potency to relatively high doses of a potent agent, as well as the use of repeated injections of a fluphenazine ester, which may induce dystonic reactions repeatedly for many months.

The pattern of high risk when tissue levels are falling early during acute exposure to a neuroleptic, the greater risk of high-potency agents, and the tendency for tolerance to develop suggest that early responses of the nervous system to potent dopamine antagonism may be important in the pathophysiology of acute dystonias. Based on studies of laboratory animals, these responses include rapid, but possibly incomplete, blockade of dopamine receptors and a marked increase in the production and turnover or release of dopamine in the forebrain and in the synthesis and release of acetylcholine in the basal ganglia. If the availability of dopamine and of acetylcholine continues while partial blockade of dopamine receptors is diminishing, it is possible that a temporary state of relative excess of both dopaminergic and cholinergic function may occur.

The main clinical problem with this syndrome is distinguishing it from a seizure disorder, tetany or tetanus, or "hysteria." Patients in dystonic reactions are typically terrified and should be forewarned about them and treated immediately as a medical emergency. Treatment by injection of an antiparkinsonism agent is usually dramatically effective and virtually diagnostic. Diphenhydramine (Benadryl, 25 or 50 mg given intramuscularly or 25 mg intravenously) and benztropine mesylate (Cogentin, 2 mg given intravenously) are currently popular choices. Some clinicians prefer to add an antiparkinsonism agent routinely when starting to treat a patient with a potent neuroleptic; recent experience suggests that a protective effect against dystonia or other acute extrapyramidal reactions by such combined therapy may occur, especially when moderate or high

Table 17 *Neurological side effects of neuroleptic-antipsychotic drugs*

Reaction	Features	Period of maximum risk	Proposed mechanism	Treatment
Acute dystonia	Spasm of muscles of tongue, face, neck, back; may mimic seizures; *not* hysteria	1–5 days	Dopamine excess? Acetylcholine excess?	Antiparkinsonism agents are diagnostic and curative (i.m. or i.v., then p.o.)
Parkinsonism	Bradykinesia, rigidity, variable tremor, mask-facies, shuffling gait	5–30 days (may persist)	Dopamine blockade	Antiparkinsonism agents (p.o.); dopamine agonists risky?
Akathisia	Motor restlessness; patient may experience anxiety or agitation	5–60 days (commonly persists)	Unknown	Reduce dose or change drug; low doses of propranolol;[a] antiparkinsonism agents or benzodiazepines may help

Tardive dyskinesia	Oral-facial dyskinesia; choreo-athetosis, sometimes irreversible, rarely progressive	6–24 months (worse on withdrawal)	Dopamine excess?	Prevention best; treatment unsatisfactory; slow spontaneous remission
"Rabbit" syndrome	Perioral tremor (late parkinsonism variant?); usually reversible	Months or years	Unknown	Antiparkinsonism agents; reduce dose of neuroleptic
Malignant syndrome	Catatonia, stupor, fever, unstable pulse and blood pressure, myoglobinemia; can be fatal	Weeks	Unknown	Stop neuroleptic; antiparkinsonism agents usually fail; bromocriptine often helps; dantrolene variable; general supportive care crucial

a. There may be an increased risk of hypotension on interacting high doses of propranolol with some antipsychotic agents; clonidine may also be effective at doses of 0.2–0.8 mg/day, but carries a high risk of hypotension (Zubenko et al., *Psychiatry Res.* 11:143, 1984).

doses of a potent neuroleptic are used. Thus, the probable benefits of routine use of moderate doses of an antiparkinsonism agent must be balanced against the possible added risk of peripheral autonomic or central neurotoxic complications of treatment. If an anticholinergic agent is given early to protect against dystonia, its need should be reevaluated within two weeks.

Drug-induced parkinsonism is similar to other forms of the disorder except that tremor is less prominent in the neuroleptic-induced form. The onset of the syndrome usually occurs within the first weeks of treatment. The risk increases with advancing age, but children may also have an increased risk of this reaction. There may be some tolerance to this effect, as the signs sometimes diminish over two or three months, but the requirement for antiparkinsonism medication is unpredictable and varies among individual patients. In some cases bradykinesia and inexpressive facies persist indefinitely and may be confused clinically with manifestation of the late "defect state" of schizophrenia or with depressed mood. Antipsychotic agents with higher milligram potency induce parkinsonism and dystonic reactions with greater frequency than less potent agents. Severe akinetic, catatonic reactions and mutism have also been associated with relatively high doses of potent antipsychotics such as the piperazine phenothiazines and thioxanthenes, haloperidol, and loxapine. With such severe reactions, the temptation is to suspect worsening functional psychosis and to give even higher doses of the offending agent, although improvement usually follows reduction in its dosage. The antiparkinsonism agents, including anticholinergics or amantadine (Symmetrel), may help. A similar but even more severe reaction ("neuroleptic malignant syndrome" or "hypothalamic crisis") is described separately in the next section.

A variety of agents are now used for the treatment of idiopathic as well as drug-induced parkinsonism, and the differential effectiveness of various classes of agents provides strong support for the theory that dopamine deficiency (and perhaps a relative excess of cholinergic function) in the basal ganglia is an important aspect of the pathophysiology of both forms of the syndrome. In addition, there is excellent neuropathological and postmortem neurochemical evidence of dopamine deficiency in idiopathic Parkinson's disease. The antiparkinsonism drugs available for psychotic patients are listed in Table 18. L-dopa and dopamine agonists are considered too likely to produce agitation for routine use in such patients.

Table 18 *Equivalent doses of agents used to treat extrapyramidal reactions to neuroleptic drugs*

Generic name	Trade name	Dosage forms (mg)	Usual daily dose (mg)
Anticholinergic agents			
Benztropine	Cogentin, Tremin, etc. (generic)	(T) 0.5,1,2; (V) 1/ml	1–6
Biperidin	Akineton	(T) 1; (A) 5/ml	2–10
Cycrimine	Pagitane (not actively marketed)	(T) 2.5	2.5–15
Diphenhydramine	Benadryl, etc. (generic)	(C) 25,50; (L) 50/ml; (A + V) 10 or 50/ml	25–100
Ethopropazine	Parsidol	(T) 10,50	50–200
Orphenadrine	Disipal, Norlex, etc. (generic)	(T) 50,100; (L) 30/10ml; (A) 60/2ml	50–300
Procyclidine	Kemadrin	(T) 5	5–30
Trihexylphenidyl	Artane, Pipanol, etc. (generic)	(T) 2,5; (L) 2/5ml	5–15
Atypical agents			
Amantadine	Symmetrel	(C) 100; (L) 50/ml	100–300
Specialized agents			
Bromocriptine	Parlodel	(T) 2.5; (C) 5	5–50
Dantrolene	Dantrium	(C) 25,50,100; (V) 20/60ml	60–600
Propranolol	Inderal	(T) 10,20,40,60,80,90; (A) 1/ml	20–120

Dosage forms: (T) tablets; (C) capsules; (L) syrup or other liquid for oral use; (A or V) ampules or vials for parenteral administration (diphenhydramine is also available in syringes, 50 mg/ml).

These agents are commonly given orally in two or three divided doses to provide the typical daily adult total doses recommended above for use in neuroleptic-induced toxic reactions (but not necessarily for other purposes). Benztropine (2 mg) or diphenhydramine (25 or 50 mg) are often given intramuscularly or intravenously to reverse acute dystonic reactions. Amantadine can be used for parkinsonism, catatonia, or akathisia but is relatively expensive and may lose effectiveness within a few weeks; it may be dopaminergic, and overdoses may respond to physostigmine even though amantadine is not strongly anticholinergic. Diphenhydramine and orphenadrine are antihistaminic and antimuscarinic; ethopropazine is a strongly anticholinergic phenothiazine. Bromocriptine may be useful for neuroleptic malignant syndrome but is not used for parkinsonism caused by neuroleptics in psychotic patients because of a possible risk of worsening psychosis; dantrolene may also benefit malignant reactions, but less consistently than the malignant hyperthermia of general anesthesia. Propranolol in low doses with little cardiovascular effect appears to be selective against akathisia (other beta-adrenergic antagonists are less effective). Most of these agents are available as HCl salts (amantadine as the longer-acting sulfate is used in Europe); orphenadrine is available as the citrate and benztropine and bromocriptine as the mesylates; dantrolene is the sodium salt. Note that most of these agents, on excessive dosing, can induce cerebral intoxication or apparent exacerbation of psychosis.

Most of the recommended antiparkinsonism drugs (except amantadine) are strongly antimuscarinic (atropine-like) and thus can induce the syndrome of *anticholinergic poisoning.* This is characterized by restless agitation, confusion, disorientation, perhaps seizures, hyperthermia, dry and sometimes flushed skin, tachycardia, sluggish and at least moderately dilated pupils, decreased bowel sounds, and often acute urinary retention. These effects are probably due to peripheral and central anticholinergic actions of these potent muscarinic blocking agents. The antiparkinsonism agents and cyclic (imipramine-like) antidepressant drugs are among the most potent centrally active anticholinergic agents used in medicine. Some antipsychotic drugs with relatively less tendency to induce acute extrapyramidal reactions (for example, clozapine and thioridazine) are also strongly anticholinergic (see Table 10). The anticholinergic intoxication syndrome is best managed by immediate removal of the offending agent (see also Chapter 4). In addition, physostigmine (Eserine, Antilirium) — the only commonly available, centrally as well as peripherally active, reversible anticholinesterase agent — may be useful in moderate degrees of intoxication. However, its usefulness and safety in more serious and life-threatening intoxications with coma and impaired vital functions (especially those associated with an acute overdose of a tricyclic antidepressant) are less likely, and emergency physicians avoid its use in comatose or otherwise dangerously intoxicated patients with unstable vital functions.

The potential of antiparkinsonism agents to induce CNS toxicity indicates caution in their use, particularly in patients treated with neuroleptics of low potency or with tricyclic antidepressants. Other problems of these drugs include the added complexity and expense of routine "polypharmacy." Dependence may occur with these agents, and they sometimes induce euphoria — effects that may contribute to the common difficulty in discontinuing them. Although the antiparkinsonism agents are sometimes given prophylactically to avoid acute extrapyramidal effects of antipsychotic agents, this practice is often unnecessary, especially given conservative dosing with the neuroleptics. It is a matter of clinical judgment to evaluate the urgency of indications and contraindications for their use. Further, sound practice includes the attempt to withdraw these drugs *gradually* after several weeks, and certainly within 4 to 12 weeks after the onset of an acute extrapyramidal reaction. This practice is often possible because of the tolerance to early neurological effects of the antipsychotic drugs that evolves in many patients.

Akathisia (motor restlessness, fidgeting, pacing, "restless legs," and a drive to move about) is a common but often overlooked early motor symptom complex of obscure pathophysiologic basis. Although the experience of anxiety is a part of the syndrome, it is often experienced as "alien" to the patient. The anxiety should not be mistaken for increasing primary psychotic anxiety or agitation or treated by increasing the dose of an antipsychotic drug. The risk of akathisia appears to be high at all ages, and especially between ages 30 and 60. The reaction can sometimes be managed by reducing the dose or changing to a different chemical class of antipsychotic agents. Antiparkinsonism drugs, including amantadine, may have a beneficial effect, as may anxiolytic-sedative agents with putative muscle-relaxing properties, such as the benzodiazepines. Moderate doses of propranolol may also be beneficial. Unfortunately, some patients respond poorly to treatment, and the distress of the akathisia must be weighed against the need for antipsychotic medication. While the timing of this reaction is generally similar to that of parkinsonism, it may emerge as the symptoms of acute psychosis abate or may reoccur or persist indefinitely, because tolerance to akathisia is less likely than to dystonic reactions or parkinsonism.

Tardive dyskinesia (late and persistent dyskinesia) is a late-developing extrapyramidal syndrome that encourages reappraisal of the benefits and risks of routine, uninterrupted, and indefinitely prolonged neuroleptic drug therapy. The syndrome consists of involuntary or semivoluntary movements of a choreiform (rapid, tic-like) nature, sometimes with an athetoid or dystonic component. These classically affect the tongue, facial, and neck muscles but often also affect the extremities and digits as well as the trunk and muscles that control breathing or swallowing. Early signs of tardive dyskinesia are unwanted movements of the tongue, face, or extremities. Oral-lingual-masticatory movements are common, especially in older patients, but it is usual to find abnormalities of posture and choreoathetotic movements of the fingers as well, especially in younger patients. The movements of tardive dyskinesia are much less voluntary and purposeful and more classically choreoathetotic than the stereotyped mannerisms and posturing that may occur spontaneously in schizophrenia. The signs of tardive dyskinesia usually become worse if the antipsychotic agent is withdrawn and can be suppressed, at least temporarily, by increasing the dose, readministering a neuroleptic drug, or adding an amine-depleting agent such as reserpine. There is no evidence that tardive dyskinesia is progressive, but continued use of a neuroleptic probably reduces the chances of spontaneous remission.

Although tardive dyskinesias are painless, the syndrome can be embarrassing and distressing, especially in relatively well functioning outpatients. In some cases the patient's skills in self-care, feeding, and swallowing, as well as vocationally or recreationally important dexterity, can be impaired; and severe cases can be as disabling as Huntington's disease. A thorough neurological evaluation of cases of tardive dyskinesia should attempt to exclude other involuntary movement disorders such as Huntington's disease, rheumatic chorea, Wilson's disease, and other rare toxic or degenerative dyskinetic syndromes (see Table 19). The prevalence of the syndrome has varied in epidemiological studies from a few percent to as many as 40 to 50% of patients "maintained" on antipsychotic medications for many years. It is unusual to develop the syndrome in less than a few months. Recent reports suggest an incidence of about 5% after a year

Table 19 Differential diagnosis for tardive dyskinesia (TD)

Alternative disorder	Familial	Psychiatric features	Specific findings
Transient dyskinesias on neuroleptic withdrawal	0	+	Recent neuroleptic treatment
Stereotyped mannerisms of schizophrenia	?	+	Psychiatric history; characteristic movements, not choreic
Oral dyskinesias of the elderly (e.g., Miege's syndrome)	0	+/−	Miege's progressive oral-mandibular dystonia with blepharospasm
Dental conditions, dentures	0	0	Dental history and examination
Torsion dystonia (dystonia musculorum deformans)	+	+/−	Early onset, progressive, no chorea
Focal dystonias (torticollis, mandibular dystonia, blepharospasm)	?	+/−	Dystonic rather than choreic
Tourette's syndrome; focal "tics" ("habit" spasm)	+/−	+/−	Vocalizations prominent, rarer in TD
Huntington's disease	+	+	Dominant inheritance; chorea early, dementia late; CT scan (caudate atrophy late)
Heavy metal intoxication (manganese, selenium)	0	+	Mining, industrial exposure; assays for specific metal
Wilson's hepatolenticular degeneration	+	+/−	Serum Cu < 80 μg/dl, ceruloplasmin < 20 μg/dl; urine Cu > 100 mg/dl; ophthalmic, hepatic, renal symptoms

of treatment with depot fluphenazine, and that the period of maximum risk may be from 6 to 24 months (see Baldessarini, 1985). Several surveys among the elderly indicate that spontaneous dyskinesias (especially oral-lingual movements) unrelated to neuroleptic treatment occur in perhaps 5 to 10% of those evaluated. The prevalence of persistent dyskinesias, corrected for the occurrence of spontaneous dyskinesias, averages approximately 15 to 20% among those exposed to a neuroleptic agent for more than a year.

The risk of tardive dyskinesia and of spontaneous dyskinesias increases strikingly with age, especially after age 50, although children and adolescents sometimes develop severe and widespread dyskinesias. Generally, too, the severity increases in elderly patients, and chances for spontaneous

Table 19 (continued)

Alternative disorder	Familial	Psychiatric features	Specific findings
Calcifications of basal ganglia (e.g., Fahr's syndrome)	+/−	0	Skull x-ray
Rheumatic chorea (Syndenham's; St. Vitus' dance)	0	0	Recent streptococcal infection
Residua of encephalitis or anoxic damage	0	+/−	Specific history; EEG
Neural aspects of systemic metabolic or inflammatory disorders	0	+/−	Tests for specific diagnoses, including hepatic, renal, hyperthyroid, hypoparathyroid, hypoglycemic, inflammatory
Dopamine agonist excess	0	+/−	Recent exposure to L-dopa, bromocriptine, amphetamine
Other drug intoxications	0	+/−	Phenytoin, lithium, antidepressants
Cerebral neoplasm (esp. basal ganglia, thalamus)	0	+/−	Focal neural symptoms, CT scan, EEG

Symbols: + indicates usually present; +/− indicates variable; 0 indicates not present; ? indicates uncertain.

Note that in most cases, the psychiatric history, exposure to neuroleptics, and pattern of symptoms are strongly indicative of TD; most of the alternatives are either rare or clearly indicated by the history and examination; the high risk of spontaneous dyskinesias, especially of tongue and jaw in the elderly can be confused with TD unless systemic choreic-dystonic symptoms are also present.

remission diminish markedly. Women may be at a slightly higher risk than men, although younger men may be at somewhat higher risk of severe and generalized forms of the condition. There is also suggestive but inconclusive epidemiological evidence of greater risk in patients with a major affective disorder and even more preliminary suggestions that intermittent dosing with neuroleptics (which may covary with affective disorders) may also increase the risk of tardive dyskinesia. Since most patients treated with neuroleptics do not develop late dyskinesias, it follows that unknown constitutional factors contributing to risk probably exist. Associations of increased risk with particular agents, such as neuroleptics of high potency or prolonged duration of action, or with the use of high doses, have been suspected but not demonstrated.

The cause of tardive dyskinesias remains mysterious. It is not even certain that it is reasonable to seek a unitary pathophysiology or etiology in view of the variable clinical manifestations and pharmacologic responses of conditions currently considered as tardive dyskinesia. Animal experimentation indicates that increasing sensitivity of dopamine receptors during prolonged neuroleptic treatment can lead eventually to a state of increased response to a dopamine agonist, even if the neuroleptic is not withdrawn, and may be associated with excessive spontaneous mouth movements in rodents or dyskinesias in monkeys. The observation of increased sensitivity to dopamine agonists after prolonged treatment of animals with a neuroleptic has suggested a "dopamine supersensitivity" hypothesis for tardive dyskinesia, but this concept has not been proved to account for all features of the clinical syndrome. Clinical support for this concept has, however, been provided by observations that tardive dyskinesia tends to be worsened by dopamine agonists and improved by antagonists. The observation that anticholinergic antiparkinsonism agents tend to worsen the movements is consistent with overactivity in the dopamine system as well.

No satisfactory treatment for tardive dyskinesia has been found. Many cases resolve slowly (months) after withdrawal of the neuroleptic treatment when the patient's psychiatric condition permits this course of management. Perhaps the best way to deal with the problem is through the thoughtful and conservative use of neuroleptic agents. Compelling indications (chronic psychosis that responds to the treatment) should be required to continue a neuroleptic for longer than 6 to 12 months. Other treatments are available for recurrent or chronic mood disorders, severe personality disorders, and conditions characterized by anxiety. Alternatives should be considered for conditions in which indications for a neuroleptic agent are not strong. Sound practice involves an empirical search with each patient for the lowest effective dose of a neuroleptic for prolonged use in a maintenance program, as well as repeated attempts to remove the drug altogether. Additional suggestions for the management of tardive dyskinesia are given in Table 20.

Sometimes transient tardive dyskinesia–like reactions occur for several days on the sudden discontinuation of a neuroleptic. These so-called withdrawal-emergent dyskinesias are especially common in young patients after discontinuation of relatively high doses of a potent neuroleptic. It is not known whether these temporary reactions are pathophysiologically identical to tardive dyskinesias or whether they represent early cases of the more prolonged variety. It is usual for tardive dyskinesia to worsen, or to become fully manifest, on withdrawal of neuroleptic treatment, and the distinction between this phenomenon and transient, withdrawal dyskinesias is sometimes unclear or arbitrary.

Table 20 Suggested guidelines for the avoidance and management of tardive dyskinesia

- Consider indications for prolonged neuroleptic therapy carefully; indications (chronic psychosis) should be compelling, with objective evidence of benefit
- Seek alternative therapies in neuroses and mood and personality disorders
- Use lower doses in elderly patients and children, strive for minimum effective doses, avoid multiple drugs, and remove antiparkinsonism agents when possible
- Advise patients and families of risks and benefits; arrive at a mutual decision when use of neuroleptic exceeds six months. Note discussion and agreement in clinical record
- Examine patient regularly for early signs of choreoathetosis and oral-lingual dyskinesia. Consider alternative neurological diagnoses
- Reevaluate and document indications and response at least every three to six months and attempt to reduce dose
- At earliest sign of dyskinesia, lower the dose, change to a less potent agent, or ideally stop treatment and await remission as long as psychiatric status permits
- Treat dyskinesia with benign agents first (diazepam, deanol, or lecithin in high doses, possibly lithium or valproate); stay alert to new experimental therapies, if only to bide time and offer hope. While reserpine may be relatively safe and at least partly effective, reinstitute a neuroleptic only as an extreme measure for disabling dyskinesias (or urgent psychiatric indications), using lowest feasible doses

"Rabbit" syndrome (perioral tremor) is another reaction associated with neuroleptic drugs which usually occurs late in therapy. This timing has led to its (probably erroneous) classification with the tardive dyskinesias. It may represent an atypical and localized variant of parkinsonism, since the rate of the mouth movements (about five per second) is similar to more typical limb tremors of parkinsonism. Moreover, the reaction sometimes responds favorably to treatment with antiparkinsonism agents and is usually reversible after the neuroleptic treatment has been discontinued.

Other Neurological Effects

In addition to the common, neuroleptic-induced neurological syndromes already described, other effects of antipsychotic drugs on the central nervous system have also been reported. They are described in the following paragraphs.

Neuroleptic malignant syndrome. This syndrome, or "hypothalamic crisis," is a group of reactions marked by extreme parkinsonism-like rigidity or catatonia and variable abnormalities of autonomic function, sometimes with striking hyperthermia. The reaction had been considered rare but is encountered increasingly commonly when large doses of the more potent neuroleptics are used. Additional risk factors may include youth or advanced age and elevated environmental temperature. The syndrome typically occurs early in treatment. The pathophysiology is not known, but it is reasonable to assume that effects which contribute to other acute extrapyramidal reactions as well as the poikilothermal or temperature-deregulating actions of many neuroleptics are involved, as well as changes secondary to hypertonic activity of skeletal muscle.

Features of this syndrome include persistent (sometimes high) fever, muscular rigidity, and catatonia (often with elevated plasma creatinine phosphokinase and myoglobin), coarse tremor, drooling, akinesia, stupor with fluctuating levels of consciousness, mutism or severe dysarthria, unstable blood pressure, and tachycardia. Dyspnea and seizures may also occur. There is a risk of myoglobinuria with renal impairment. This severe reaction has a significant mortality rate, possibly as high as 20%, and its treatment is unsatisfactory. Antiparkinsonism agents usually are not beneficial. There are a few case reports of beneficial effects with the muscle relaxant dantrolene sodium (Dantrium), typically in oral doses of 200 mg/day, by analogy to the use of intravenous dantrolene to interrupt the malignant hyperthermia rarely associated with general anesthesia and based on altered calcium transport in skeletal muscle that is not found in the neuroleptic syndrome. The dopamine-agonist ergoline drug bromocriptine mesylate (Parlodel) in divided oral doses of 5–30 mg/day may also be helpful and is remarkably well tolerated by psychotic patients in the presence of a neuroleptic agent. Management of the malignant neuroleptic syndrome includes intravenous fluids, control of the fever, and other supportive measures after immediate discontinuation of the neuroleptic. The reaction usually subsides gradually within a week or two. Especially prolonged and dangerous reactions have occurred following a depot injection of fluphenazine.

Seizures. Neuroleptic drugs, and perhaps especially low-potency phenothiazines and loxapine, may increase the incidence of seizures in epileptic patients. The piperazines and haloperidol possibly have less tendency to do this, and molindone may be especially unlikely to do so. (Antidepressants and lithium salts can also have this effect.) These impressions, however, are based on clinical anecdotes and indirect evidence from animal or other laboratory experiments rather than on controlled clinical studies. Usually, clinical judgment is required to balance the patient's need for antipsychotic medication with the need for an anticonvulsant. The dosage of the latter may need to be increased to counter the potentially increased risk of seizures. On the other hand, anticonvulsants often increase metabolic inactivation of neuroleptics and may diminish their effectiveness.

Acute intoxication. In contrast to almost all other CNS depressants, the lethality of antipsychotic agents on acute overdose and their potential for inducing deep and prolonged coma and respiratory depression are limited; that is, they have a very high *therapeutic index* (ratio of toxic or lethal to therapeutic doses). The clinical half-maximally effective lethal doses (LD_{50}) for these agents are not known but can be 20 to over 1,000 times higher than behaviorally effective doses in laboratory animals. Patients have survived ingestions of many grams of chlorpromazine, and it is virtually impossible to commit suicide by taking an overdose of an antipsychotic agent alone. It is essential, however, to consider the simultaneous presence of more lethal or treatable forms of acute intoxication, since ingestions are often mixed. For example, comatose psychiatric patients may also have taken alcohol, a barbiturate, an agent with strong anticholinergic activity, or an antidepressant or lithium salt. Dialysis can be used to remove barbiturates, lithium, and some other central depressants, but it is not effective in removing antipsychotic or antidepressant agents because of their strong affinity for protein and lipids in blood and tissues. The reversible anticholinesterase agent physostigmine (Eserine or Antilirium) penetrates the blood-brain diffusion barrier and can be administered cautiously for the central anticholinergic syndrome uncomplicated by coma or severe cardiovascular dysfunction. Attempts to induce vomiting after overdoses of antipsychotic agents may be unsuccessful, owing to the strong antiemetic effects of most of them (thioridazine and clozapine are exceptions). One implication of the limited acute toxicity, as well as the lack of addiction potential, of antipsychotic agents is that large quantities of these drugs can be prescribed with relative impunity, even for patients with impaired judgment or impaired impulse control.

Psychiatric Complications

With the increased interest in tardive dyskinesia and other possible late complications associated with long-term use of neuroleptic agents, there has been some speculation about the potential for patients' mental status worsening after prolonged treatment. Support for such speculation includes the plausible, but unproved, hypothesis that there may be a "limbic" equivalent to supersensitivity to dopamine in the basal ganglia and that this might become manifest as psychiatric disturbances. This concept has already been mentioned with respect to the point that neuroleptic discontinuation studies have not ruled out a slow withdrawal reaction to the loss of medication (see Figures 6 and 7), and to observations of rising requirements of neuroleptic doses in a minority of chronically psychotic patients (see Table 16). Since there is little evidence of new, iatrogenic disturbance in these latter cases, however, it seems more parsimonious to interpret them as an example of late *tolerance* to the antipsychotic effects of the treatment. It has been suggested, moreover, that some patients when rapidly withdrawn from relatively high doses of a neuroleptic may experience transient psychiatric disturbances dissimilar in quality and severity from their previous condition. Finally, there have been similar suggestions concerning some children whose behavior became more disturbed following prolonged neuroleptic treatment. These intriguing and potentially serious possibilities require further investigation and add to the necessity of using long-term neuroleptic treatment thoughtfully and only with compelling indications, minimum effective doses, and gradual changes in dose.

General Toxicity of Antipsychotic Agents

Peripheral actions presumed to represent anticholinergic effects are modest with most antipsychotic agents and are usually limited to annoying symptoms such as dry mouth and blurred vision, although ileus and urinary retention can occur, particularly in older patients. Precipitating an attack of acute *glaucoma* with any agent having anticholinergic activity is a possibility; but with antipsychotic agents and even with antidepressant drugs, this event is rare and is usually associated with narrow-angle glaucoma, which itself is not common. Acute glaucoma is an emergency calling for immediate ophthalmologic treatment with a cholinergic or other miotic agent such as pilocarpine. Chronic glaucoma can almost always be managed with cholinomimetic eyedrops, even while anticholinergic psychotropic agents are being used. Occasionally cholinergic agents have also been given in eyedrops (such as pilocarpine nitrate, 1% ophthalmic solution) to overcome cycloplegia and impaired visual accommodation, in a mouthwash to increase salivation, or orally (in daily doses of 5 to 10 mg of pilocarpine, 5 to 15 mg of neostigmine, or about 75 mg a day of bethanechol [Urecholine]) to counter these or other systemic anticholinergic side effects of the antipsychotic or antidepressant agents, such as constipation or urinary hesitation. In general, however, this approach is not consistently effective and it is not usually used.

Other ophthalmologic problems can also occur with the antipsychotic agents. The most serious is a rare, irreversible, degenerative *pigmentary retinopathy* following large doses of thioridazine (above 900 mg/day) and possibly other low-potency neuroleptics. In addition, prolonged high doses of low-potency phenothiazines and thioxanthenes have been associated with deposits of drug substances and pigment in the cornea and lens as well as in the skin. The deposits in the eye can be visualized best with a slit lamp, rarely impair vision, and disappear over many months after withdrawal of the medication. Although penicillamine and other agents have been advocated to hasten the removal of phenothiazines from the eye or skin, there is little evidence that they help.

Skin reactions include photosensitivity early in treatment and later a blue-gray discoloration. The latter has most often been associated with prolonged high doses of chlorpromazine. Maculopapular rashes occur on occasion, and there is some risk of contact dermatitis among nurses handling solutions of antipsychotic agents.

The risk of severe cardiovascular toxicity due to antipsychotic agents is not high. Although sustained hypotension is not frequently encountered, *orthostatic hypotension* can be a problem, especially when the less potent phenothiazines are given to elderly patients. The hypotensive effects of these agents are rather idiosyncratic and inconsistently correlated with doses; thus the formerly common ritual of giving small test doses of intramuscular medication is poorly founded. An important practical reason for avoiding large intramuscular doses, especially of the less potent agents, is that they are painful and may lead to elevated serum levels of transaminases or lactic dehydrogenase from local necrosis, *not* liver damage. If severe hypotension does develop, it can usually be managed by bed rest or elevation of the legs and use of elastic stockings. If a vasoactive agent is required, the rational choice is a purely alpha-adrenergic pressor amine such as metaraminol (Aramine; rarely is the more potent agent l-norepinephrine, Levophed, required) to reverse the modest alpha-antagonistic effects of phenothiazines. The beta-agonistic cardiac stimulants such as epinephrine or isoproterenol (Isuprel) would increase pooling of blood in the splanchnic and peripheral areas to worsen the hypotension and thus are contraindicated.

In addition to the unpredictable effects of antipsychotic agents on blood pressure in certain vulnerable patients, they may increase the risk of potentially lethal *ventricular arrhythmias,* partly because they decrease intracardiac conduction time and may prolong ventricular repolarization. These hazards may be greatest with thioridazine and pimozide among the antipsychotic agents, but the risk with any antipsychotic agent appears to be small. With pimozide, it is recommended that the dose be decreased or the drug stopped if the Q-T interval on electrocardiogram exceeds 520 msec in adults or 470 msec in children. Haloperidol, the potent piperazine phenothiazines, and molindone appear to be relatively safe for cardiac patients and unlikely to interact badly with digitalis or other cardiovascular and diuretic agents. Because of their potential cardiovascular effects, as well as the possibility of undesirable drug interactions, it is considered good practice to reduce or omit the use of low-potency neuroleptics for a day or two prior to electroconvulsive treatment with barbiturate anesthesia and prior to surgery. Alternatively, small divided doses of high-potency agents can be used when required in such circumstances.

Other annoying side effects of antipsychotic agents include presumably autonomic or hypothalamic effects such as changes in appetite, *weight gain,* fluid retention, *breast enlargement* and engorgement (in men as well as women), and even galactorrhea, decreased libido, and *ejaculatory incompetence* in men, and delayed ovulation and amenorrhea in women.

These effects are most often associated with the less potent phenothiazines and particularly with thioridazine. (Thioridazine has even been advocated as an adjunct in the treatment of premature ejaculation.) Such sexual effects are sometimes overlooked by clinicians but can represent serious problems to patients.

A sustained *prolactin-increasing action* is characteristic of most antipsychotic agents (largely mediated by the antagonism of effects of hypothalamic dopamine on the anterior pituitary) and even of small doses of reserpine as used to treat hypertension. This response represents a theoretical risk in patients with an occult or identified carcinoma of the breast. However, there is at present no compelling evidence that antipsychotic agents have a breast-tumor-inducing effect or that they increase the risk of any carcinoma. Nevertheless, regular breast examination should be a routine part of the medical management of female patients treated with a prolactin-elevating agent for more than six months. Antipsychotic agents can mildly depress testosterone output, but this is of doubtful physiological or psychosexual significance. It has been reported that antipsychotic agents have inhibitory effects on the output of growth hormone, opposite to the releasing action of L-dopa. This effect is also of doubtful physiological importance, and antipsychotic drugs are not useful as a treatment of acromegaly. There is no evidence that antipsychotic agents retard the growth and development of psychotic children to a clinically important extent, although growth should be monitored closely in young patients exposed to any psychotropic agent for more than six months.

Although there has been a great deal of concern about jaundice and agranulocytosis being caused by antipsychotic agents, these problems are encountered infrequently. The *jaundice* is almost always of a cholestatic, presumably allergic, type and is usually transient. It was formerly more common, particularly in association with chlorpromazine, and it may have become less frequent (incidence not more than 2%) because of factors related to pharmaceutical formulation. It usually appears within the first month of treatment. Many CNS depressants can worsen hepatic encephalopathy, partly owing to their direct actions on the brain but also because of their tendency to diminish hepatic function by competition with hepatic microsomal oxidases. Subclinical biliary obstructive effects may be common; liver biopsies have revealed an incidence of mild obstructive changes in as many as 25% of patients treated with an antipsychotic agent.

Agranulocytosis is rare (incidence less than 0.01%); it has a peak incidence within the first two months of treatment, and has been encountered particularly in older women. This reaction has almost always been associated with low-potency phenothiazines and thioxanthenes as well as clozapine and is virtually unknown with haloperidol, fluphenazine, or thiothixene. Agranulocytosis is a potentially catastrophic and often rapidly developing medical emergency with a high mortality rate. It can be predicted only in rare instances from occasional routine white blood cell counts and *must be suspected* and promptly evaluated in cases of malaise, fever, or sore throat that occur early in the course of antipsychotic chemotherapy. Frequent leukocyte counts in the first two months of treatment may reveal a downward trend predicting agranulocytosis, although early, moderate, transient reductions in white cell levels of little significance are not unusual. Some hematologists advise weekly leukocyte counts for at least eight weeks after initiation of therapy, particularly with chlorpromazine, clozapine, or other low-potency agents.

Defensive rituals of little value have developed in the medical management of patients receiving antipsychotic agents for prolonged periods; these include occasional routine liver function tests and blood counts, which contribute little other than a false sense of security and possibly some decreased risk of malpractice charges. Laboratory tests cannot substitute for an alert and well-informed physician.

The safety of antipsychotic agents in *pregnancy and lactation* is not well established. These agents do pass the blood-placenta barrier as well as the blood-brain barrier, and they are secreted in human milk in very low levels. They can induce a mild degree of sedation followed by motor excitement in the newborn if the mother has recently been treated with a neuroleptic. Evidence of sustained neurotoxic actions in newborn laboratory animals born to mothers exposed to a neuroleptic is tentative and inconsistent; there is no evidence that antipsychotic agents are responsible for an increased incidence of fetal malformations. Low, divided doses of the high-potency neuroleptics may be relatively safe during pregnancy. Nevertheless, the current consensus is that the use of antipsychotic agents should be avoided as far as possible during pregnancy and lactation, and especially in the first trimester of pregnancy. As a general principle, it is probably wise to avoid the use of single high doses and of low-potency agents during pregnancy to minimize exposure to potentially toxic foreign molecules. Despite the need for a conservative approach to antipsychotic medication during pregnancy, clinical judgment must be exercised when the indications for medical treatment or psychiatric hospitalization during pregnancy are compelling.

Elderly patients treated with antipsychotic agents are particularly likely to be troubled by toxic effects of all types, and unwanted effects on the brain and behavior may be especially striking. Generally, except for the increased incidence and seriousness of effects in the elderly, the qualitative nature of the side effects of antipsychotic agents does not change with advancing age. Although there is a tendency to keep doses of antipsychotic agents low because of the intolerance of older patients to side effects, daily doses less than the equivalent of 200 or 300 mg of chlorpromazine are often ineffective in the control of psychotic thought, affect, and behavior. Thus, minimum effective doses of antipsychotic agents are probably not much lower than those estimated for younger adults or adolescents, but the margin of safety is significantly reduced in the elderly. *Low, divided,* and *gradually increased doses* of the *more potent agents* are currently preferred over low-potency phenothiazines or thioxanthenes for elderly psychotic patients.

Interactions with Other Agents

Antipsychotic agents can have additive central-depressant effects when administered with other agents with such actions, including sedatives, hypnotics, opioids, or alcohol. The low-potency antipsychotic agents can add to central and peripheral anticholinergic actions of antiparkinsonism, antidepressant, or other drugs with antimuscarinic activity. Toxic, confusional states are common when antipsychotic and other psychotropic agents, including lithium salts, antidepressants, and sedatives, are combined. Some neuroleptics have been reported to increase plasma levels of tricyclic antidepressants. Chlorpromazine and some of its N-desmethylated metabolites appear to have sufficient ability to block uptake into noradrenergic neurons that they can be expected to interfere with the antihypertensive actions of guanethidine (Ismelin) and other postganglionic blocking agents that act by local accumulation in such neurons. Most neuroleptic agents can be expected to worsen idiopathic Parkinson's disease and to diminish the efficacy of its treatment. Blood levels of amantadine may rise with the addition of some diuretics.

Alternative and Investigational Treatments

There is no longer any doubt that adequate treatment with antipsychotic agents is a cornerstone to the medical management of acutely psychotic patients. Evidence of useful long-term effects in schizophrenia or other disorders with sustained psychotic manifestations is also strong, as has been discussed earlier. It is less clear, however, that the use of antipsychotic agents is adequate or sufficient treatment for patients with acute or chronic psychotic disorders. A particularly complicated question is whether other forms of treatment contribute importantly to the management of chronic schizophrenic psychoses. The evaluation of the role of psychotherapies in schizophrenia has been much less rigorous than that of the chemotherapies. However, there is some information based on comparisons of chemotherapy with psychosocial forms of treatment. Research at the Massachusetts Mental Health Center and the extensive studies of P. R. May in California support the conclusion that the presence or absence of an antipsychotic agent made a marked difference in the clinical outcome in schizophrenia, whereas supportive milieu treatment and rehabilitation efforts, or intensive psychotherapy even when conducted by experienced therapists, contributed very little and were largely ineffective when used without medication. In a similar study of nearly 400 chronic schizophrenics, G. E. Hogarty and his colleagues (1977) evaluated the rate of relapse after one year of treatment and found that only 26% of the patients treated with chlorpromazine plus supportive psychotherapy relapsed (and perhaps nearly half of those who relapsed did not take the medication regularly), whereas 63% treated with identical support plus placebo relapsed (see Figure 7); the withholding of psychotherapy (drug treatment alone) increased the relapse rates by only another 10%.

The importance of psychotherapy in the treatment of schizophrenia remains a controversial topic, and one that is heavily influenced by traditions, schools of thought, and practice rather than scientific evaluation. Clearly, psychoanalysis and dynamic psychotherapy have contributed a great deal to an appreciation of the psychotic experience and to hypotheses about the intrapsychic dynamics and possible influences of early and current life experiences on the development and course of schizophrenia. Moreover, a few very dedicated analytic therapists have invested enormous efforts in treating a few chronic schizophrenics; their results have occasionally been encouraging, but uncontrolled and anecdotal. There seems to be a fair consensus among experienced psychotherapists that probing and uncovering techniques are contraindicated in the treatment of schizophrenia. Additional research is now emerging on this topic. Two important studies reported in 1984 from the Chestnut Lodge Hospital in Maryland (McGlashan, 1984) and McLean Hospital in Massachusetts (Gunderson et al., 1984) sustained the impression that intensive, psychoanalytically-oriented psychotherapy, even when conducted for years by experts, has little impact on the course of schizophrenia or adds little to a supportive, medically-oriented approach. These studies are somewhat inconclusive in that critical control conditions were not included, sharp distinctions between forms of treatment were not always maintained, and patients with dissimilar illnesses may have been included but not randomly assigned. The studies do appear to support the impression that intensive psychotherapy is not an economical or routine alternative in the treatment of schizophrenia. Indeed, psychotherapy alone without medication is rarely attempted at the present time; a confused and incoherent patient is not an optimal candidate for rational verbal psychotherapy, and there is evidence that the antipsychotic agents can facilitate the relationship and verbal interchanges between patient and therapist. Even though the efficacy of these efforts has not been rigorously demonstrated, on clinical and humanitarian grounds most psychiatrists reasonably combine supportive and rehabilitative efforts with medications in working with chronically psychotic patients. The hypothesis that thorough and lasting change in schizophrenia can only be gained by prolonged, intensive, and expensive attempts to bring about characterological change through self-understanding must be judged unproved. Moreover, the idea cannot be supported that medications are merely palliative or that they deprive patients of a positive or "growth-promoting" experience of "working through" a psychosis in psychotherapy. Psychosis is painful, and its early termination or alleviation should be the desired and appropriate goals of management.

A curious source of suspicion about the use of medication in schizophrenia has come from some particularly zealous psychosocially or community-oriented professionals and from certain "antipsychiatrists" critical of the medical model of schizophrenia. They have asserted that medications are used by agents (medically trained psychiatrists) of an oppressive society to control eccentric or sensitive individuals, and to impose on them a medical label for what is really an idiosyncratic lifestyle or highly personal point of view. While such a point of view has its appeal, if only to diminish responsibility for the care of some of the most severely ill and incapacitated psychiatric patients, it does not offer a reasonable alternative.

One of the risks in dealing with a pervasive and severely disruptive chronic illness that is also idiopathic and essentially incurable, particularly if it involves mental and social function, is that unusual and offbeat proposals may arise. Over the centuries there have been many examples of this phenomenon in proposals for the treatment of schizophrenic patients. Recent examples include an unusual set of hypotheses and practices that have become something of a cult in North America. Nevertheless, it can be stated categorically that the use of "orthomolecular" or "megavitamin" treatments of chronic schizophrenia, including special diets and extraordinary doses of vitamins, minerals, or other chemicals, have not been demonstrated to offer a viable alternative to usual psychiatric treatments based on scientifically acceptable evidence.

An imaginative approach that has undergone a fair degree of testing in recent years is the use of hemodialysis to treat schizophrenia, perhaps to remove an endogenous, unidentified toxin. This approach has not been strongly or consistently supported in several controlled studies. A hypothesis associated with this endeavor, which accompanied the nearly revolutionary rise of interest in peptides in neuroscience in the past decade, was that peptide molecules might be responsible for some features of schizophrenia and could be removed by dialysis. Other related therapeutic proposals that have included attempts to treat psychotic patients with opioids, opioid antagonists, or natural or chemically modified synthetic peptides have so far been unsuccessful in small numbers of controlled trials. Nevertheless, the general idea may have merit beyond fashionable attempts to apply the latest technology to a difficult unsolved problem. As effective methods are developed to alter peptide metabolism or activity pharmacologically, additional treatments of this type may become available in the future.

Novel but more conventional pharmacologic therapies have also been considered, but remain unproved or ineffective. The attempt to modify psychosis by the use of large doses of beta-adrenergic antagonists or of benzodiazepines has not been successful in schizophrenia. The potentially useful short-term sedative actions of benzodiazepines in cases of acute psychosis, as well as the promising actions of low doses of propranolol against neuroleptic-induced akathisia, have already been mentioned.

There is some evidence that lithium salts or other antimanic agents may have beneficial effects in some patients who may meet diagnostic criteria for schizophrenia. Nevertheless, the characteristics of those who respond favorably are similar to patients with manic-depressive illness. Many are "schizo-affective," typically excited and agitated as well as psychotic. The distinction between this syndrome and the major affective disorders is difficult, if not impossible, at the present time. Occasional reports of favorable effects of carbamazepine or other anticonvulsants may reflect a similar diagnostic overlap with major affective disorders, cases of occult cerebral dysrhythmia (similar to temporal lobe epilepsy), or simply chance associations with spontaneous remissions.

Other interesting proposals have emerged recently, including a possible role for calcium channel blocking agents, which are commonly employed in cardiology. For example, there are a few reports of favorable responses, at least in acutely disturbed patients (most of whom were probably manic), to verapamil (Calan, Isoptin). It has also been noted that certain older antipsychotic agents, including thioridazine and diphenylbutyl-piperidines, also have effects on calcium transport at neuronal and other excitable cell membranes. Whether such observations may lead to useful new treatments for psychotic patients remains a topic for future research.

One of the most provocative concepts in this field in recent years is the increasing skepticism concerning the requirement for antidopaminergic actions of an effective antipsychotic agent, and concerning the inevitability of association of neurotoxic extrapyramidal effects and desirable antipsychotic effects. Atypical agents such as clozapine, fluperlapine, an experimental piperazinyl-propylcarbazole (BW-234U), and perhaps sulpiride encourage the search for new principles of antipsychotic drug action. Nevertheless, such a search is still severely limited by the lack of understanding of the pathophysiology or etiology of the idiopathic psychoses or a coherent theory to account for the actions of the more atypical antipsychotic agents. It is very likely that further progress will require greater reliance on empirical, clinical trial and error, or continued readiness for chance observations and a repetition of serendipitous advances like those of the 1950s.

Summary and Conclusions

The availability of modern, effective, and safe antipsychotic drugs has contributed to an almost revolutionary change in the pattern of delivery of psychiatric care to the most severely disturbed patients. These agents have supported and reinforced the melioristic expectations of modern hospital and community psychiatry. Most psychotic patients can be managed in open psychiatric hospitals or in general hospitals, and the duration of hospitalization has been markedly reduced. Many psychotic patients can be maintained in day-care or foster-care programs or at home, and many incipient attacks of acute psychosis can be managed by psychiatrists or other physicians without the need for hospitalization.

Many antipsychotic drugs are now available to the physician; most are "neuroleptic" or more or less neurotoxic. Although there are several chemical types of antipsychotic drugs, they are pharmacologically similar, partly because the methods of predicting antipsychotic activity of new agents have usually depended on observing their neurological actions in animals or their interactions at dopamine receptors in laboratory tests. The main shortcoming of the available antipsychotic agents is their regular tendency to produce acute and sometimes long-lasting or even irreversible neurological disorders of the extrapyramidal motor system. A second shortcoming of these drugs is that their efficacy is easiest to demonstrate in patients with the best prognosis; results are more disappointing as the chronicity of psychosis increases. Despite these shortcomings of the currently available antipsychotic agents, they are clearly effective in the treatment of a broad range of severe psychiatric and neuropsychiatric disorders, and there is reason to hope that better agents can be found to produce antipsychotic effects with minimal neurological toxicity.

3

Lithium Salts and Antimanic Agents

The lithium ion is a unique agent with considerable selectivity in the treatment of mania. In addition, it may have beneficial effects on certain acute psychoses (formerly sometimes called "acute schizophrenic reactions") or so-called excited schizoaffective states in which an affective or mood disturbance is very prominent, some of which may represent atypical forms of mania. Lithium salts also have a unique place in the long-term maintenance of patients with a variety of severe, recurrent mood disorders. Lithium is inferior to the antipsychotic agents, however, in the treatment of other forms of psychosis, particularly schizophrenia. The differential effectiveness of antipsychotic agents and lithium salts has led to a much-needed reawakening of interest in the careful diagnostic differentiation of acute psychoses and to a reconsideration of the former tendency in American psychiatry to use the term *schizophrenia* inappropriately, almost as a synonym for *psychosis.*

Lithium had been used in American medicine in the nineteenth century for the treatment of gout, because lithium urate is very soluble. In that era, lithium bromide was also considered a superior sedative and anticonvulsant. In the late 1940s the solubility of lithium urate led John Cade in Australia to give animals a lithium salt to decrease the nephrotoxicity of uric acid, with which he was experimenting, in his search for a connection between purine metabolism and behavior. Serendipitously, he noted that the lithium salt produced a quieting effect in the animals and decided to try lithium clinically as a sedative. In 1949 he reported several striking anecdotes of favorable responses among severely disturbed manic patients. This report led to an intense investigation of the biology and clinical actions of lithium salts in Europe, notably by Mogens Schou in Denmark in the 1950s and 1960s. The results of several studies led to the early acceptance of lithium in European and English psychiatric practice as a highly effective and safe treatment for manic-depressive illness, both for the treatment of acute mania and for reducing the frequency and severity of recurrent mania and depression.

For a number of reasons, lithium salts were not accepted into American medical practice until 1970. One reason was the strong skepticism felt by American physicians about the safety of lithium salts after several cases of severe intoxication and even death were reported in 1949–1950 among patients using large, uncontrolled amounts of lithium chloride as a salt substitute, while on a sodium-restricted regimen for cardiac or renal failure. It is now known that congestive heart failure or other conditions associated with retention of fluid and salt, as well as sodium restriction and diuresis, markedly increase the retention and toxicity of the lithium ion and that lithium salts cannot be used safely in gram quantities without careful monitoring of blood levels. This high risk of intoxication reflects the very narrow margin of safety (low therapeutic index) of this agent, in contrast to most other psychotropic agents. Another factor contributing to slow development of lithium therapy was the lack of commercial interest in this inexpensive, unpatentable mineral and, consequently, the lack of industrial support to demonstrate the efficacy and safety of its use. However, an overwhelming amount of evidence accumulated to support the usefulness and safety of lithium, and it was finally accepted in American psychiatric practice.

Other metal ions have also been investigated partially for their potentially useful behavioral effects: *cesium* produces behavioral quieting in animals, and *rubidium,* which has many characteristics similar to those of potassium, can produce behavioral stimulation in animals. Rubidium has already been given to man safely and appears to have some stimulatory or antidepressant activity. Its clearance from tissue is extremely slow, however, and the potential toxicity of rubidium and cesium is not well evaluated. Neither agent has been accepted for clinical use. Several additional agents have recently been proposed for the treatment of mania and are discussed at the end of this chapter.

Pharmacology

Preparations of Lithium Salts for Clinical Use

At present there are more than 50 preparations of lithium salts available worldwide, most of which are carbonates (Li_2CO_3). Commonly, tablets are prepared containing 300 mg of the carbonate. Each gram–molecular weight contains two equivalents of lithium, and each 300-mg tablet contains 8.12 milliequivalents (mEq) of lithium; or 1 mEq of lithium is equal to 37 mg of the carbonate salt. Since salt forms and dosage preparations may vary in their content of lithium and in the number of molar equivalents per milligram of salt, it is usual to compare the preparations on the basis of their content of lithium itself in milliequivalent terms. Similarly, blood levels are usually standardized and reported as milliequivalents per liter (mEq/L) of plasma or serum (essentially equivalent). The preparations of lithium salts that are used clinically include acetate, citrate, glutamate, gluconate, orotate, and sulfate salts as well as the carbonate, but currently only carbonate tablets and capsules and citrate syrup are available in this country. A summary of the preparations available in the United States is provided in Table 21.

Because of the low therapeutic index, or safety margin, of lithium salts, daily doses are not set in terms of milligram quantities given but in terms of blood levels of free lithium ion (mEq/L), determined and defined by convention as the levels obtained at 12 hours after the previous dose. Safe and recommended blood concentrations are discussed further in the section on clinical uses of lithium.

Table 21   Lithium preparations in the United States

Salt form	Commercial names	Dosage forms	
Lithium carbonate	Eskalith, Lithane, Lithonate, Lithotabs, and generic	(T),(C) 300 mg (8.1 mEq)	
Lithium carbonate, slow release	Eskalith	(T) 450 mg	(12.1 mEq)
	Lithobid	(T) 300 mg	(8.1 mEq)
Lithium citrate	Cibalith-S and generic	(S) —	(8 mEq/5 ml)

Dosage forms: (C) = capsules; (S) = syrup; (T) = tablets.

Note: Comparisons are best made between preparations and salts on the basis of their content of lithium (expressed as milliequivalents, mEq). Thus, one teaspoon (5 ml) of lithium citrate and one 300-mg tablet or capsule of lithium carbonate contain the same amount of lithium (about 8 mEq) and thus are equivalent for dosing. Daily doses can vary from 300 to over 3,000 mg of lithium salt, and safe dosing requires meeting individual needs to produce a therapeutic blood level (typically about 1 mEq/L of serum at 10–14 hours after the last daily dose), commonly reached on a three-times-per-day dosing regimen. The slow-release preparation of lithium carbonate, Eskalith, contains 450 mg for simplification of its most common use on a twice-daily schedule, in which a total of 900 mg per day is a frequently employed dose to attain a therapeutic blood concentration of lithium.

Absorption, Metabolism, and Elimination

Lithium is readily absorbed after oral administration, and injectable forms are not used. It is easily measured by flame-photometric or atomic-absorption techniques used to assay sodium and potassium. Unlike sodium and potassium ions, lithium lacks a strongly preferential distribution across cell membranes and tends to distribute evenly throughout the total body water space. There is some lag in penetration into the cerebrospinal fluid (CSF), but there is no absolute barrier to its entry into the brain; equilibration between blood and brain is nearly complete within 24 hours. Although assay of lithium concentration in the erythrocyte has been suggested as a superior index of brain levels, this approach has no special advantage in routine clinical practice over the monitoring of serum or plasma levels.

The "metabolism" of lithium ion is almost entirely by renal excretion. As with sodium, 70 to 80% of the lithium ion, which readily passes into the glomerular filtrate, is reabsorbed in the proximal renal tubules and loop of Henle of the nephron. Although there is further absorption of sodium distally (15 to 20%), there is almost no absorption of lithium in the distal renal tubules. Because the proximal reabsorption of these two ions is competitive and distal uptake is not, sodium diuresis and a deficiency of sodium tend to increase the retention of lithium, and hence to increase its toxicity. The renal excretion of lithium is maximal within a few hours and then proceeds more slowly over several days. The average half-life of lithium in the body varies with age, from about 18 to 20 hours in young adults to as long as 36 hours in elderly patients. The pharmacokinetic characteristics of the lithium ion are summarized in Table 22. An important feature of the renal excretion of the lithium ion is that its rate of removal cannot be increased appreciably by the administration of most diuretic agents; similarly, additional sodium input has little effect on the excretion of lithium, while sodium deficiency has a large effect. These physiological facts therefore have important implications for the medical management of patients intoxicated by overdoses of lithium salts.

While most of absorbed lithium is eliminated in the urine, some also appears in other body fluids. For example, levels in saliva are about twice those in plasma; levels in tears are about equal to plasma concentrations. Both fluids have been proposed for clinical monitoring of lithium levels as an alternative to blood samples, but are not frequently employed at the present time. Although it had been believed that loss of water and salt by profuse sweating might lead to retention of lithium, recent investigation

Table 22   Pharmacokinetic parameters for lithium salts

Measurement	Mean ± S.D.
Oral bioavailability	ca. 100%
Distribution volume	0.79 ± 0.34 L/kg
Plasma binding	ca. 0%
Half-life[a]	22 ± 8 hr
Plasma clearance[b]	0.35 ± 0.11 ml/min/kg
Urinary excretion	95 ± 15%
Effective plasma level	0.75–1.25 mEq/L
Toxic plasma level	over 2.0 mEq/L

Note: These characteristics are based mainly on short-term studies, but the rate of elimination tends to decrease over time, and half-life may double after more than a year of treatment. There is also an aging effect, in which half-life may double between ages 20 and 70.
   a. Increased greatly in uremia and increased moderately with aging (to ca. 30–40 hr).
   b. Decreased in uremia and with aging.

reveals that lithium is preferentially secreted in sweat in concentrations about four times in excess of sodium levels, on the basis of ratios to their respective plasma concentrations. Thus, sweating can actually lead to increased *losses* of lithium rather than to retention and increased plasma levels. Evidently as a reflection of the relative nonequilibrium of lithium ion across cell membranes, erythrocyte concentrations average 45% of plasma concentrations in man. CSF levels are also somewhat lower than plasma levels of lithium. Evidence that regulation of the distribution of lithium across cell membranes may be altered in patients with major affective disorders has been reported, but it remains inconsistent and unconvincing.

Because of lithium's low therapeutic index, it is possible to encounter toxic effects even when the blood level, as typically determined clinically, is in the nominally "therapeutic" range (ca. 1 mEq/L). Assays are usually obtained in the morning before the first dose of the day, and at about 12 hours after the last dose of the previous day. This is done for convenience and also to avoid times when plasma levels are rising and falling rapidly, in order to increase the reliability of the measurement. Nevertheless, peak levels are higher than those determined clinically. The potential dangers of high peak concentrations of lithium can be seen by considering the consequences of dosing with the same amount of lithium carbonate (900 mg/day) on a once, twice, or three times daily, divided basis (Table 23). At once-a-day dosing, the peak plasma concentration of lithium can be nearly four times higher than that at the daily nadir. If the latter is

Table 23 Variations in plasma lithium concentration by treatment schedule or formulation of lithium carbonate

Dosage form	Dose/24 hrs (mg)	Dosing interval (hr)	Peak : trough ratio[a]	Mean daily fluctuation (%)[b]
Standard tablet	900	24	3.7	±57.3
	900	12	1.9	±32.0
	900	8	1.7	±25.0
Slow-release tablet	900	12	1.6	±22.5

Source: Data have been reanalyzed after Amdisen, Danish Med. Bull. 22:277, 1977.

Note: While multiple daily dosing or use of a slow-release formulation provides the smoothest delivery of lithium, the peak plasma levels may be considerably higher than the nominal lithium level as typically obtained clinically. For example, on a 300 mg t.i.d. schedule, a nominal level of 0.75 mEq/L might correspond to a peak level of 1.3 mEq/L.

a. Indicates peak level if trough (e.g., at morning blood sampling) = 1.0 mEq/L.

b. Indicates mean variation around mean plasma level.

1 mEq/L, the peak level is almost certain to be associated with toxicity. Even at twice or three times a day dosing, the peak levels may be nearly twice those assayed clinically near the daily lowpoint. These too may be associated with toxicity in some susceptible patients, especially in the elderly.

One means of minimizing the effect of high peak levels of lithium, even on divided dosage schedules, has been the development of slow or controlled release preparations of lithium salts. Two are currently available in the United States (see Table 21). Such preparations can reduce the daily fluctuations of plasma lithium concentrations significantly (see Table 23) and thus may be better tolerated by some patients. Their bioavailability (amount of total dose absorbed) is high and generally similar to that of regular preparations of lithium salts, although this requires verification with blood assays when the preparation is changed. Some patients complain of lower abdominal cramps or diarrhea with such preparations, evidently as a reflection of their delayed absorption in the gut.

A practical consequence of the low therapeutic index of lithium is that once-daily dosing schedules are not used, even with slow-release preparations. Even though the rate of elimination of lithium is similar to that of many neuroleptic and antidepressant agents, which are sometimes given once a day, the low margin of safety precludes this practice with lithium salts. This point was illustrated earlier in Table 5.

In the clinical use of lithium salts, because of their low therapeutic index and the broad range of individual differences in tolerance and excretion of lithium ion, it is usual to determine individual requirements by a close adherence to blood levels of lithium ion. These are often determined daily or every few days early in treatment, as daily oral doses are gradually increased. However, it is possible to determine individual dosage requirements more precisely and quickly by the use of test doses of a lithium salt. Typically, 600 mg of the carbonate is employed, since this dose is rarely toxic in relatively healthy young adults; however, smaller doses are appropriate for elderly or infirm patients, especially those with impaired renal function. In one method, average predictive data (as summarized in Figure 8) can be used to predict individual dosage requirements, based on a single blood assay of lithium ion at 24 hours after the test dose. A somewhat more complex method can give an estimated dosage requirement within 12 hours of the test dose, and requires assay of urine volume for 4 hours as well as the lithium concentration in urine and plasma during the urine collection to permit computation of clearance of lithium ion from the plasma into the urine. Given an estimate of lithium clearance and the desired morning level of plasma lithium concentration, one then

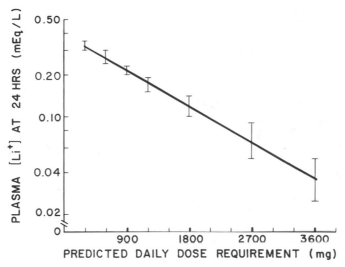

Figure 8 Prediction of approximate total daily dose requirement for lithium carbonate from the plasma lithium level observed 24 hours after a 600-mg oral test dose of the salt. Doses below 600 mg/day or above 3600 mg/day are rarely required. Data are adapted by permission from T. B. Cooper et al., Am. J. Psychiatry 130:601, 1973; and Am. J. Psychiatry 133:440, 1976.

Table 24 Predicting daily dosage of lithium from clearance

To compute daily dose:

Dose (mg/day) = (clearance, L/h)

$\times$ (desired morning plasma [Li$^+$], mEq/L) $\times$ (1.25)

$\times \dfrac{(300 \text{ mg})}{(8.1 \text{ mEq})} \times$ (24 h/day)

To compute lithium clearance:

Clearance (L/h) = (urine [Li$^+$], mEq/L) $\times$ (urine flow, L/h)

$\div$ (observed plasma [Li$^+$], mEq/L)

Source: Norman et al., *Am. J. Psychiatry* 139:1625, 1982.

Protocol: Take 600 mg of lithium carbonate orally; void in 8 hours and collect urine for 4 hours, with plasma (or serum) [Li$^+$] assayed at 2 hours and urine volume and concentration of lithium assayed at the end of the 4-hour collection. The blood and urine samples can also be used to assay sodium and creatinine to monitor renal function prior to initiating lithium treatment. For the computations above, 1.25 corrects the clinical plasma concentration of lithium obtained at 12 hours after the final dose of the day, to the daily mean plasma level; 8.1 = mEq of Li in 300 mg of lithium carbonate (Li$_2$CO$_3$).

computes the required daily dose of lithium carbonate by the methods given in Table 24.

Mechanisms of Action

The mechanisms underlying the effects of lithium ion in affective disorders are not established, although several interesting aspects of its effects have been elucidated. Most attention has been directed to the effects of lithium on electrolyte balance across cell membranes or on the functions of membranes, including those of neurons. Since lithium cannot act as a substrate for the sodium pump, the complete replacement of sodium by lithium leads to the failure of neuronal membranes to maintain their polarization and to conduct action potentials; however, these effects do not explain the actions of lithium concentrations, on the order of 1.0 mEq/L, encountered clinically.

Even though significant alterations in action potentials do not occur at pharmacologic concentrations of lithium ion, there might be more subtle changes in the distribution of ions, including potassium and calcium, as well as sodium. For example, there is some evidence of a temporary increase in intracellular sodium in major affective disorders, and it is possible that lithium might tend to normalize this distribution. However, the basic pathophysiological concept is not established. In general, the lack of a coherent theory of the cause or even of the pathophysiology of mania, bipolar illness, or other major affective syndromes makes it difficult to pose questions that might lead to enlightenment on the clinical actions of lithium.

A recurring theme among hypotheses concerning altered cerebral biochemistry in major affective disorders has been that of increased functional activity of monoamine neurotransmitters in mania and underactivity in depression. Most attention has been directed to the catecholamines and serotonin, with some consideration of acetylcholine as well. Lithium is not known to have significant effects on cholinergic transmission. It does interact at pharmacologic concentrations with catecholamine neurotransmission. For example, significant inhibition of the release of norepinephrine has been reported, and a similar inhibition of the release of dopamine can occur. Serotonin is not affected in the same way; in fact, there is evidence that the release of serotonin can actually be increased in some regions of the brain, notably the hippocampus. There are also reports of subtle alterations in the uptake, intracellular storage, and turnover of catecholamines and of serotonin, but their possible significance is unclear. These findings, overall, tend to support the hypothesis that mania may reflect overactivity of catecholamine neurotransmission or underactivity of serotonin in the brain. Nevertheless, they leave unexplained the mood-stabilizing effects of lithium on depression as well as mania in recurrent affective disorders—actions that are by now rather well established.

Another level of activity of the lithium ion, which might be important in accounting for side effects if not its main clinical effects, is at the function of receptors for neurotransmitters and hormones at cell membranes. There is good evidence of the ability of clinically attained concentrations of lithium to block the stimulation of adenylate cyclase by several hormones at their receptors. Such cyclic-AMP-mediated hormonal actions include the effects of antidiuretic hormone (ADH) of the pituitary on tubular cells of the nephron, where interference by lithium may contribute to the diabetes insipidus syndrome sometimes associated with the use of lithium salts. There may be a similar antagonistic effect at the thyroid gland to interfere with the actions of thyroid-stimulating hormone (TSH). There is also less consistent evidence of an interaction with thyroid hormone. Effects on the stimulation of adenylate cyclase systems in some cells by prostaglandins of the E type (PGE), as well as of catecholamines, have also been reported. However, the evidence for such actions in the central nervous system is weak.

A particularly attractive hypothesis advanced in recent years is that of a "receptor-stabilizing" action of lithium which promised to account for the mood-stabilizing effects of lithium treatment. Evidence for this concept arose from neurophysiological and receptor assay experiments involving catecholamines, mainly dopamine, in the mammalian brain. It is well known, for example, that repeated treatment with an agent that deprives receptors of their endogenous agonist can lead to increased sensitivity or abundance of the receptors at the surface of responsive cells. This effect is usually termed *disuse supersensitivity* and has been found to follow treatment of animals with neuroleptics, reserpine, and methyltyrosine — drugs that block receptors, interfere with presynaptic storage, and inhibit synthesis of dopamine, respectively. Cotreatment with such an agent (for example, a neuroleptic) and lithium was reported to prevent emergence of supersensitivity of dopamine receptors in some experiments. However, these results have not been replicated consistently, and the status of this interesting concept is now uncertain. The neurotransmitter and receptor systems involved were discussed in Chapter 2 in the section on the pharmacology of neuroleptic agents (see Figures 3 and 4).

Another concept related to receptor function in neuronal and other cell membranes for which there is good evidence is that lithium can interfere with the synthesis of certain phospholipids that are important in the structure and function of membranes. A specific effect has been proposed that involves blockade of the enzyme inositol phosphatase. The polyphosphoinositides that are derived from this metabolic pathway are believed to be important in the membrane actions of neurotransmitters, including acetylcholine, and norepinephrine in its alpha-adrenergic actions. These several proposals concerning the actions of lithium are summarized in Table 25.

Lithium ion can also bring about subtle and poorly characterized changes in the cellular uptake and oxidation of glucose. A number of other reported effects of high concentrations of lithium ion on behavior and neuronal function probably are not related to its clinical actions.

Clinical Use

Lithium carbonate was not licensed in the United States for the treatment of mania until 1970. Because some fear continued to exist about its toxic potential, it was only gradually accepted into general psychiatric practice

Table 25   Pharmacologic actions of the lithium ion

- Blocks release of norepinephrine and dopamine in brain
- May increase release of serotonin in some brain regions (e.g., hippocampus)
- May increase neuronal uptake but decrease intracellular storage of catecholamines
- Blocks receptor-mediated actions of several hormones on adenylate cyclase (e.g., antidiuretic hormone, thyroid-stimulating hormone, prostaglandins E, with less certainty about catecholamines and thyroxin)
- Inhibits inositol phosphatase in membranes to inhibit formation of polyphosphoinositides that may mediate actions of some neurotransmitters (e.g., acetylcholine, and norepinephrine at alpha receptors)
- May alter distributions of other ions (e.g., Mg^{++}, Ca^{++}, K^+, and Na^+)
- Experimental data are mixed regarding stabilization of catecholamine and acetylcholine receptors during altered neurotransmitter availability; the importance of these effects is thus uncertain

outside teaching centers in the United States, although its use was widespread in other countries in the 1960s. It was estimated that only about 50,000 American patients were receiving this agent in the early 1980s, although perhaps a million or more Americans with severe recurrent mood disorders could be so treated. A large number of controlled studies demonstrate the efficacy of lithium carbonate in hypomania and acute mania, with improvement rates typically 70–80% in 10 to 14 days.

Short-Term Treatment

One of the problems in evaluating lithium's spectrum of effectiveness in psychiatric illness is the differential diagnosis of the psychoses and the severe mood disorders. Whereas lithium salts are a poor treatment for chronic schizophrenia, they might have beneficial effects in some atypical forms of acute psychosis, particularly "schizoaffective" disorder and dysphoric or paranoid forms of mania, which can be even more florid than an acute exacerbation of a schizophrenic illness.

When lithium treatment is initiated in mania it is usual to hospitalize the patient, although treatment can sometimes be started on an outpatient basis for cooperative hypomanic patients. In the first days of treatment a neuroleptic or sedative agent is often used while awaiting the attainment of therapeutic blood levels of lithium, antimanic effects, and relatively stable fluid and electrolyte balance (typically in 5 to 10 days).

Lithium can also be started during the depressed phase of a bipolar illness.

The initial medical evaluation includes a physical examination and laboratory tests of renal, electrolyte, and thyroid function, fasting blood sugar, complete blood count, and electrocardiogram (ECG). Although lithium has been used safely and successfully in patients with coexisting severe cardiovascular and renal disease, these conditions require close monitoring of electrolyte balance and close medical supervision. The requirements for repeated laboratory and medical evaluations are not clearly established, but sound practice calls for later reevaluation of renal, electrolyte, cardiac, thyroid, and general medical status at least two to four times a year, as well as knowledge of pregnancy in women.

When the administration of lithium carbonate is started in manic patients, the initial daily intake is usually 600 or 900 mg in divided oral doses. Guidelines to predicting dosage requirements based on blood levels or clearance after a small test dose were discussed in the preceding section. The goal is to increase the dose gradually over several days to attain blood levels above 0.9 mEq/L, ideally between 1.0 and 1.25 mEq/L. Although blood levels as high as 1.5 mEq/L have been accepted, this is in general an unnecessarily risky practice; toxic effects are common at levels of 2.0 mEq/L or more, and are usually severe above 3.0 mEq/L. Rapid increases in the dose and blood levels of lithium ion often produce gastrointestinal distress and nausea, which can usually be avoided by increasing the dose *gradually* and administering the medication three or four times a day with, or just after, a meal. The final oral dose required to attain the desired blood level varies considerably among individuals: younger and larger patients require larger doses. Typically, daily doses range between 1,200 and 2,400 mg of lithium carbonate for manic patients, but requirements can vary from 300 to 3,600 mg.

The most important principle in the use of lithium is that, in contrast to most other medications used in psychiatry, the oral dose is not an adequate guideline, and the proper maintenance of *blood concentrations* of the agent is crucial. Because of the low therapeutic index of the lithium-ion, peak blood levels can attain toxic concentrations over the 24-hour cycle, as discussed in the preceding section. Therefore, doses are divided and blood levels are assayed according to a strict protocol: the appropriate blood levels are defined as those measured at approximately 12 hours after the final dose of the day and prior to the first morning dose. In the early period of treatment of manic patients, daily and then every-other-day blood assays should be obtained if lithium is given immediately; twice-weekly assays are adequate if lithium is deferred until immediate control of mania is obtained by antipsychotic or sedative agents. An antipsychotic drug is often required in the first week of treatment. Electroconvulsive treatment is rarely necessary. Once the appropriate dose of a lithium salt is known, it can be continued until the mania begins to abate. At that point there is a risk of change in the fluid and electrolyte balance, as well as an increased chance of intoxication with lithium, so the dose should be gradually reduced to maintain the blood concentration at about 1.0 mEq/L.

For prophylaxis after discharge from hospital, blood levels of 0.75 to 1.0 mEq/L are adequate and safe. Each patient usually has a stable requirement for a total daily dose that provides the desired blood level of lithium (typically between 600 and 1,500 mg, and most often 900 mg/day), although there is considerable variation among patients. After a few weekly blood assays to establish the appropriate maintenance dose for an individual patient, blood assays can be performed infrequently, perhaps monthly or even less often, with random and unannounced blood samples taken as a check on the reliability of the patient. After treatment with lithium is established, there is ordinarily no need to prescribe salt supplements, but the maintenance of *normal sodium intake and output* is important. Patients have been maintained on stable doses of lithium carbonate with reduced risk of recurring episodes of mania and depression for many years without serious problems.

Attempts have been made to specify factors in a patient's clinical history or symptomatic presentation that might predict a favorable response to lithium treatment. Other than a clinical diagnosis of mania and an adequate plasma level of lithium ion, none has been clearly established. Factors such as the age of onset of bipolar illness, rate of recurrence, severity of attacks, and family history of similar illnesses have not differentiated lithium-responsive and unresponsive patients, although there is a suggestion that nonspecific abnormalities in the electroencephalogram (EEG) may predict an unfavorable response. A relationship between outcome of lithium treatment and the ratio of lithium ion concentration between plasma and erythrocytes has been suggested, but evidence for this is weak. There is preliminary evidence that an acute antimanic or behavior-quieting effect of physostigmine (a centrally active, reversible anticholinesterase agent that diminishes the inactivation of acetylcholine in the central nervous system) may predict an antimanic effect of lithium treatment within two weeks.

Lithium can be used to treat geriatric patients with severe, recurrent manic-depressive mood disorders. It should be noted that older patients have a decreased ability to clear and excrete the lithium ion and are less tolerant of it chemically (higher blood levels) and functionally (greater risk of intoxication). Lithium has also been tried in a number of other psychiatric disorders, which are discussed in the following section. Thus, short-term lithium treatment may be of value in conditions that do not clearly resemble mania but may include acute psychoses and other excited "schizoaffective" states that have not yet been evaluated adequately in controlled trials.

Long-Term and Alternative Uses of Lithium

The usefulness of lithium carbonate in acute mania is based solidly on experimental evidence. In fact, however, the response to lithium by itself is usually impractically slow, and it is generally necessary to add an antipsychotic or sedative agent within the first few days of treatment to bring about prompt behavioral control of mania, particularly in a general hospital or an open psychiatric unit. The more promising feature of lithium therapy is that it can diminish the rate and severity of recurrences of major mood disorders.

If lithium is started mainly for its prophylactic actions in a period of normal mood, or if its use is to be continued indefinitely after an acute attack of mania or bipolar depression, two important guidelines should be followed: the indications should be *convincing,* and the patient should be *reliable* enough to follow the required medical regimen. Thus, infrequent episodes of even severe mania or depression separated by several years or relatively frequent episodes of milder abnormalities of mood require that clinical judgment balance the inconvenience and risk of the treatment against the indications for it. Very impulsive or suicidal patients are not good candidates for the sustained use of lithium treatment on an outpatient basis, because the acute ingestion of even a few days' supply of lithium carbonate can be highly toxic or even lethal. One advantage of lithium in prophylactic treatment is that many bipolar or recurrently manic patients who are reluctant to be inhibited by antipsychotic agents or to engage in prolonged contact with a psychiatrist or psychotherapist will accept the almost imperceptible subjective effects of lithium and will comply with medical supervision and blood tests.

In a review of ten controlled studies of the long-term treatment (typically for one year) of patients with a variety of major affective disorders, most of whom had recurrent episodes of mania or hypomania, a total of 367 patients had been treated with a lithium salt and 372 with an inactive

Table 26 Prevention of bipolar relapse by lithium

Study	Year	Total N	Relapse rate (%)		Protection ratio
			Placebo	Lithium	
Baastrup et al.	1970	50	45.5	0.0	>45
Persson	1972	24	91.7	41.7	2.2
Prien et al.	1973	236	79.5	39.5	2.0
Coppen et al.	1978	38	100.0	17.6	5.7
Fieve et al.	1978	53	86.2	58.3	1.5
Quitkin et al.	1978	6	66.7	0.0	>67
Quitkin et al.	1981	11	71.4	25.0	2.9
Total or mean (7 studies)		—	78.5	34.3	2.3

Sources: Review and references cited therein by Appleton and Davis, *Practical Clinical Psychopharmacology* (Williams and Wilkins, Baltimore, 1980), p. 126; and Quitkin et al., *Psychopharmacol. Bull.* 17:142, 1981. These studies included bipolar cases with mania (type I) and mild hypomania as well as recurrent major depression (type II bipolar disorder). Patients were followed typically for about one year. Means are weighted by the number of patients per study.

Additional information is provided by Davis, *Am. J. Psychiatry* 133:1, 1976 in a review of nine controlled studies involving 659 patients in whom relapses due to major affective illness of all types decreased 2.3-fold with lithium versus placebo treatment (35.6% vs. 79.4% relapse); and in five studies of bipolar patients, lithium treatment was associated with a 3.2-fold sparing of relapse versus placebo treatment (25.1 ± 7.6% versus 79.8 ± 7.8% relapse rates ± S.D., respectively). The same literature was also reviewed and updated by Appleton and Davis, *Practical Clinical Psychopharmacology,* p. 125; they again found a more than 2-fold reduction in risk of recurrent major mood disorders during treatment with lithium versus placebo. Similarly, in a study of the risk of yearly morbidity due to recurrent affective illness (mainly major depression) in bipolar type II patients, a sparing effect due to lithium over placebo of 2.4-fold was found by Dunner et al., *Arch. Gen. Psychiatry* 39:1344, 1982.

placebo (Appleton and Davis, 1980, p. 125). The weighted mean relapse rate of acute major affective disorder was 79.3% with a placebo and only 36.6% with lithium treatment, for a reduction in morbidity of 2.2-fold. A summary of modern studies of 418 bipolar patients is provided in Table 26, which shows that treatment with lithium reduced the attack rate of affective episodes by 2.3-fold, from 79% to 34%. Similar levels of partial protection have been reported in a smaller number of studies of patients with severe, recurrent depression but only mild, subclinical hypomania (either spontaneous or induced by an antidepressant or electroconvulsive treatment), sometimes referred to as type II bipolar disorder (whereas recurrences of mania and major depression represent type I bipolar disorder). The impression that lithium treatment can benefit the type II bipolar disorder, which is significant clinically mainly for major depressive episodes, raises the question of whether lithium is beneficial for the depressed phase of all bipolar disorders. Although only a limited number of studies specifically address this question, the strong impression arising from available research as well as clinical experience is that both manic and depressed phases of bipolar disorders are benefited, and probably to a similar extent, as indicated in Table 27.

It is important to realize, and to advise patients, that the protective effect of lithium in recurrent major affective disorders is rarely absolute. In an average response, the attack frequency is reduced by about half and severity is also modified. Because of this partial protection and the risk of toxicity of lithium salts, careful clinical judgment is required to balance the risks and sometimes limited benefits of treatment against the potentially catastrophic risk of avoiding treatment. The most compelling indication for prolonged use of lithium is a proven history of bipolar manic-depressive illness with marked severity and disruption of functioning, perhaps with hospitalizations, and at least a moderate rate of recurrence, perhaps every year or two. Less severe illness or a low rate of recurrence calls for a more cautious decision. In some patients with very severe bipolar illness and rapid fluctuations of mood over periods of weeks or months (sometimes called "rapidly cycling" manic-depressive illness),

Table 27   Rate of recurrence of mania or depression in bipolar manic-depressives with lithium or placebo

Treatment	Relapse rate (%) by type of episode[a]	
	Manic episodes (120)	Depressive episodes (63)
Lithium	29.2	36.5
Placebo	70.8	63.5
"Protection ratio" (Placebo : Lithium)	2.4	1.7

Source: Davis, Am. J. Psychiatry 133:1, 1976.

a. Data are mean percentage of patients relapsing in the manic or depressive phases of bipolar affective illnesses during approximately one year of treatment with lithium or placebo. Results are derived from the only two controlled studies that provided sufficient data to evaluate the differential effects of the treatment on the two phases of the illness. Lithium appears to produce a protective effect against both types of relapse, but there are too few results to permit statistical analysis. It is interesting to note that about two-thirds of all 183 relapses were manic in type regardless of the treatment.

In another recent study, Prien et al. (1984) found that lithium treatment gave similar effects on depressed and manic phases of bipolar illness (29% and 26% relapse rates, respectively) in 42 patients followed for 2.5 years.

Table 28 Effect of lithium on rapidly cycling bipolar illness

	Proportion of time in mood state (%)		Benefit ratio
Mood of patients	Placebo	Lithium	
Euthymic	35.1	63.3	1.8
Manic	20.0	8.1	2.5
Depressed	44.8	28.6	1.6

Source: Dunner et al., *Comprehen. Psychiatry* 18:561, 1977. Data were obtained from 29 bipolar patients followed for one year before and one year during treatment. The increases of normal mood and decreases of pathological mood are all highly significant statistically, with a slightly smaller effect on depression among patients with several episodes of major affective disorder per year prior to treatment with lithium carbonate.

even though the benefits of lithium treatment may not be obvious, there is evidence that substantial benefit may still be found, especially in the manic phase (Table 28). There is also a clinical impression that, in addition to modifying the instability of mood in rapidly cycling bipolar illness, lithium may have a long-term effect of reducing the risk of recurring bouts of such rapid fluctuations over years of treatment.

Other potential long-term uses of lithium are less well established. For example, it is customary at the present time to be cautious about treating patients in the depressed phase of bipolar syndromes with an antidepressant or electroconvulsive treatment (ECT) alone, because of a suspected risk of inducing a rapid shift of mood into mania or psychosis (known as the "switch process" in manic-depressive illness). Although there is abundant clinical experience to sustain the impression that mania is common following treatment of bipolar depression without lithium, well-controlled research to document a suspected increase in risk of mania is sparse (Table 29) and does not consistently demonstrate a marked increase in risk of mania following the use of an antidepressant alone. On average, however, the reported risk of mania in bipolar patients treated with an antidepressant plus lithium is only slightly higher than with lithium alone. For this reason, as well as the strong clinical impression that the risk of mania is increased by the use of an antidepressant alone for bipolar patients, it is common and sound practice to add lithium to antidepressant or ECT therapy of a patient with known bipolar illness. In addition, such combined therapy is often considered in patients with suspected bipolar characteristics (including those with bipolar type II disorder and cyclothymic patterns by past history, as well as those who

Table 29 Risk of mania and treatment of bipolar illness

Study	Year	Total N	Rate of mania or hypomania (%)			
			Placebo or no treatment	Antidepressant	Antidepressant + lithium	Lithium
Prien et al.	1973	35	33.0	67.0	—	12.0
Bunney	1978	2,346	—	8.6	—	—
Bunney	1978	1,577	—	11.1[a]	—	—
Wehr and Goodwin	1979	26	—	69.2	—	—
Akiskal et al.	1980	18	—	50.0	—	—
Quitkin et al.	1981	75	—	—	24.0	10.5
Lewis and Winokur	1982	93	41.0	28.0	—	15.0
Prien et al.	1984	114	—	53.0	28.0	26.0
Mean or total (8 studies)		4,284	37.0	41.0	26.0	15.9
Risk ratio vs. spontaneous rate			1.0	1.1	0.7	0.4

Source: Review and citations therein by Goodwin, *McLean Hosp. J.* 8:1, 1983; the data from Prien et al. are in *Arch. Gen. Psychiatry* 41:1096, 1984.

a. A review of patients treated with a monoamine oxidase inhibitor; other studies involved a tricyclic antidepressant. In a related study, Wehr and Goodwin, *Arch. Gen. Psychiatry* 36:555, 1979, found that the cycle length (time between onset of episodes of major mood disorder) in five rapidly cycling female bipolar patients decreased from 127 ± 22 to 33 ± 6 days (means $\pm$ S.E.M.; 3.85-fold change) when a tricyclic antidepressant was added to lithium treatment. In addition, Kane et al., *Arch. Gen. Psychiatry* 39:1065, 1982, found, even among a group of 49 initially *nonbipolar* patients, that the rate of manic switches during more than 18 months of follow-up varied with treatment as follows: imipramine, 18.2%; placebo, 7.7%; lithium, 0%.

The results support the antimanic effect of lithium treatment, but fail to provide consistent support for the common clinical impression that there is an increased risk of "switching" mood into mania with antidepressant treatment. There is a notable lack of appropriate control rates on a placebo, but the comparison of rates with an antidepressant alone versus an antidepressant plus lithium may suggest a mania-inducing effect of antidepressants.

Table 30 Prevention of nonbipolar relapse by lithium

Study	Year	Total N	Relapse rate (%)		Protection ratio
			Placebo	Lithium	
Baastrup et al.	1970	34	52.9	0.0	>53
Persson	1972	42	66.7	28.6	2.3
Prien et al.	1973	43	87.5	48.1	1.8
Coppen et al.	1978	26	80.0	9.1	8.8
Fieve et al.	1978	28	64.3	57.1	1.1
Quitkin et al.	1978	10	80.0	40.0	2.0
Peselow et al.	1981	77	84.3	62.2	1.4
Quitkin et al.	1981	13	100.0	28.6	3.5
Kane et al.	1982	24	76.9	27.3	2.8
Prien et al.	1984	71	65.0	57.0	1.1
Total or mean (10 studies)		445	75.5	43.5	1.7

Sources: Review and references cited therein by Appleton and Davis, *Practical Clinical Psychopharmacology* (Williams and Wilkins, Baltimore, 1980), p. 126; and Peselow et al., *Psychopharmacol. Bull.* 17:53, 1981; Quitkin et al., *Psychopharmacol. Bull.* 17:142, 1981; Kane et al., *Arch. Gen. Psychiatry* 39:1065, 1982; and Prien et al. *Arch. Gen. Psychiatry* 41:1096, 1984). Treatment lasted 6 months to 3 years; means are weighted by the number of patients per study.

previously switched from depression into mania with antidepressant treatment).

In addition to lithium's main use in the treatment of patients with various forms of bipolar major affective disorders, there has been a growing interest in the possible efficacy of lithium in either short-term or long-term management of patients with recurrent, nonbipolar affective syndromes (so-called unipolar depression). The most substantial body of data exists for the long-term prevention of recurrences of major depression, by analogy to the preventive actions of lithium in bipolar syndromes. Although the results to date are encouraging, they are inconsistent and not compelling (Table 30). One of the problems in this area of investigation is the difficulty of defining nonbipolar illnesses, which may be biomedically heterogeneous. At the present time, a guideline that seems rational is to consider the use of lithium alone or with an antidepressant for severe and frequently recurring major depression when there is some suggestion in a patient's past or family history of similarity to more clear-cut bipolar illness (for example, strong family history of affective illness, recurring psychosis, or alcoholism; past history of cyclothy-

Table 31 Acute antidepressant effects of lithium

Study	Year	Total N	Response rates	
			Bipolar	Nonbipolar
Goodwin et al.	1969	18	10/13	2/5
Goodwin et al.	1972	52	32/40	4/12
Johnson	1974	5	—	5/5
Noyes et al.	1974	22	6/6	7/16
Baron et al.	1975	23	7/9	3/14
Mendels et al.	1975	21	9/13	4/8
Totals (6 studies)		141	64/81	25/60
Means		—	79.0%	41.7%

Source: Review and citations therein by Goodwin, *McLean Hosp. J.* 8:1, 1983.

mia; early onset and rapid recurrence of depressions, especially with psychotic features).

In the short-term treatment of an episode of major depression, the evidence of an antidepressant action of lithium is even less clear than for prevention of recurrent attacks of nonbipolar depression. A survey of recent studies on this point (summarized in Table 31) suggests that the overall short-term response rate to lithium in nonbipolar depression (42%) was not much higher than that expected with an inactive placebo (perhaps 20–30%), whereas in the depressed phase of bipolar illness a clear-cut response, similar to that found in the treatment of mania, was found (79% response rate). A small number of studies exist of the antidepressant effects of lithium in comparison to a tricyclic antidepressant. Although three out of four studies concluded that the two forms of treatment were indistinguishable, the studies were not optimally designed. A placebo group is also desirable to support the conclusion that the standard antidepressant was performing at an expected level of efficacy; that is, "not different from" is sometimes *not* equivalent to "as good as." There are also several anecdotal reports of patients who improved when lithium (and more time for spontaneous remission) was added following poor responses to an antidepressant or even to ECT (see Table 32), but these findings are difficult to interpret. Overall, it is tempting to speculate that some patients, even without obvious characteristics of bipolar affective illness, may experience an antidepressant as well as a mood-stabilizing effect of lithium. On the other hand, support for such treatment is not

Table 32 Comparison of lithium to standard antidepressants in the treatment of acute major depression

Study	Year	Total N	Outcome
Fieve et al.	1968	29	Imipramine better than lithium
Mendels et al.	1972	12	Lithium equal to desipramine
Watanabe et al.	1975	45	Lithium equal to imipramine
Worrall et al.	1979	63	Lithium equal to imipramine
de Montigny et al.	1981	9	Lithium + antidepressant better than previous treatment with antidepressant or ECT alone

Source: Review and citations therein by Goodwin, *McLean Hosp. J.* 8:1, 1983.

sufficient to encourage routine use of lithium in nonbipolar depression, either short-term or long-term.

In addition to their use in treating bipolar and other major mood disorders, lithium salts have been reported to have beneficial effects in a variety of other disorders. Most of the experience with such conditions has been in short-term treatment for a few weeks or months; controlled, long-term treatment aimed at preventing recurrences has not been studied adequately. Table 33 provides a summary of conditions in which research reports and clinical experience suggest possible efficacy, equivocal results often due to inadequate testing, or conditions in which lithium is unlikely to produce consistent benefit. Clear and generally accepted indications are for treatment of acute mania and for prevention or recurrences of mania and depression in bipolar disorder. Efficacy is also probable or strongly suspected in other conditions that may represent or resemble bipolar affective illness, including bipolar type II disorder. Mania and bipolar conditions are increasingly recognized or suspected in school-age children, who may also respond to lithium, although this use is not yet well studied or widely accepted. There is also a growing suspicion that certain acute psychotic illnesses that may or may not arise in patients with an unequivocal history of bipolar illness may also respond to lithium, at least in the short term. These conditions include excited, so-called schizo-affective states, which are poorly defined currently and may include psychotic affective disorders, including cases of bipolar disorder. This group of conditions may meet current diagnostic criteria for schizophrenia and thus contribute to an impression that some "schizophrenic" patients may respond to lithium. It is unlikely, however, that classic,

Table 33 Conditions in which lithium treatment has been investigated

---

Treatment effective
- Acute mania (but slow)[a]
- Prevention of recurrence of mania and depression in bipolar illness[a]

Treatment probably effective
- Recurrence of depression in bipolar type II disorder (with mild hypomania)

Treatment possibly effective or insufficiently investigated
- Mania or bipolar variants in children
- Recurrent nonbipolar major depression
- Acute or recurrent schizoaffective (excited) or recurrent atypical psychotic disorders (may be bipolar variants)
- Some cases of recurrent paranoid disorder (uncommon)
- Emotionally unstable character
- Repeated impulsive-aggressive behavior (including the mentally retarded)
- Acute major depression
- Cyclothymic personality disorder
- Alcoholism or substance abuse disorder with affective disorder
- Cluster headache
- Periodic hypersomnia and hyperphagia of Kleine-Levin syndrome[b]
- Euphoria induced by stimulants
- Syndromes of inappropriate secretion of antidiuretic hormone (ADH)

Treatment probably ineffective
- Anxiety disorders
- Phobias
- Obsessive-compulsive disorder
- Chronic schizophrenia
- Attention deficit disorder with hyperactivity
- Tardive dyskinesia
- Huntington's disease
- Spasmodic torticollis
- Premenstrual tension
- Ménière's syndrome
- Thyrotoxicosis
- Bone marrow hypoplasia (as in cancer chemotherapy)
- Gout

---

a. Indicates conditions for which lithium is "officially" recommended by manufacturers and the U.S. Food and Drug Administration, although empirical clinical use for conditions in the "probably" and "possibly" effective categories is not unusual at this time, especially when alternatives have been unsuccessful.

b. Lithium is considered excessively dangerous for routine use in the treatment of bulimia or other eating disorders, which are typically associated with unstable balance of fluid and electrolyte concentrations (e.g., hypokalemia) and poor cooperation.

chronic schizophrenic patients are benefited by lithium treatment. An apparently diverse group of other conditions, typically marked by an episodic course and periods of acute agitation and dysphoria, have also been proposed as possible indications for lithium treatment, although they have not yet been adequately investigated, especially in the long term (see Table 33).

In order to maximize the safety of lithium treatment for long-term use, several guidelines are suggested, including close attention to the indications for such treatment; consideration of alternatives for disorders in which effective alternative treatments are available; the use of moderate plasma levels of lithium below 1.0 mEq/L, perhaps as low as 0.5–0.75 mEq/L for some patients; and regular surveillance of renal and thyroid function as well as pregnancy, based on considerations of potential toxic effects of lithium. These guidelines are summarized in Table 34.

Influence of Age on Lithium Treatment

Lithium has not been studied adequately for use in children, although there is a growing, largely uncontrolled, clinical experience with it in episodic disorders of school-age and adolescent children that resemble adult bipolar illness. In such children, or those with acute mania-like

Table 34 Recommended guidelines for long-term lithium therapy

- Review indications rigorously (not only according to Table 33 and comparable reviews, but also by severity and frequency of major episodes of bipolar major affective disorders)
- Consider alternative treatments for other disorders (e.g., antidepressants in unipolar major depression)
- Seek the lowest apparently effective plasma concentration of lithium below 1.0 mEq/L to minimize toxicity
- Monitor serum creatinine levels approximately monthly for a year and quarterly thereafter, watching for evidence of a steady increase, even if below 1.2 mg/dL
- Monitor 24-hour urine volume yearly; if over 3 L, check creatinine clearance and rule out other renal disorders (associated with toxins, chronic analgesic treatment, infections, obstructions, hypertension, etc.)
- Monitor other potential targets of toxic effects, including CNS, skin, thyroid (monitor TSH and T_4 as well as thyroid size at least twice yearly), and electrolytes (including calcium)
- Avoid pregnancy in women of child-bearing age

Table 35 *Effects of lithium in disorders of children*

Disorder	N	Response rate (%)
Apparent bipolar disorder	61	65
Major depression	41	27
Conduct disorders	17	23
Attention deficit disorder with hyperactivity	12	0[a]

Source: Clinical experience of DeLong and Nieman (personal communication, 1984). A total of 131 children (mean age 9.8 years) were given lithium carbonate in doses of 600–1,200 mg/day (with blood levels of 0.5–1.2 mEq/L) for an average of 30 months.

a. Some hyperactive children worsened with this treatment.

episodes, responses to lithium appear to be similar to those in comparable adult patients. On the other hand, responses of acute depression to lithium in young patients are not demonstrated to be above levels expected with an inactive placebo. Results in conduct disorders and in attention deficit disorder with hyperactivity are poor, and the latter may even worsen. A recent large series of uncontrolled clinical experiences with 131 children is summarized in Table 35. Apparently effective blood levels as well as total daily doses were similar to those typical in adult patients. Since the significance of major mood disorders in young children is only beginning to be understood, the use of lithium and other mood-altering agents in young patients urgently requires further study, with careful attention to possible toxic or untoward developmental effects that may be unique to growing children.

The manic-depressive syndrome in children may have a somewhat different appearance from that in adults. Although the onset has been described as young as 4 years, an age of about 10 years is a typical time of onset. There may be a family history of affective illness, acute psychosis, or alcoholism. The past history often includes episodes of severe tantrums, aggressive or hostile behavior, cruelty to siblings or pets or other antisocial behaviors, as well as distractability and hyperactivity that are not improved by stimulants. Withdrawn, mute, dysphoric, and self-abusive phases may alternate with periods of hyperactivity, grandiosity, intrusive overtalkativeness, silliness, and variable changes in sleep. Episodes of bulimia and food stealing, as well as salt craving and profuse sweating, have also been described. The long-term effects of lithium on the health and development of younger children have not been adequately investigated. If such treatment is given to a school-age child, it is wise to follow skeletal development as well as neurological and renal function and to watch for changes in the function of thyroid and parathyroid glands.

Lithium can also be used safely and effectively in elderly patients, although systematic evaluation in this population has not yet been undertaken. Although the ability to eliminate lithium ion diminishes to some extent with aging in patients with apparently normal renal function, this is usually not a major consideration in the use of lithium. On the other hand, tolerance of plasma levels that may be benign in younger adults is often limited in the elderly. The risk of cerebral intoxication is especially high in the elderly, particularly if lithium is combined with other centrally active agents or if dementia is present. Although lithium can be used cautiously for elderly bipolar patients, it has not been established that lithium is either effective or safe in the treatment of fluctuation of mood and behavior in demented patients. In general, careful adjustment of dosage and blood levels in order to minimize fluctuations of tissue concentrations and risk of intoxication is especially necessary in the use of lithium salts in the geriatric population.

Toxicology

The most common problems associated with the use of lithium salts are mild or occasionally distressing nausea, vomiting, and diarrhea, usually when doses are rapidly increased. Effects on the nervous system may also occur, including light-headedness and some confusion, but typically the subjective effects of lithium are minimal and patients rarely complain of feeling "medicated" or mentally dull. A fine resting tremor is common and is of no particular importance, although a clear increase in the tremor or the appearance of unsteady handwriting can be an important early clue to incipient intoxication. More severe tremor not associated with acute intoxication occurs occasionally and in some cases has been reported to respond favorably to propranolol in moderate doses.

The most important early means of detecting *serious intoxication* are the clinical signs, and blood assays should only be considered as secondary and confirmatory; when signs of intoxication are observed, the intake of lithium should be decreased or stopped without waiting for results of the blood lithium assay. Early signs of intoxication include increasing tremor, weakness, ataxia, giddiness, drowsiness or excitement, slurred dysphasic speech, blurred vision, and tinnitus. More severe intoxication produces increased neuromuscular irritability, increased deep tendon reflexes, and nystagmus; increasing confusion, lethargy, and stupor may lead to coma, sometimes with generalized seizures. Extrapyramidal reactions are rare with ordinary doses of lithium, but choreoathetosis or other bizarre dyskinesias can occur with severe intoxication. The electroencephalogram (EEG) ordinarily reveals generalized slowing, with a prominent 4–6 Hz (cycles/second) activity, even without toxic levels of lithium. Toxicity can be expected at blood levels of 2–4 mEq/L, and levels much above 5 mEq/L may be fatal. In acute overdoses of lithium, the usual causes of death are the secondary complications of coma, including pneumonia and shock.

A small number of cases of uncertain significance have been reported which suggest the possibility that the combination of lithium in high doses with haloperidol may produce severe forms of irreversible and even fatal CNS intoxication, although this combination has been safely used for many years throughout the world and continues to be used today. Irreversible CNS deficits can also occur after acute intoxication with lithium alone. Generally, the risk of acute excess sedation or toxic confusion is greater when other psychotropic agents are added to lithium salts and in the elderly. It is particularly important to watch for subtle features of an organic mental syndrome (delirium) in elderly patients receiving prolonged lithium treatment. Moreover, patients with systemic disorders (such as congestive heart failure, hepatic ascites, nephrosis) associated with retention of fluid, salt, and lithium are at increased risk of intoxication and require very cautious treatment with reduced doses of lithium and close monitoring of clinical status and plasma levels of lithium.

In the medical management of acute intoxication with lithium, it is essential to discontinue lithium treatment immediately (without risk of a withdrawal reaction). Usually, sufficient treatment consists of gastric lavage, the support of vital functions and electrolyte balance, and careful nursing care in a specialized medical toxicology unit while awaiting the spontaneous elimination of lithium. An important implication of the renal excretion of the lithium ion is that its rate of removal cannot be increased by the administration of most saluretic drugs; the thiazide diuretics or spironolactone, by preferential removal of sodium, may even increase the retention and toxicity of lithium. There is little evidence that intravenously administered solutions of sodium chloride appreciably increase the removal of lithium, but the management of lithium intoxication should include normal availability of sodium; the administration of sodium bicarbonate is also helpful. Fluid loading, solute-induced diuresis, as with mannitol, and theophylline can all contribute to some increased renal excretion of lithium in cases of intoxication, and dialysis techniques are very effective in serious overdosage. The use of lithium in patients with salt restriction or sodium wasting requires extra caution in monitoring blood levels of lithium and avoiding intoxication.

Cardiovascular problems are unusual in patients given controlled quantities of lithium salts. Hypotension and arrhythmias are rare, although electrocardiographic changes can occur. At doses that are likely to be encountered clinically, the most typical changes are similar to those associated with hypokalemia, even though blood levels of potassium are almost always normal. These changes include flattening and even inversion of the T waves; the effects are dose-dependent and reversible. In experimental animals, extraordinarily high concentrations of lithium (above 10 mEq/L, levels unlikely to be encountered clinically) have been reported to produce changes resembling those of hyperkalemia: high, peaked T waves; T-wave inversions; depressed S-T segment; widened QRS complex; and evidence of atrioventricular dissociation and conduction blockade. Depressed or absent P waves, atrial fibrillation, and standstill with independent ventricular responses also occur.

Severe *renal tubular damage* resulting from lithium treatment was formerly a concern, mainly because pathologic changes in the kidney of uncertain significance were reported in early cases of gross overdosage with lithium chloride given to patients with preexisting circulatory, renal, or hepatic disorders associated with retention of fluid and sodium (and lithium as well). Similarly, reports of renal tubular damage in the rat are hard to relate to the clinical use of lithium in psychiatry, inasmuch as these studies have used toxic doses of lithium salts. A more likely clinical problem with kidney function is a form of nephrogenic *diabetes insipidus* characterized by the intake of many liters of water per day and the output of huge quantities of very dilute urine. This syndrome is believed to result from the ability of lithium ion to interfere with the activity of antidiuretic hormone (ADH) on the renal tubules, either by preventing its access to the appropriate membrane site or by blocking the response of an ADH-sensitive adenylate cyclase. While mild or transient *polyuria* is not unusual early in lithium therapy, severe diabetes insipidus later in the course of prolonged treatment is a less common but potentially more serious complication.

Since polyuria and diabetes insipidus are so commonly encountered during treatment with lithium, their management requires special consideration. Up to half of patients treated with lithium experience some polyuria of up to 3–4 liters per day. Such responses are not clearly related to the plasma concentration of lithium, and thus appear to be more idiosyncratic than dose-dependent. Simple, practical steps in management include reducing the dose of lithium when possible (despite the lack of ability of dose to predict the response in groups of patients) and reducing the solute load (salt restriction and reducing intake of urea-producing foods such as protein). In about 5% of cases, a more severe diabetes insipidus syndrome that includes output of more than 5 liters of urine per day may require more vigorous treatment, or even interruption of lithium therapy. Cautious use of a thiazide diuretic which acts on the distal nephron (where resorption of sodium and lithium are dissociated, in contrast to the proximal nephron and loop of Henle) can successfully reduce urine output, but also decreases the daily requirement for lithium.

There have been several reports of degenerative, granulomatous *changes in renal biopsies* from patients exposed to lithium salts for prolonged periods, usually for several years. In a recent series of 49 such cases in Denmark, only 8% were considered clearly pathologic, while 30% were uncertain and 62% were considered within the range of normal variation (Rafaelsen et al., 1979). These biopsies were obtained after 1 to 15 years of treatment with lithium; all patients biopsied had serum creatinine levels within the normal range, and 24-hour urine volumes were below 3 liters in two-thirds of the patients. Abnormal findings were more common among those with high urine volumes. In another recent Scandinavian study, only 4% of 272 patients treated for several years had reduced creatinine clearance, and 8% had increases of serum levels of creatinine of more than 0.3 mg/dL (Vestergaard et al., 1979). Moreover, when well-matched groups of patients treated with lithium and without lithium were compared in this and several other American and European studies (Lipmann, 1982), there were only minor, insignificant differences between them among several measures of renal function, with the notable exceptions that urinary ADH levels were elevated by nearly fourfold among those treated with lithium, and urine volumes above 4.0 liters/24 hours were reported in 10–20% of cases. There have also been reports of pathologic changes in renal biopsy material from bipolar patients who had not been treated with lithium, raising questions about an association between the psychiatric diagnosis and renal pathology or, more likely, about the nonspecificity of the histological observations associated with lithium treatment.

A recent American report from Johns Hopkins Hospital (De Paulo et al., 1981) noted that the duration of exposure to lithium correlated with urine volume and, inversely, with urine concentration, but only weakly with creatinine plasma levels or clearance. Thus, it is possible that long-term changes in renal function can occur in association with lithium treatment. The most frequently documented changes, however, appear to be extensions of common effects of lithium on the function of ADH, and include diabetes insipidus which may respond poorly to trials of exogenous, synthetic ADH-like peptides, and which in some cases may be associated with relatively nonspecific pathologic changes in renal tissue at histological examination. These latter changes are not specific to lithium treatment and can occur in many other chronic illnesses and drug treatments. The evidence so far suggests that progressive, irreversible loss of renal function is rare even after sustained use of lithium for more than a decade. However, in order to minimize any potential risk, it is good practice to monitor serum levels of creatinine and lithium regularly and to suspect renal changes if these indexes start to increase consistently, and especially if signs of diabetes insipidus arise late in the course of treatment. If renal toxicity is suspected at that point, further evaluation of renal function, possibly with a renal biopsy, should be considered with expert consultation.

Another metabolic abnormality is the development of a form of benign, diffuse, nontoxic *goiter* in as many as a third of patients receiving ordinary doses of lithium salts for prolonged periods. These patients almost always remain euthyroid or only marginally hypothyroid, although there is usually an increase in the circulating levels of thyroid-stimulating hormone (TSH). Significant biochemical hypothyroidism occurs in fewer than 5% of cases. The risk may be higher in women, who may also have a higher risk of carrying antithyroid autoantibodies, which can be assayed as part of an initial screening evaluation. Significant neonatal hypothyroidism has also been reported after use of lithium late in pregnancy. There is experimental evidence for the ability of lithium to interfere with thyroid metabolism at several points, including the iodination and release of iodinated tyrosine, and some evidence of its interference with the actions of thyroxin on target tissues, much as the actions of ADH seem to be impaired. There is usually no serious danger from the goiter, but judgment must be exercised, with the help of endocrinological consultation, as to whether to continue the lithium treatment. Rarely does serious functional hypothyroidism or myxedema occur. In many cases treatment with thyroxin (typically in daily doses of 50 – 200 μg) leads to regression of the goiter and permits maintenance of a euthyroid status while lithium therapy is pursued.

Other toxic effects of lithium include the occasional development of localized edema, eruptions (especially a reversible but potentially recurrent form of folliculitis that resembles keratosis pilaris), or even ulcerations of the *skin*. An antihistaminic agent may be helpful for the rashes, and topical steroids are useful for the rare skin ulcers. A particularly common dermatological problem is the worsening of *acne vulgaris,* which may require vigorous treatment with an antibiotic or other antiacne agents after consultation with a dermatologist. This effect occurs in adult patients as well as adolescents. Thinning and loss of hair may also occur during treatment with lithium, although this loss is rarely severe.

Hepatic and bone marrow toxicity are rarely associated with lithium therapy. Although it is not unusual to observe a mild elevation of the peripheral leukocyte count, its significance is uncertain. Lithium has been reported to worsen myasthenia gravis in rare instances.

A great deal of concern surrounds the use of lithium in *pregnancy and lactation,* partly because studies in classical embryology revealed grossly teratogenic effects of very high concentrations, and because more recent evidence in experimental animals indicates that very high doses of lithium are associated with fetal wastage and anomalies of the central nervous system. There are also reports of uncertain significance that lithium can alter the metabolism of the rat testis, as well as the motility of human sperm. Together with other alterations in fluid and electrolyte metabolism, there is an increased clearance of lithium during pregnancy; with the diuresis after delivery there may be an increased *retention* of lithium and consequently an increased risk of intoxication. Fetal distress may occur when lithium is used near term, and there may be hypotonia, listlessness, lethargy, cyanosis, and decreased suck response and Moro reflex in the newborn infants of mothers taking lithium, as well as hypothyroidism. In nursing mothers, breast milk lithium concentration is about 30–50% of the mother's blood level. A small number of reports have associated human fetal anomalies with the use of lithium in pregnancy, and suggest that the rate of such occurrence may be increased over that expected in the general population (Table 36). A reasonable position is that there is enough circumstantial evidence about the potential fetal toxicity of lithium to urge avoidance of its use in the early months of pregnancy, to advise caution and discontinuation of lithium before term, and to permit the use of lithium in pregnancy only for the most urgent indications.

The possible toxic effects associated with lithium treatment are summarized in Table 37. In addition, several interactions of lithium with other agents are noteworthy; these are summarized in Table 38. It is especially important to reemphasize that many diuretic agents with distal

Table 36 Outcome of pregnancy with lithium treatment

Category	Outcome among births to women treated with lithium (%)	Incidence in pregnancies in the general population (%)
Stillborn infant	3.6	13.0
All malformations	10.8	5.0
Down's syndrome	1.0	0.08
Cardiovascular malforma-tions	8.2	0.65
Ratio of cardiovascular to all malformations	76.0	10.0
Ebstein's cardiac malforma-tions	2.8	0.005
Induced abortions	2.6	14.0

Source: L. Weinstein, Langley-Porter Neuropsychiatric Institute Lithium Birth Registry data, 1977 (personal communication), and various other U.S. Public Health Service sources for the general population. Another potential risk is neonatal hypothroidism after fetal exposure to lithium late in pregnancy. The data above suggest that the risk of cardiac malformations is especially high with lithium (about 13 times above that of the general population), particularly in the case of Ebstein's malformation of the tricuspid value and cardiac septal defect (ca. 560-fold increase in risk; this latter malformation is sometimes diagnosed in utero and may be surgically correctable). These data should be interpreted with great caution, however, because of the high risk of biased sampling in the Registry data and the possibly unreliable estimates in the general population. The Registry data included a total of 194 births to mothers who used lithium at some point during pregnancy. All experiences with lithium in pregnancy should be reported to the Langley-Porter Lithium Registry in San Francisco and to the Lithium Information Center at the Department of Psychiatry, University of Wisconsin in Madison.

actions on sodium transport in the nephron tend to retain lithium and to increase its plasma levels, and thus to decrease dosage requirements for lithium salts. Since lithium is secreted preferentially over sodium in the sweat, heavy perspiration is probably not an important source of lithium retention and intoxication, as was formerly believed. Several antibiotics and many nonsteroid antiinflammatory agents can lead to retention of lithium, presumably by actions on the nephron. There are a few case reports suggesting an increased risk of confusion when lithium and ECT are combined.

Medical conditions in which special caution is required in the use of lithium include hypothyroidism and osteoporosis. There have been a few reports of worsening of myasthenia gravis with lithium treatment. Any

Table 37   Toxic effects of lithium salts

Nervous system

  Light-headedness, lethargy, weakness, mild confusion, tremor
  Severe intoxication on overdose, occasionally with irreversible damage
  Myasthenia gravis may worsen

Kidney

  Early polyuria and thirst; later tolerance usual (weight gain may occur if large
    amounts of high-calorie beverages are consumed)
  Later diabetes insipidus with elevated levels and poor response to ADH (if
    24-hour urine volume exceeds 5 L and there is a gradual rise in serum creati-
    nine or lithium, suspect granulomatous tubular degeneration and obtain
    renal biopsy)
  Serum levels of bromide ion have been reported to increase

Thyroid-parathyroid

  Occasional diffuse, nontoxic, non-premalignant goiter
  Borderline or mild hypothyroidism; TSH often elevated
  Mild changes in serum calcium or worsening of osteoporosis

Development

  Possible cardiovascular malformations, especially Ebstein's tricuspid valve and
    cardiac septal defects

Hematopoiesis

  Mild nonleukemic neutrophilia with relative lymphocytopenia

Skin

  Marked worsening of acne vulgaris
  Variable alopecia
  Mild fluid retention or local edema
  Rare eruptions, folliculitis (resembling keratosis pilaris), or ulcerations

---

debilitating illness, especially conditions associated with retention of fluid
and sodium (such as congestive heart failure, ascites, and nephrosis),
increases the risk of intoxication by lithium resulting from its retention
and requires a decrease in dosage.

It is also important to note that the effects of lithium can sometimes
cause confusion in the differential diagnosis of psychiatric conditions,
especially if a patient is encountered who is already responding to the
effects of lithium treatment. For example, the lethargy or hypothyroidism
sometimes associated with lithium intoxication may be mistaken for
recurrence of depression, and mania modified by lithium treatment may

Table 38 Drug interactions with lithium salts

Agent	Effect
CNS depressants	
Alcohol, sedatives, antidepressants, neuroleptics, antihypertensives	Excessive sedation, confusion
Agents with probable renal actions	
Sodium-losing diuretics	
Thiazides, ethacrynic acid, triamterene, spironolactone (but not furosemide; variable with amiloride)	Increase in plasma lithium level
Antibiotics	
tetracyclines, metronidazole (Flagyl)	Increase in plasma lithium; may also induce diarrhea
Nonsteroid antiinflammatory agents	
Indomethacin, ibuprofin (Motrin, Rufin and others), mefanamic acid (Ponstel), naproxin (Naprosyn), piperoxicam (Feldene), suldinac (Clinoril)	Increase in plasma lithium level
Low-potency neuroleptics	
Chlorpromazine, thioridazine, and others	May cause decrease in plasma clearance and increase in plasma level of lithium
Sodium-sparing diuretics	
Theophylline, caffeine, acetazolamide	Decrease in plasma lithium level

be mistaken for other forms of psychosis, such as schizophrenia or agitated major depression.

Alternative and Experimental Treatments

Because the efficacy of lithium in preventing recurrences of mania and depression is imperfect, and because lithium is a potentially toxic substance, especially on acute overdose in patients at high risk of suicidal behavior, there is intense interest in possible alternatives to sustained maintenance treatment with lithium salts. One alternative is to treat bipolar illness, as discussed in the previous chapter for schizophrenia, on an intermittent basis early in recurrences or at times of increased likelihood of recurrence. However, it is difficult to predict the timing of recurrences of mania or major depression or to define risk factors, and the impact of recurrences is potentially serious or even personally and financially catastrophic for some patients who may function well between episodes of acute illness.

The role of psychotherapies or other nonpharmacologic treatments in bipolar illness is only starting to be evaluated scientifically. Although there is some evidence that various forms of psychotherapy may add to the benefit of medication in the long-term treatment of patients with relatively mild or moderate depressive illnesses, possible benefits of psychotherapy in mania or in the course of severe bipolar manic-depressive illness are not known. Nevertheless, it is usual to combine psychotherapeutic methods to increase cooperation with medical treatment of this disorder, and it is well known that denial of illness and striving for autonomy are frequently encountered in bipolar patients and can make treatment difficult.

Among alternative medical treatments, the most commonly employed and best investigated alternative is the use of the anticonvulsant *carbamazepine* (Tegretol). This agent appears to have an antimanic action and possibly an effect like that of lithium salts to prevent recurrences of bipolar disorder. As in the treatment of seizure disorders, it is used in affective disorders in doses that provide plasma levels of 6 to 12 μg/ml, typically in the range of 600 to 1,200 mg/day given orally. Although there are several studies that support the antimanic and prophylactic actions of carbamazepine given with lithium or alone (see Post et al., 1982), this indication is still not "officially recommended" by its manufacturer or by the U.S. Food and Drug Administration. Nevertheless, it is used in this way increasingly commonly, especially in combination with a lithium salt when the latter proves inadequate alone. There is no evidence that the risk of toxicity of this combination exceeds that of either agent given alone. Since carbamazepine has occasionally been associated with suppression of bone marrow function and aplastic anemia, it is good practice to monitor the complete blood count regularly when this agent is employed, especially early in treatment and when high doses are required. Although there is a need for further studies of this use of carbamazepine and possibly other anticonvulsants, especially to verify the long-term efficacy and safety of treatment in psychiatric patients, there is sufficient experience with carbamazepine with neurological patients and sufficient research data in bipolar patients in North America, Europe, and Japan (see Post et al., 1982) that this option can now be recommended when lithium therapy has proved unsatisfactory or is considered too dangerous because of a coexisting medical condition.

Another line of investigation includes the evaluation of structural analogues of carbamazepine, including its keto-congener, *oxycarbamazepine.* Recent studies of this agent in Germany indicate that it has useful antimanic actions and may be associated with a decreased risk of toxic effects compared to carbamazepine. It has been used in doses between 600 and 3,000 mg/day, which were well tolerated alone and in combination with lithium salts and antidepressant or antipsychotic agents. Other anticonvulsants are also under investigation for use in mania and bipolar disorder, including *dipropylacetamide.* This drug has been well tolerated and found similar in efficacy to lithium in several recent short-term and long-term studies in Europe. It is claimed that this agent, too, is relatively free of side effects such as polyuria that complicate the use of lithium. Another anticonvulsant that might have antimanic and long-term preventive effects is *sodium valproate,* given in divided daily doses of 900 to 3,600 mg. Recent experience in Germany suggests that some patients who responded inadequately to lithium did well when treated with valproate for up to three years of follow-up. A congener of this agent, *valproic acid amide,* is also being evaluated, with encouraging early results in mania and in recurrent bipolar disorder.

The benzodiazepine *clonazepam,* which is also an anticonvulsant, has been claimed to have selective antimanic properties in early investigations of the use of doses of 4 to 16 mg/day in combination with lithium. This effect may not be unique, however, since earlier studies and much recent clinical experience indicate that other benzodiazepines, such as diazepam and lorazepam, as well as short-acting barbiturates such as amobarbital, also have useful but probably nonspecific or sedative effects in manic and other acutely psychotic patients. It remains to be seen whether benzodiazepines have useful and well-tolerated actions in the long-term treatment of recurrent major affective disorders.

A different strategy has been the attempt to increase the CNS actions of acetylcholine. The phospholipid *lecithin,* a common dietary source of phosphatidylcholine and hence of choline, the immediate precursor of acetylcholine, has been tested for its antimanic effects. Although there may be some added antimanic benefit of high doses of relatively pure lecithin in combination with lithium, this effect is not striking. An antimanic effect has not been shown to occur with lecithin alone, and the agent is not convenient to administer. Typically, lecithin is given in doses on the order of 10–20 grams per day added to food or beverages. *Choline* itself has also failed to prove effective and is not well tolerated in gram doses, especially since it produces a "fishy" odor of the breath and body because of its metabolic products. In addition, experience with parenterally administered *physostigmine* has not been encouraging in the treatment of mania, although injections of physostigmine can exert a sometimes striking, short-lived (60- to 90-minute) sedative or depressant effect in some susceptible manic patients. The status of oral physostigmine is uncertain, especially because its pharmacologic (potentiation of acetylcholine) and clinical (antimanic) efficacy are insecure, and its actions are probably not much longer than the injected agent. Indeed, evidence that any of these putative acetylcholine-potentiating treatments leads to significant and sustained increases of cholinergic activity in the CNS under clinical conditions is weak, even though choline and lecithin can produce significant increases of plasma levels of choline, and injections of physostigmine can induce short-lived cholinergic actions.

Another therapeutic approach has been to use small doses of the potent direct dopaminergic agonists *apomorphine* and *N-propylnorapomorphine,* both of which have beneficial effects in Parkinson's disease when given in high doses (below those that induce nausea and vomiting). Low doses of these agents are believed to have paradoxical antidopaminergic actions, supposedly because of selective agonistic effects at dopamine "autoreceptors" which are believed to be located at dopamine nerve terminals as well as dendrites and cell bodies, and capable of throttling the synthesis and release of dopamine. These agents have given inconsistent and unconvincing results in the treatment of schizophrenic patients, but they may have useful effects in some manic or acutely psychotic patients. However, these effects are not strong, are very short-lived (30 to 60 minutes), and may undergo tolerance with repeated treatment; the oral bioavailability of these agents is also poor. Nevertheless, experimentation with other congeners of this type continues and could lead to the development of useful psychopharmacologic agents.

There have been repeated clinical suggestions that monoamine oxidase (MAO) inhibitors may have special effects in bipolar patients, particularly in the depressed phase, although this point has not been investigated adequately. A recent novel addition to this idea is that certain MAO inhibitors not only may be effective in the short-term treatment of bipolar major depression, but also may have a low risk of inducing a "switch" of mood into mania or psychosis. Moreover, there are some preliminary data to suggest that a selective inhibitor of MAO type A, *clorgyline* (discussed further in the next chapter), may have prolonged mood-stabilizing actions similar to those of lithium in bipolar affective disorders. There is also a recent report of similar mood-stabilizing effects of the new atypical antidepressant bupropion (Wright et al., 1985). These interesting leads require further investigation in controlled, prospective therapeutic trials.

Yet another line of investigation is the use of antiadrenergic agents with CNS activity for the treatment of mania. Anecdotal experience is emerging to indicate that the antihypertensive alpha-2 agonist *clonidine* (Catapres) may have useful antimanic actions. On the other hand, this agent is also sedating and may induce hypotension in doses that are effective in mania (typically 0.1 – 0.2 mg/day). Moreover, there may be tolerance to its sedative as well as its antimanic effects, and it is not known whether this agent or other antiadrenergic compounds have long-term prophylactic benefits in bipolar or other recurrent major psychiatric disorders. The potential uses of such antiadrenergic agents require further evaluation. Since clonidine is generally available for clinical use and has been found to be effective in other neuropsychiatric disorders, including Gilles de la Tourette's syndrome, it can be considered for cautious trials if other treatments for mania have been found to be ineffective or poorly tolerated, even though its specific utility in mania has not been rigorously demonstrated scientifically.

The possible antimanic or antipsychotic effects of calcium channel blocking agents such as *verapamil* (Calan, Isoptin) have already been mentioned in the preceding chapter on antipsychotic agents.

Summary and Conclusions

Lithium ion provides a useful and specific form of chemotherapy for manic and hypomanic episodes. Since its clinical actions may be delayed for a week or more, the use of an antipsychotic or sedative agent may be required in the initial period to control the behavior of very disturbed patients. The main limitation of lithium is its narrow therapeutic index and requirement for close medical supervision. The most promising aspect of the use of this agent is its prophylactic effect in reducing the frequency and severity of manic and depressive attacks in bipolar affective illness. Several promising alternatives to lithium salts include anticonvulsant and centrally antiadrenergic compounds.

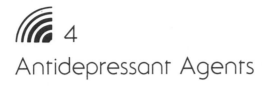 4

Antidepressant Agents

Prior to the 1950s, the physical treatment of severe depression included the use of various "shock" treatments, notably hypoglycemia induced by large doses of insulin and convulsive treatments based on the use of chemicals (camphor and later the inhaled convulsant gases such as flurothyl, or Indoklon) or electrical currents applied directly to the head (electroconvulsive treatment, or ECT). Of these, all but ECT are now only of historical interest and have been replaced by the modern antidepressant chemotherapies.

ECT still has an important place among modern medical therapies for major psychiatric disorders, despite an undeservedly poor reputation owing to its inconvenience, risks of side effects and physical trauma, and overly enthusiastic application to conditions in which its effectiveness is minimal and its use unjustified. As currently practiced, modern ECT is not only safe but also highly effective in severe depressions—in fact, consistently more effective than any antidepressant chemical treatment. Modifications in technique have reduced most of the untoward effects of ECT, with little if any loss in efficacy, and have added only slight additional risks due to anesthesia and neuromuscular blockade. Ultra-short-acting barbiturates used for anesthesia and paralyzing doses of succinylcholine eliminate orthopedic damage from seizures (except occasionally in the jaw, where local, direct electrical stimulation of muscle can still produce strong contractions), and application of the electrodes over the nondominant cerebral hemisphere probably reduces postictal confusion with little, if any, loss in efficacy. ECT is still the treatment of choice for certain patients with severe retarded or agitated depressions, including those with striking insomnia, withdrawal, and weight loss, or patients who are severely suicidal, for whom ECT may be lifesaving. It is often the best choice when therapeutic doses of antidepressant agents for several weeks prove to be ineffective. Because there are few absolute contraindications to ECT, short of increased intracranial pressure, it can be a safe form of treatment in patients who may be at high risk of toxicity from antidepressant chemicals (especially the elderly, those with severe cardiovascular disease, and pregnant women). Moreover, ECT still has a place in the treatment of manic or catatonic patients or others with atypical psychoses marked by profound agitation or mood change, and it is still occasionally considered for chronic schizophrenics who respond poorly to antipsychotic medications.

Before the 1950s the medical treatment of depression employed the stimulant amphetamines for psychomotor retardation and barbiturates for agitation. Although stimulants are still occasionally used for mild, short-lasting depression, particularly in apparent reaction to stressful circumstances or medical illness, there is little reason to use these drugs in most cases of major depression. Their use in severe depression is not indicated and may even worsen agitation and psychosis.

It was discovered in the late 1940s that several structural analogues of nicotinic acid had bacteriostatic properties and were particularly useful in the treatment of tuberculosis. The hydrazine derivative of isonicotinic acid, or isoniazid (INH), is still used for this purpose. Isoniazid, and more importantly its isopropyl analogue *iproniazid* (Marsilid), were found to have euphoriant or mood-elevating and behaviorally activating properties in some tuberculous patients. In 1952 iproniazid was reported by Ivan Selikoff, Jean Delay, and their collaborators in Europe to have useful antidepressant properties in psychiatric patients; similar findings were reported several years later by George Crane and Nathan Kline in the United States. Iproniazid was discovered to be a potent and irreversible inhibitor of the amine-catabolizing enzyme monoamine oxidase (MAO). Since that time other hydrazine compounds and nonhydrazines with MAO-inhibiting properties have been introduced into psychiatric practice; they are discussed in a separate section of this chapter. A few years later the second important, and now dominant, class of *tricyclic antidepressant* compounds was introduced.

Pharmacology

Types of Molecules with Antidepressant Activity

The tricyclic antidepressant compounds have two benzene rings joined through a central seven-member ring (see Figure 9). The first compound of this class was *imipramine* (originally Tofranil, but now available under several trade names and as a generic compound). Compounds of this type (dibenzazepines) contain two benzene rings linked through a central nitrogen (azo)-containing seven-membered central ring and are structurally analogous to the phenothiazines, with which they were compared initially, as well as the antipsychotic dibenzazepines loxapine and clozapine. *Trimipramine* is also a dibenzazepine. In the 1950s imipramine was found to have behavioral effects on animals superficially resembling some of those of the phenothiazines, and it had been known since the 1940s that imipramine and a structurally related group of agents had antihistaminic and sedative properties, as well as considerable anticholinergic activity. Because many of these properties and the general structure of imipramine were apparently similar to those of the phenothiazines, a prediction was made that imipramine might have antipsychotic properties. In one of the initial clinical trials of the new drug in Switzerland in 1957 – 1958, Roland Kuhn found that it had little antipsychotic efficacy but seemed to have mood-elevating and behavior-activating properties. Since that time, imipramine and the structurally related tricyclic agents have been found repeatedly in controlled comparisons with a placebo or a stimulant to be effective in the treatment of major depression. Although these clinical effects have not always been easily demonstrated, in contrast to most trials of the antipsychotic agents and lithium salts, and despite the considerable toxicity and side effects of this class of drugs, they have become by far the most popular and common medical treatment for depressions, particularly severe depressions with prominent pathophysiological features.

The search for chemically related compounds has led to more than 50 agents with pharmacologic properties resembling those of imipramine, many of which have useful antidepressant and other psychotropic actions, including sedative-hypnotic and antianxiety effects. Most of these agents were developed by making relatively minor alterations in the dibenzazepine molecular structure or by seeking agents with preclinical, behavioral, and biochemical actions similar to those of imipramine. Several additional agents are atypical in their pharmacologic properties, as discussed in the last section of this chapter, particularly in that they do not appear to block the inactivation of norepinephrine by neuronal uptake — a property common to most of the imipramine-like agents. Some of these newer, atypical antidepressants were discovered by serendipitous clinical observations suggesting their mood-elevating effects, whereas their initial evaluations suggested that they had mainly sedative or antianxiety effects. Examples include the phenylpiperazine-triazolopyridine *trazodone,* and the triazolo-benzodiazepine, *alprazolam.* Yet another agent with some atypical characteristics is *nomifensine,* which is a tetrahydroisoquinoline, and thus dissimilar structurally to older tricyclic antidepressants; while it inhibits the uptake of norepinephrine like the tricyclic agents, it also has stimulant-like effects and inhibits the uptake of dopamine. The status of the nearly 75 putative antidepressant agents that have been evaluated worldwide is uncertain, since evidence for their efficacy in major depression is variable and not always convincing. The United States has been particularly slow to accept new antidepressants, including some in routine clinical use for many years in other countries. Most of the agents in clinical use in this country are similar to imipramine, have only recently been accepted, or are continuing to gather support for their efficacy in severe depression and their safety in comparison with older agents. The structures of antidepressant agents currently approved by the U.S. Food and Drug Administration and in current clinical use in the United States are shown in Figure 9.

In addition to the dibenzazepines imipramine and trimipramine and the secondary amine congener (and active metabolite) of imipramine, *desipramine,* other agents in clinical use include *amitriptyline* and its N-desmethylated (nor-) product *nortriptyline* (a benzoxazepine) and *protriptyline* (a potent and long-acting dibenzocyclohexylheptatriene). Two other compounds with more unusual variations on the basic tricyclic structure of many antidepressants are *maprotiline* and *amoxapine,* which have been introduced into American medicine in the 1980s. Maprotiline contains an additional ethylene bridge across a central six-carbon-atom ring, which has suggested the misleading appellation "tetracyclic," although it is pharmacologically and clinically similar in many ways to imipramine and its congeners, and especially to other N-desmethylated tricyclic compounds such as desipramine and nortriptyline (secondary amine agents). Amoxapine (which can also be called nor-loxapine) is an N-desmethylated dibenzoxazepine, closely related to the typical neuroleptic agent loxapine, and possessing neuroleptic as well as antidepressant properties that include risk of extrapyramidal neurological toxicity. Other N-desmethylated derivatives of neuroleptic agents (for example, nor-chlorpromazine) share with amoxapine its potent activity against the uptake of norepinephrine but have not been evaluated as possible antidepressants.

Despite the variations in structure of this entire group of antidepressant agents, the general, trivial term "tricyclic" antidepressants can be retained. Alternatives, such as the use of "tetracyclic" for maprotiline

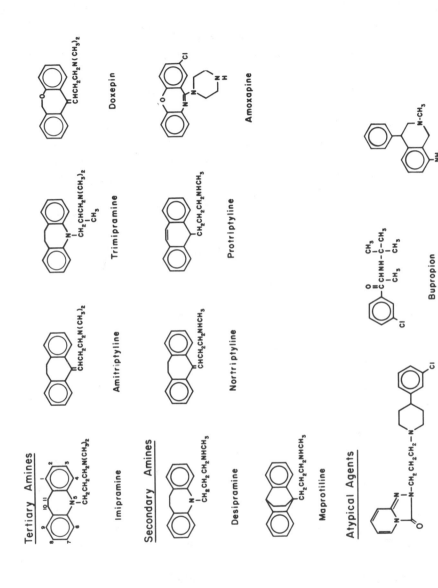

Figure 9 Chemical structures of antidepressants.

and amoxapine or the use of the terms "cyclic" or "heterocyclic" are chemically imprecise (for example, amitriptyline, nortriptyline, maprotiline, and protriptyline contain only carbon atoms in their three-ring cores but no "hetero" atom, and thus can not be called heterocyclic). The term "atypical antidepressant" is often employed to refer to *trazodone, bupropion* (see Figure 9), and other experimental agents whose structures and pharmacology are dissimilar to those of the tricyclic antidepressants. An additional alternative is to refer to the entire group as "non-monoamine-oxidase-inhibitors," but this term is awkward (and imipramine has weak inhibitory effects on this enzyme).

Preparations and Dosing

The available forms and suggested doses of tricyclic and atypical antidepressant agents currently in clinical use in the United States are given in Table 39. (The MAO inhibitors and stimulants are discussed in a separate section later in the chapter.) As the oldest antidepressant of this type, and one of the most intensively studied, imipramine is sometimes cited as a standard agent, much as chlorpromazine represents the neuroleptics. Doses are thus sometimes compared to the approximately equivalent amount of imipramine, although in contrast to the antipsychotic agents, the usual daily doses of most antidepressants are rather similar, typically 100–200 mg of imipramine or its equivalent for medically healthy young adult patients.

Absorption, Metabolism, and Elimination

Imipramine and other tricyclic antidepressants are well absorbed after oral administration and are rarely given by injection. Only amitriptyline and imipramine are available for intramuscular injection in the United States; 3-chloroimipramine (*clomipramine,* Anafranil), which is not available in the United States but is used clinically in Canada and many other countries, has been employed intravenously. Oral doses usually are divided into two or three portions, at least initially until some tolerance to the side effects of the antidepressants has developed. Many patients eventually tolerate and prefer once-daily dosing, especially for long-term treatment, but this practice is safest with doses not greater than the approximate equivalent of 150 mg of imipramine. Since insomnia is often a symptom of major depression and since most tricyclic antidepressants

Table 39 Tricyclic and atypical antidepressant drugs: Preparations and doses

Agent	Trade names	Dosage forms[a]	Usual dose (mg/day)	Extreme dose (mg/day)[b]
Tricyclic agents				
Amitriptyline hydrochloride[c]	Amitril, Elavil, Endep (and generic)	(T) 10, 25, 50, 75, 100, 150 mg (V) 10 mg/ml in 10 ml	100–200	25–600
Amoxapine hydrochloride[d]	Asendin	(T) 50, 100, 150 mg	200–300	50–600
Desipramine hydrochloride	Norpramin, Pertofrane	(C) 25, 50 mg; (T) 25, 50, 75, 100, 150 mg	100–200	25–300
Doxepin hydrochloride	Adapin, Curetin, Sinequan	(C) 10, 25, 50, 75, 100, 150 mg (S) 10 mg/ml	100–200	25–300
Imipramine hydrochloride[e]	Janimine, SK-Pramine, Tofranil (and generic)	(T) 10, 25, 50 mg; (A) 25 mg/2ml	100–200	25–300
Nortriptyline hydrochloride	Aventyl, Pamelor	(C) 10, 25 mg; (S) 10 mg/5ml	75–150	20–150
Maprotiline hydrochloride	Ludiomil	(T) 25, 50 mg	100–150	25–225[f]
Protriptyline hydrochloride	Vivactil	(T) 5, 10 mg	15–40	10–60
(+)Trimipramine maleate	Surmontil	(C) 25, 50, 100 mg	75–250	25–300
Atypical agents[g]				
Bupropion hydrochloride	Wellbutrin	(not yet released in U.S.)	450–600	100–750
Nomifensine maleate	Merital	(C) 50 mg	100–200	50–300
Trazodone hydrochloride	Desyrel	(T) 50, 100 mg	150–200	50–600

a. C = capsule, T = tablet, A or V = ampule or vial for intramuscular injection, S = oral solution or concentrate.
b. Low extreme doses are for very young and elderly patients; high doses are for hospitalized patients when low doses are not adequate.
c. Amitriptyline-HCl is also available mixed with fixed doses of perphenazine (Etrafon, Triavil), or with chlordiazepoxide (Limbitrol); these mixtures are not recommended for routine use.
d. Amoxapine has neuroleptic-like actions and side effects.
e. Imipramine is also available as the pamoate (Tofanil-PM), but its advantages over the hydrochloride are not established.
f. Maprotiline should be used very cautiously in doses above 200 mg/day because of the risk of seizures.
g. Atypical agents lack imipramine-like antagonism of the uptake-inactivation of norepinephrine, and their action mechanisms are uncertain; nomifensine does block uptake of norepinephrine but is atypical in structure and effects, with amphetamine-like properties.

have sedative and hypnotic effects, it is customary to provide most of the daily dose at bedtime.

Peak concentrations of imipramine and its congeners are typically attained after a single oral dose within 2 to 8 hours, but may require as long as 10 to 12 hours in some patients. Although parenteral administration offers the theoretical advantage of more rapid attainment of therapeutic tissue levels of antidepressants, it has not been proved that the typically slow onset of therapeutic benefits over several days or more is shortened by such administration. Nevertheless, intramuscular dosing is used occasionally for severely depressed and anorexic or poorly cooperative patients who may refuse oral medication, especially early in hospital treatment, and clomipramine has been used intravenously.

High doses of these strongly anticholinergic agents can slow gastrointestinal activity and gastric emptying time, with slow or erratic absorption of these and other drugs taken simultaneously. This effect on gastrointestinal motility can also complicate the management of acute overdoses of antidepressants.

Once absorbed, these compounds are widely distributed and exhibit pharmacokinetic properties resembling those of the chemically similar antipsychotic agents, such as chlorpromazine. They are relatively lipophilic and are strongly bound to plasma proteins (more than 85%) and to tissues, leading to high volumes of apparent distribution in the range of 10 to 50 L/kg. Their avid binding to tissue and plasma proteins makes it virtually impossible to remove imipramine-like agents by hemodialysis, adding to the danger of acute overdoses.

Like the phenothiazine antipsychotic agents, the tricyclic antidepressants are dealkylated and oxidized by hepatic microsomal enzymes, followed by conjugation with glucuronic acid. The major route of metabolism of imipramine and amitriptyline (with tertiary amine terminals on their side chains) is by initial N-dealkylation by microsomal enzymes to yield the active secondary amine products desipramine and nortriptyline (see Figure 9). It was proposed that such active metabolites might mediate the actions of antidepressants or might act more rapidly than the parent drug molecules, but neither proposal has found substantial support, although it is likely that the N-desmethylated products contribute to pharmacologic activity in many patients. The ratio of parent tricyclic agent to the active secondary amine products varies markedly among patients, by as much as 50-fold, although this ratio appears to be a relatively stable characteristic of each person over time. In many patients the amount of desmethylated product may exceed that of the administered precursor.

Once desmethylated, imipramine is usually further oxidized to form ring, 2-hydroxylated metabolites, which may then be conjugated to form glucuronides. Amitriptyline and its major N-desmethylated product nortriptyline are oxidized preferentially at the 10-position in the central ring (see Figure 9), and then conjugated. The 2-hydroxy metabolites of imipramine and desipramine, and possibly the 10-hydroxy metabolites of amitriptyline and nortriptyline, are biologically active; for example, they have potent activity against the neuronal uptake of norepinephrine, like that of the parent molecules. Doxepin is probably also converted to an active N-desmethylated product, nordoxepin.

The production of desmethylated and other metabolites of tricyclic antidepressants and the blood levels attained after a specific dose appear to be relatively stable characteristics of individual patients, presumably under genetic control. This characteristic individual difference in metabolism and clearance of antidepressants has been used experimentally to predict individual dosage requirements. Although this strategy for dosing, like that discussed in the preceding chapter concerning lithium salts, should increase the safety and reliability of administering antidepressants — especially to patients at high risk of intoxication (such as the elderly or those with hepatic or cardiovascular disease) — it has not been widely accepted in clinical practice. Two examples of clinical experience with this dosing strategy are provided in Table 40 and Figure 10, illustrating individual differences in blood levels of nortriptyline or the sum of im-

Table 40 Prediction of dosage requirement from blood concentration after a test dose of nortriptyline

Plasma concentration (ng/ml)	Predicted dosage (mg/day)
<12	150
13–19	100
20–24	75
25–34	50
35–40	30
>41	20

Source: Cooper and Simpson, *Am. J. Psychiatry* 135:333, 1978. A group of depressed patients were given a test dose of nortriptyline (50 mg by mouth); 24 hours later, blood was obtained for assay of plasma concentrations of nortriptyline. The dosage predictions were made so as to provide plasma levels of approximately 100 ng/ml, a clinically appropriate level.

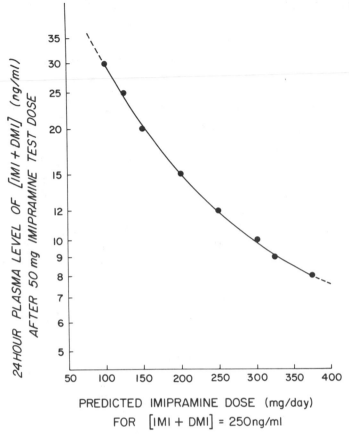

Figure 10 Prediction of therapeutic dose of imipramine based on blood levels following a test dose. A group of depressed patients were given a test dose of 50 mg of imipramine orally, and plasma levels of imipramine (IMI) and desipramine (DMI) were assayed in blood samples obtained 24 hours later. The patients were then treated clinically and plasma levels were monitored for several weeks. The data obtained permitted this predictive relationship of a clinical dose required to attain a plasma level at steady state of approximately 250 ng/ml. The data have been reanalyzed after Brunswick et al., Clin. Pharmacol. Ther. *25:605, 1979.*

ipramine plus desipramine following small test doses of nortriptyline or of imipramine, respectively.

Not only does the proportion of N-desmethylated to tertiary amine antidepressant vary markedly among individual patients, but the plasma levels of active agents attained after a fixed dose of an antidepressant drug also vary by 10-fold to 20-fold among individuals. Correlations between plasma concentrations of tricyclic antidepressants and clinical antidepressant or toxic effects have been investigated intensively in recent years, but the conclusions and clinical guidelines arising from this research remain incomplete and tentative. A general impression is that concentrations below 50 ng/ml (ng, or nanogram, $= 10^{-6}$ mg) are likely to be ineffective, while levels above 500, and certainly above 1,000 ng/ml of most antidepressants are likely to be associated with toxic effects, especially on the nervous system and cardiovascular tissue. It is suspected, but still unproved, that concentrations of the parent drug molecule and the important, active N-desmethylated metabolites of imipramine and amitriptyline above 100 ng/ml are most likely to be associated with therapeutic, antidepressant benefits with a limited risk of toxicity. It is further proposed that increases in levels between approximately 100 and 300 ng/ml may correlate with increased benefit, with little additional benefit found at higher levels, where toxicity is more likely. Such generalizations have not been established for other tertiary amine antidepressants, including doxepin and trimipramine.

It has also been proposed that in the case of some secondary amine antidepressants, most notably nortriptyline, there may be a more complex relationship between increasing blood levels and clinical effect. That is, several investigators have reported that optimal antidepressant effects of nortriptyline were found when plasma levels ranged from about 60 to 150 ng/ml, while lower levels are, and higher levels may be, associated with lesser benefits. The loss of effect at high levels is not necessarily because of increased toxicity. It has not been proved that other secondary amine tricyclic antidepressants follow a similar pattern, although clinically effective doses of desipramine and maprotiline are often associated with plasma levels of about 100–200 ng/ml. Such relationships are difficult to establish with reliability, particularly if the experimental protocol permits some adjustment of doses upward for patients who do not seem to respond well to a lower dose, leading to an artifactual association of higher blood levels with inferior clinical response. A tentative summary of typically encountered plasma levels of tricyclic and atypical antidepressants, as well as their average half-life, is provided in Table 41.

Although many commercial laboratories now offer assays of tricyclic antidepressants, the general and routine clinical utility of such measurements is not firmly established, and the precision or reproducibility of measurements by some laboratories has been found to be unreliable. Such measurements can help to confirm patients' compliance with medication and may be useful in the evaluation of unexpected clinical outcomes (such as severe toxicity after a low dose, or poor response and few

Table 41 Clinical pharmacokinetic characteristics of antidepressants

Agent	Elimination half-life (hours)[a]	Typical plasma concentrations (ng/ml)[b]
Tertiary amine		
Amitriptyline	16 + 30	100–250
Doxepin	16 + 50	100–250
Imipramine	12 + 30	200–300
Trimipramine	?	200–300
Secondary amine		
Amoxapine	8 + 30[c]	150–500
Desipramine	30	100–250
Maprotiline	48	200–300
Nortriptyline	30	50–150
Protriptyline	80	100–250
Atypical		
Bupropion	12	50–100
Nomifensine	3[d]	150–300
Trazodone	5[d]	800–1600

a. Half-life is only an approximate mean, varies markedly among individuals, and tends to increase with age; generally, the secondary-amine metabolites or agents are somewhat more slowly eliminated and are unusually potent as well. The two values for tertiary amines represent the half-life of the parent compound and the major active secondary-amine metabolite.

b. Plasma concentrations are those typically encountered with effective doses of antidepressants, and are not recommended as guidelines to optimal levels in treatment; except for nortriptyline, imipramine, desipramine, and amitriptyline, these values have not been evaluated adequately to guide treatment. Commercial laboratory assays of antidepressant levels may not be as reliable as for other therapeutic agents. The concentrations stated include the active secondary-amine metabolites as well as the tertiary-amine compounds administered. Serum levels may be lower than plasma levels.

c. Amoxapine itself is rapidly metabolized and eliminated (8 hours) to ring-hydroxylated metabolites (30 hours) which account for 80–90% of the total material in plasma; in man, the 8-OH metabolite predominates over the 7-OH analogue, which, like loxapine, has neuroleptic activity.

d. The short half-life of trazodone and nomifensine makes once-daily dosing impractical; nomifensine is also given more than once daily, but not at bedtime due to its stimulant-like effects.

side effects with high doses of an antidepressant), or to assist in the cautious dosing of infirm or elderly patients.

The process of metabolism of tricyclic antidepressants, like that of antipsychotic agents, leads to by-products that are more water-soluble and thus more easily eliminated by renal excretion, and, ultimately, biologically less active. The processes of metabolism and elimination of tricyclic antidepressants occur over several days. The elimination half-life ranges from about 20 hours for imipramine to an extreme of about 126 hours for protriptyline, with intermediate values for other agents (see Table 41). Metabolism and elimination, as well as tolerance of the effects

Table 42 Effect of aging on metabolism and elimination of antidepressants

Measurement	Under 65 years	Over 65 years	Change in elderly (%)
Imipramine dose (mg/day)	150	92	61
Total plasma [TCA] (ng/ml)	52	141	271
[TCA]/dose (ng/ml/mg)	0.35	1.52	434
[DMI] : [IMI] ratio	0.66	0.68	103
Half-life, imipramine (hours)	19	24	126
Half-life, desipramine (hours)	34	76	224

Source: Data adapted from Nies et al., Am. J. Psychiatry 134:790, 1977. Depressed adults were tested in a steady state of drug metabolism after at least a week of treatment; data are means for groups of about six patients. Similar results were obtained with amitriptyline. There was a significant correlation of total tricyclic antidepressant (TCA) plasma level (imipramine [IMI] + desipramine [DMI]) versus age ($r = 0.54$).

of tricyclic antidepressants, diminish in the elderly (Table 42). Half-life is longer following overdoses, but with ordinary clinical doses most of the tricyclic agents should be eliminated within a week after termination of treatment (with the exception of protriptyline). In cases of severe intoxication with acute overdoses, cardiac and other toxic effects may occur as late as 10 to 14 days afterward, in part because of prolonged retention of drug molecules in tissue. Systematic studies aimed at detecting tissue levels of tricyclic antidepressants at times long after their prolonged administration, comparable to those discussed in the previous chapter for the antipsychotic agents, are not available. Nevertheless, it is not safe scientifically or clinically to assume a return to the drug-free state after discontinuation of an antidepressant for a few weeks.

There have been several attempts to alter the rate of metabolism of antidepressants with agents competing for hepatic microsomal enzymes. Phenothiazines and stimulants including methylphenidate (Ritalin) increase blood levels of tricyclic antidepressants, as do certain antibiotics and possibly aspirin. In contrast, contraceptive hormones, other steroids, and barbiturates are capable of inducing increased amounts of several liver enzymes and decreasing the levels of antidepressants, presumably by increasing their hepatic metabolism. Although this work has been scientifically interesting, it has not yet led to convincing evidence that the clinical efficacy or safety of the tricyclic antidepressants can be altered by administering agents that interact with the hepatic microsomal enzymes. Moreover, the same ends might be achieved more simply by adjusting the dose of tricyclic drug.

Tolerance to some side effects of antidepressants, including sedation and autonomic effects, is usual; dry mouth, constipation, blurred vision, and tachycardia usually diminish within several weeks of treatment. Occasionally symptoms suggestive of physical dependence on tricyclic antidepressants are encountered, especially following abrupt discontinuation of prolonged high doses. A withdrawal syndrome consisting of malaise, chills, coryza, and muscle aches has been described. Therefore, gradual withdrawal is considered good practice. There are sporadic reports suggesting tolerance to the main, antidepressant effects of tricyclic antidepressants (and MAO inhibitors), leading to a requirement for increasing doses to regain clinical benefit, typically following months of maintenance treatment of patients with severe and rapidly recurring or chronic depression. The frequency of this phenomenon is not known but appears to be low.

Mechanisms of Action

It was believed initially that the tricyclic antidepressants and the phenothiazines were pharmacologically as well as structurally similar. The fact that the tricyclic antidepressants have acute sedative effects in animals and man points out one of the important problems that has limited the development of effective new antidepressants. In the case of the MAO inhibitors and imipramine, their identification as antidepressants depended on fortuitous clinical findings not predicted by preclinical screening. Since the 1950s, attempts to improve prediction of antidepressant activity in new compounds have had limited success. Some sophisticated forms of self-stimulatory behavior electrically induced with intracerebral electrodes, as well as responses in certain conditioning paradigms or endurance of stress (such as forced swimming, unavoidable shock, or early separation of primates from their mothers or peers), have shown promise, but they are relatively expensive and complicated for routine pharmaceutical screening tests and vary in their specificity for antidepressants. More often, the behavioral interactions of new agents with reserpine or tetrabenazine (amine-depleting agents), their cardiovascular interactions with various pressor amines, or their ability to block uptake of radiolabeled amines by isolated nerve endings or other tissue preparations in vitro have been utilized as relatively simple and inexpensive predictive tests or models of the clinical condition for which treatment is being sought. These tests are based on the observations that most stimulants and antidepressant agents have some ability to reverse or modify behavioral sedation induced by reserpine or by tetrabenazine. These and other amine-depleting agents (such as alpha-methyldopa, Aldomet) are themselves sometimes associated with clinical depression in susceptible patients. Furthermore, the tricyclic agents enhance the actions of directly sympathomimetic agents, notably norepinephrine, and block the effects of many indirectly sympathomimetic agents such as tyramine, whereas the MAO inhibitors enhance the actions of both types of sympathomimetic amines.

These pharmacological observations and their interpretation have given the most important support to the *amine hypothesis* of affective disorders, which suggests that major depression is associated with a relative lack of activity of certain amine neurotransmitters in the brain, most probably the catecholamine norepinephrine, while mania may be an expression of overactivity of norepinephrine or of dopamine. Furthermore, other amines including acetylcholine and serotonin may modify the effects of altered catecholamine neurotransmission and have been proposed to contribute to the pathophysiology of major depression.

A major limitation to understanding the actions of antidepressant or other mood-altering agents is the lack of knowledge of the causes of the major mood disorders. In the past two decades there has been intensive study of the physiological changes that occur in the depressed state. These investigations have given a partial picture of changes that sometimes accompany depression but are not proved to be related to the causes of depression; they may or may not be an expression of essential biological differences in patients susceptible to major depression that are strongly suggested by evidence of a genetic contribution to the risk of major affective disorders. However, there are many reasons for doubt concerning cause-and-effect relationships, including the fact that most biological changes that have been described (including altered metabolism of monoamines, altered timing and patterning of sleep stages and other biological rhythms, and disregulation of adrenal corticosteroids and other hormone functions regulated ultimately by the central nervous system) tend to return to normal upon remission of acute affective illness. Metabolic and physiological changes found in patients with acute major depression might be secondary to or concomitant with the state of depression, and not necessarily a cause of depression or a specific indication of a biological vulnerability to it. Yet another difficulty is that most patients available for investigation have been exposed to medical treatments known or suspected to have long-term effects on neuronal metabolism and function, leading to the risk of drug-induced artifacts in such studies. A few observations (including altered neuroendocrine functions and possible alterations of muscarinic acetylcholine receptors in peripheral tissues) have been proposed as more stable traits of patients susceptible to recurrent major mood disorders, which are not dependent on the state of active depression or recent drug treatment. Nevertheless, these findings remain preliminary and tentative. Metabolic evidence to support the hypothesis that depression is associated with a deficiency of monoamine neurotransmission remains weak and inconsistent, despite many years of investigation.

It remains uncertain whether the amine-potentiating actions of antidepressants of the tricyclic and MAO-inhibiting types are either necessary or sufficient to account for their clinical actions. There is a considerable risk that the process of developing new antidepressants by screening for ability to inhibit uptake of norepinephrine or otherwise to alter monoaminergic transmission has encouraged circular reasoning about the apparent association of amine-potentiating effects and clinical antidepressant actions. The development of newer, atypical antidepressants such as trazodone, bupropion, iprindole, opipramol, S-adenosylmethionine, and possibly some triazolobenzodiazepines, as well as others with little effect on amine inactivation by neuronal uptake, encourages a broader perspective concerning drug actions that might lead to mood-elevating actions. A broad perspective is especially appropriate because the basic premise that severe depression is a state of monoamine deficiency has not been proved. There is even evidence that late effects of many antidepressants (which may correspond temporarily with their typically slow onset of clinical antidepressant effects) may include decreased sensitivity in some neurotransmission systems. There is also evidence that, paradoxically, some depressed patients may be characterized by having an increased output and production of catecholamines.

Given these caveats concerning the relationships between the known actions of antidepressants and the biology of major mood disorders, these actions can be summarized as follows. First, it is useful to have a scheme of organization of monoaminergic neurotransmission in the mammalian nervous system as a framework for studying the pharmacology of antidepressants. Since the 1950s a great deal of information has been produced to describe the anatomical and metabolic organization of central monoamine-containing neuronal circuits. Much less is known about the functions of these systems, although they are strongly implicated in activities known to be deranged in major depression, including activity, arousal, affect, sex drive, appetite and eating, sleep, neuroendocrine functions,

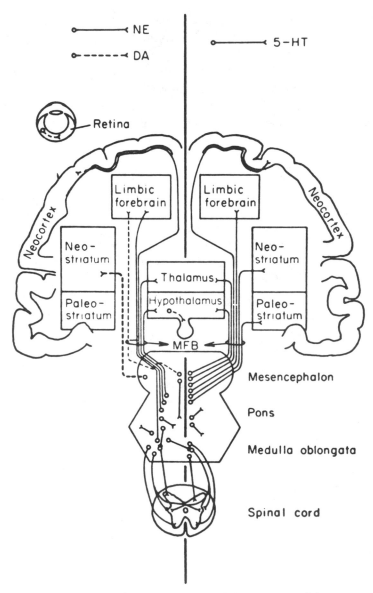

Figure 11 Organization of monoamine-containing neurons of the mammalian central nervous system. This diagram is organized with catecholamine systems on the left and indoleamine systems on the right. The catecholamines are norepinephrine (NE) and dopamine (DA), and the indoleamine is 5-hydroxytryptamine (5-HT). Cell bodies of NE neurons are few in number (thousands) and localized to the locus ceruleus and nearby sites of the pons and medulla. They project to the spinal cord and the diencephalon and forebrain relatively diffusely. DA projections are more selective to a midbrain-to-basal ganglia (nigrostriatal) projection, as well

and autonomic functions, as well as the rhythmic regulation of all of these functions on an hour-by-hour (ultradian) and daily (circadian) basis.

An organizational scheme for the major monoamine-containing systems in the mammalian central nervous system is shown in Figure 11. The following series of diagrams (Figures 12–15) provide schematic summaries of the metabolic pathways for the synthesis and metabolism of norepinephrine and serotonin (5-hydroxytryptamine), as well as current concepts of the organization of typical aminergic nerve terminals. Similar schemes for dopaminergic neurons were presented in Figures 3 and 4 in Chapter 2.

It has been known since the work of Julius Axelrod and his colleagues in the early 1960s that imipramine and other typical, tricyclic-type antidepressants block the inactivation of norepinephrine by uptake at adrenergic nerve terminals in the peripheral sympathetic and central nervous systems (see Figure 13). Many studies have added to the evaluation of this phenomenon and extended it to measurements of the transport of other monoamine neurotransmitters in the brain, particularly serotonin (see Figure 15). Relatively few laboratories, however, have systematically evaluated large numbers of antidepressants and other agents under similar conditions, so it is difficult to compare them by their activity against the uptake of various amines. A summary of representative data is provided in Table 43, which indicates that most of the typical tricyclic-type antidepressants have activity against the uptake of norepinephrine but have variable effects against serotonin, and relatively little activity against the uptake of dopamine.

Generally, the N-desmethylated compounds (secondary amine antidepressants) are somewhat more potent and more selective against the uptake of norepinephrine. Thus, protriptyline, desipramine, maprotiline, amoxapine, and the newer agents nomifensine, nisoxetine, and oxaprotiline have high potency against norepinephrine, and much less against serotonin uptake. Selectivity for norepinephrine uptake generally also corresponds with lower anticholinergic, antiadrenergic, and antihista-

---

as from midbrain to limbic structures and mesiofrontal and temporal cerebral cortex, and within the hypothalamus and retina (see also Figure 3). 5-HT projections are even more widespread than those of NE and arise from a series of midline nuclei in the pons and brainstem (raphe nuclei). This schema is based on the work of Anden et al., Acta Physiol. Scand. *67:313, 1966, as reviewed in Baldessarini,* Biomedical Aspects of Depression and Its Treatment *(American Psychiatric Association Press, Washington, D.C., 1983).*

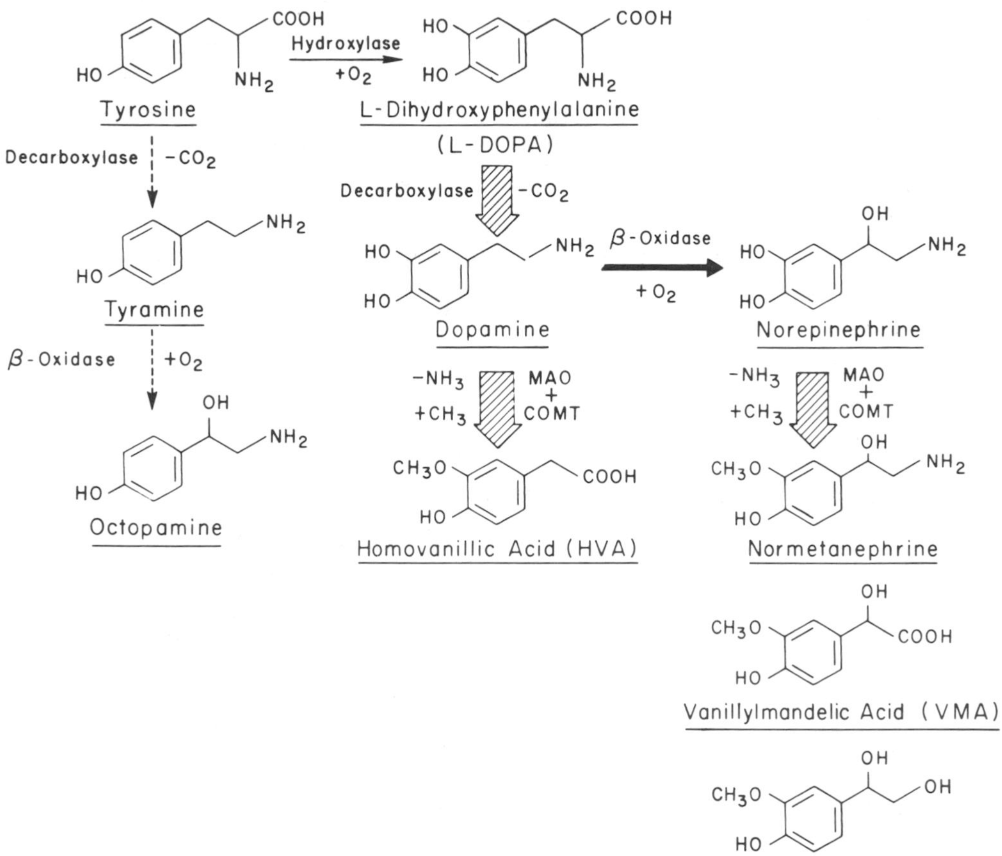

3-Methoxy-4-Hydroxyphenethyleneglycol (MHPG)

Figure 12 Metabolism of catecholamines. Catecholamines and other related phenethylamines are produced from phenylalanine and tyrosine. The sizes of the arrows suggest the relative magnitude of activity through each enzymatic step here and in Figures 13, 14, and 15. The hydroxylation of tyrosine is rate-limiting because of the small amount of hydroxylase only in catecholamine cells and its near-saturation with substrate under normal conditions. Decarboxylation occurs through a widely distributed aromatic amino acid decarboxylase enzyme, which is probably similar, if not identical, for most aromatic amines. In norepinephrine cells only, dopamine can be further oxidized at the 2 (β) position of the side-chain by dopamine-β-oxidase (or "hydroxylase," "DBH") to yield norepinephrine. Metabolic inactivation occurs through the actions of monoamine oxidase (MAO) and catechol-O-methyl-transferase (COMT), which uses S-adenosylmethionine (a putative antidepressant) as a cofactor. The deaminated and O-methylated products include normetanephrine, vanillylmandelic acid (VMA), and 3-methoxy-4-hydroxy-phenethyleneglycol (MHPG) from norepinephrine, as well as 3-methoxy-tyramine, 3,4-dihydroxy-phenylacetic acid (DOPAC), and homovanillic acid (HVA) from dopamine. In addition, some cells also produce epinephrine (N-meth-

minic activity and may also correspond with a lower likelihood of sedation and autonomic side effects.

Of the clinically available antidepressants, trimipramine and doxepin are among the least potent against norepinephrine uptake and thus should interfere least with the hypotensive actions of postganglionic sympathetic blockers such as guanethidine. However, in vivo desmethylation of these agents or other factors may alter this suggestion. For example, doxepin can antagonize guanethidine, especially after several days of treatment with effectively antidepressant doses. A related phenomenon is the interaction with indirectly sympathomimetic amines, such as tyramine, which are taken up by sympathetic nerve terminals to release norepinephrine. For example, in contrast to amitriptyline, a potent blocker of amine uptake into sympathetic terminals, trimipramine failed to block the pressor effect of intravenous infusions of tyramine given to patients pretreated with an MAO inhibitor to protect tyramine from degradation. This observation suggests that coadministration of an amine-uptake-inhibiting tricyclic antidepressant with an MAO inhibitor might protect against hypertensive reactions to tyramine-rich foods, although it should not alter the risk of other toxic interactions of MAO inhibitors and tricyclic antidepressants.

Several experimental agents, such as fluoxetine and its congeners, have relative selectivity against the uptake of serotonin. The in vivo selectivity

---

ylated norepinephrine). Other trace amines, including tyramine and octopamine, may arise separately in other cells or with catecholamines and may be released with them as cotransmitters; certain peptides may also be produced in catecholamine cells, including cholecystokinin in dopamine cells, as additional cotransmitters, "neuromodulators," or neurohormones that modify the activity of other cells. It was formerly proposed that peripherally sampled MHPG may be uniquely representative of CNS metabolism of norepinephrine, but it is clear that much urinary and plasma MHPG arises from peripheral metabolism, and that much of the MHPG from brain is converted in the periphery to VMA to contribute to its appearance in the urine.

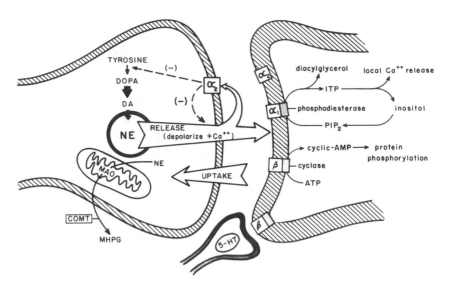

Figure 13 Organization of a norepinephrine synapse. The metabolic apparatus depicted in Figure 12 is located in specific portions of the presynaptic neuron at varicosities along the terminal portion of the axon. These varicose terminal axons course through target tissues and appear to provide norepinephrine (NE) to adrenergic receptors on responsive cells in a somewhat diffuse manner on a relatively prolonged time base. The amine neurotransmitter is released by depolarizing nerve impulses in the presence of calcium ion (Ca^{++}) by a process of exocytotic fusion of presynaptic vesicles and cell membrane to provide amine in the synaptic cleft. The transmitter is recognized by specific macromolecular receptor complexes at the postsynaptic cell surface. In the mammalian CNS, these include beta (β) receptors associated with adenylate cyclase stimulation in the case of norepinephrine (and probably beta receptors for the few epinephrine neurons of the brainstem and hypothalamus). The beta receptors facilitate the conversion of adenosine-triphosphate (ATP) to cyclic-adenosine-monophosphate (cyclic-AMP), which in turn initiates a complex series of reactions leading to altered phosphorylation of intracellular proteins, and ultimately to a change in the ion-permeability and neurophysiological activity of the receptive neurons by biochemical mechanisms that remain obscure. The alpha receptors of type 1 (α_1) are not directly associated with adenylate cyclase but are believed to act on the metabolism of phospholipids (including polyphosphoinosotides, PIPs, produced from inositol, and notably diphosphoinositide, PIP_2, which is converted to inositol-triphosphate, ITP, by the action of α_1 receptors in receptive cell membranes) to alter intracellular levels of calcium ions, and thus to influence neuronal functional activity. It is also likely that autoreceptors occur for norepinephrine (α_2 receptors); they may influence adenylate cyclase and intracellular levels of calcium and serve to throttle synthesis and release of catecholamines. Serotonin neurons are also implicated in modulating the abundance or activity of beta-adrenergic receptors. Inactivation of released transmitter occurs through the actions of the enzymes MAO and COMT (with its cofactor S-adenosylmethionine, S-AMe), to yield the O-methylated and oxidatively deaminated metabolites outlined in Figure 12. However, physiological inactivation occurs mainly by a process of high-affinity active uptake linked to the sodium transport system and sensitive to the actions of many stimulants (such as d-amphetamine and cocaine) and antidepressants of the tricyclic type.

of fluoxetine against serotonin uptake is reported to be even greater (more than a hundredfold) than its in vitro selectivity (about threefold), suggesting that pharmacologically active metabolites may play a role in vivo. Several agents of this type are undergoing clinical trials and may have useful antidepressant or antianxiety effects. Paradoxically, some putative antidepressants (mianscrin, cyproheptadine) have antiserotonin, receptor blocking effects, so the role of facilitating serotonin in the actions of fluoxetine, citalopram, and other newer antidepressant candidates remains unclear. Most clinically employed antidepressants with serotonin-uptake-inhibiting actions are also active against the uptake of norepinephrine. An example is clomipramine, an effective antidepressant that may also have selective beneficial effects in obsessive-compulsive disorder.

Several exceptions to the general rule that blockers of norepinephrine uptake are usually antidepressant can be cited: amphetamines, cocaine, methylphenidate, and mazindol. Yet these agents do have short-lasting stimulant actions in man. Chlorpromazine is also about as effective against norepinephrine uptake as doxepin; the former agent, an effective dopamine receptor antagonist, has antiagitation effects and is antipsychotic, but its status in nonpsychotic depressions is obscure. The stimulants are effective against the uptake of dopamine as well as norepinephrine, but their rapid and short-lived behaviorally activating effects are not therapeutically useful in typical cases of major depression, in which they can even worsen agitation and psychosis. Furthermore, dopamine agonists such as L-dopa and bromocriptine are not useful in depression. At least two newer antidepressants, nomifensine and bupropion, have some effect against the uptake of dopamine. Bupropion is structurally related to the amphetamines (see Figure 9) and may be metabolized to amphetamines. This drug and nomifensine have stimulant-like actions. However, nomifensine is also an extremely potent blocker of norepinephrine uptake, and the contribution of dopamine-facilitating actions to the clinical effects of this agent and those of bupropion are uncertain.

Most of the newer or experimental antidepressants are pharmacologically similar to older agents. The actions of a few, however, are obscure. These "atypical" antidepressants are not blockers of the uptake of monoamines, nor are they MAO inhibitors. The atypical agents iprindole and mianserin have been suggested to have subtle influences on the neuronal release of norepinephrine. Mianserin also has some effect against the uptake of norepinephrine in vitro, and a weaker effect in vivo. Trazodone may also have some serotonin-uptake-blocking effect, at least in vitro (see

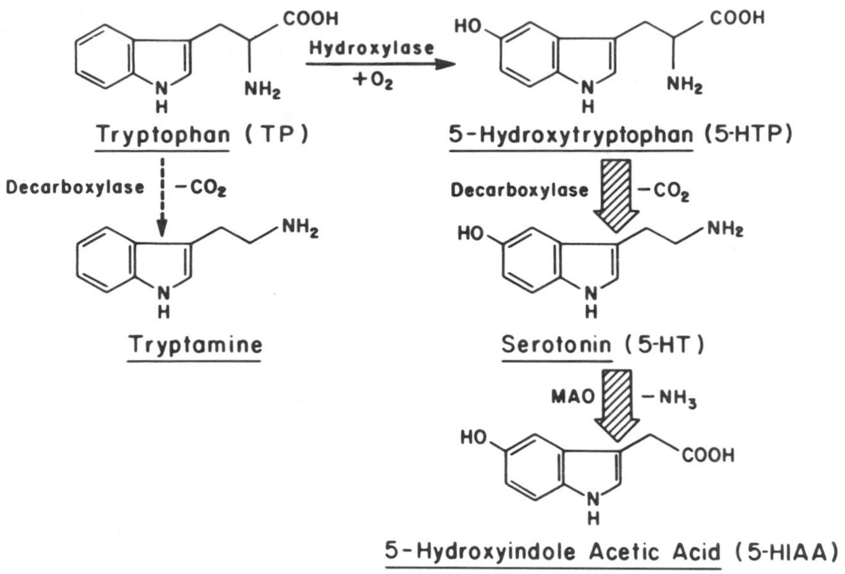

Figure 14 Metabolism of indoleamines. The arrangements at indoleamine (mainly serotonin)-producing nerve terminals are similar to those for catecholamine cells, as depicted in Figure 12. Thus, tryptophan (TP), the precursor amino acid, is first ring-hydroxylated to 5-hydroxytryptophan (5-HTP) which, in turn, is decarboxylated to the amine 5-hydroxytryptamine (5-HT, serotonin). The major route of metabolic inactivation is by mitochondrial MAO (mainly type A, as in catecholamine nerve terminals) to yield the deaminated product 5-hydroxyindole-acetic acid (5-HIAA). This and other acid by-products of catecholamine metabolism (such as HVA and VMA) are removed into the venous blood at the choroid plexus by a probenecid-sensitive transport process. Minor pathways for indoleamines also occur in the mammalian CNS, including the production of small amounts of tryptamine directly from tryptophan; the indoleamine tryptamine normally is rapidly oxidized to indoleacetic acid, except following treatment with an MAO inhibitor.

Table 43). These agents thus raise doubts about the generality of the monoamine uptake blockade hypothesis of the action of tricyclic antidepressants, assuming that the clinical efficacy of the newer, atypical antidepressants in major depression is sustained with further experience.

The effects of antidepressants on the uptake of monoamine neurotransmitters appear to persist with repeated treatment and are not known to undergo tolerance. On the other hand, many other complex changes occur in the metabolism and function of monoamines during continued treatment with these drugs, corresponding in time with the typically slow onset of clinical effects over days or weeks of treatment.

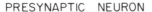

PRESYNAPTIC NEURON   POSTSYNAPTIC NEURON

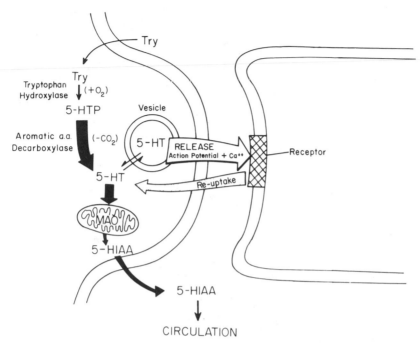

*Figure 15   Organization of a serotonin synapse. The presynaptic terminals con-
tain the metabolic system described in Figure 14. Release, uptake, and inactivation by MAO are similar to those steps described for norepinephrine in Figure 13.
The arrangement of receptors and their precise characterization in the serotonin
system are not as well developed as in adrenergic systems. The precursor tryptophan (Try) is converted to 5-hydroxytryptophan (5-HTP) and thence to 5-hydroxy-
tryptamine (5-HT, serotonin), which can then be deaminated by MAO to yield
5-hydroxyindoleacetic acid (5-HIAA). A peptide, substance P, may also be produced with serotonin in some cells and may be released with the indoleamine as a
cotransmitter or additional neurohormone. Substance P is a potent neuron-depo-
larizing agent whose physiology and pharmacology remain undeveloped.*

Recent evaluations of antidepressant agents have greatly extended understanding of their actions. Such studies have provided information on
the neurophysiological activity of monoaminergic neurons, the rates of
turnover and release of transmitters, biochemical responses and behavioral effects of their agonists, and electrophysiological responses to mi-
croapplication of amines to neurons in the central nervous system. In
addition, there has been intensive study of binding sites that are thought to
represent receptors for neurotransmitters in the nervous system. These

Table 43 In vitro inhibition by antidepressants and other agents of uptake of amines in brain tissue

Agent	Potency (IC_{50}, nM)[a]			Potency ratio (NE : 5-HT)
	NE	5-HT	DA	
Typical tricyclic-type				
Norclomipramine	0.5	40	2,200	80
Desipramine	1.2	1,100	9,000	916
Protriptyline	1.4	1,000	5,200	714
Nisoxetine	8	200	2,900	25
Oxaprotiline	8	—	—	—
Amoxapine[b]	14	570	46	40
Maprotiline	14	13,500	9,300	960
Nortriptyline	20	1,000	5,300	50
Dothiepin	34	—	—	—
Imipramine	30	260	16,000	9
Amitriptyline	50	170	5,800	3
Clomipramine	60	16	5,000	0.3
Doxepin	100	1,850	7,700	18
Viloxazine	840	40,000	56,000	48
Butriptyline	1,200	6,000	5,200	5
Trimipramine	1,875	3,750	6,700	2
Atypical				
Nomifensine	20	9,000	100	450
Fluoxetine	740	6.9	12,000	0.009
Mianserin	425	37,500	30,000	88
Iprindole	1,650	24,000	12,500	14
Bupropion	3,000	19,000	1,800	6
Citalopram	8,800	1.8	41,000	0.0002
Trazodone	10,000	760	60,000	13
Stimulants				
d-Amphetamine	78	21,000	280	270
l-Amphetamine	150	77,000	1,300	500
Cocaine	170	600	350	4
Methylphenidate	200	81,000	700	400
Others				
Benztropine	450	14,000	270	31
Chlorpromazine	150	10,000	12,000	67
Thioridazine	4,000	5,500	3,500	1.4

Source: Data are pooled from a previous review and references cited therein (Baldessarini, Biomedical Aspects of Depression and Its Treatment, American Psychiatric Press, Inc., Washington, D.C., 1983) and

include sites believed to represent traditional α_1 (postsynaptic), α_2 (partly presynaptic), and β noradrenergic receptors, dopamine receptors (of types D-1 and D-2), histamine receptors (H_1 and H_2), and serotonin receptors (types 5-HT_1 and 5-HT_2), as well as muscarinic acetylcholine (ACh_m) receptors. A summary of representative findings concerning receptor-directed activity of antidepressants is provided in Table 44. In addition, the binding of labeled antidepressants has been partially evaluated; although such labeling may represent membrane macromolecules involved in amine transport rather than receptors, its significance remains unclear.

There are few consistent relationships between the in vitro potency of interaction of antidepressants with various receptor sites and their clinical potency, even among agents that are similar chemically or similar in an independent pharmacologic characteristic such as ability to inhibit uptake of norepinephrine. In part this lack of correlation reflects the limited range of clinical potencies of antidepressants, which are typically given in clinical doses between 30 and 300 mg per day. In addition, however, it may be possible that receptor interactions are not crucial to the clinical antidepressant actions of these drugs. On the other hand, some of the effects at receptors appear to correlate with or to predict certain side effects of antidepressants and may contribute to a more complete characterization of their range of activities.

A particularly important receptor interaction that has some limited success in predicting clinical side effects and toxicity is the apparent anticholinergic activity of antidepressants, usually as assayed by competing with the binding of a potent muscarinic antagonist, such as tritiated quinuclidinyl benzilate (^{3}H-QNB) or ability to stimulate synthesis of cyclic-guanosine-monophosphate (cyclic-GMP) by neural tissue (see Table

---

from data concerning uptake of norepinephrine by human cerebral cortex provided by E. Richelson of the Mayo Clinic (personal communication, 1984). Data are based on the uptake of low concentrations of radiolabeled norepinephrine (NE), serotonin (5-HT), or dopamine (DA) by isolated nerve-ending preparations (synaptosomes) of cerebral cortex (rat and human, as well as mouse heart, for NE; rat brain for 5-HT and DA).

a. IC_{50} = half-maximally effective drug concentration in nM.

b. Both 7-OH- and 8-OH-amoxapine had similar activity against uptake of NE and 5-HT. Note that clomipramine and fluoxetine are selective against uptake of 5-HT, and that stimulants (and nomifensine) are active against uptake of DA as well as NE. In an analysis of comparable data obtained by in vivo experiments on the blockade of uptake of ^{3}H-NE or the selective neurotoxin 6-OH-dopamine into cardiac tissue as an index of NE uptake and of the uptake of p-Cl-amphetamine in mouse brain as an index of 5-HT uptake, clomipramine was less selective against 5-HT, amitriptyline was more selective against NE, and fluoxetine was more selective against 5-HT. Despite these shifts in absolute potency, the potencies in vitro and in vivo with respect to NE uptake were closely correlated ($r = 0.91$, slope $= 1.16$), as reviewed by Baldessarini, *Biomedical Aspects of Depression,* 1983).

Table 44 Potency of antidepressants and other agents for amine receptors (IC$_{50}$, nM)

Agent	Cholinergic ACh$_m$	Adrenergic			Dopaminergic (D-2)	Serotonin		Histamine	
		α$_1$	α$_2$	β		5-HT$_1$	5-HT$_2$	H$_1$	H$_2$
Typical tricyclic-type									
Amitriptyline	34	26	765	6,800	290	1,480	13	0.1	54
Butriptyline	36	560	4,800	—	—	—	—	—	—
Protriptyline	70	200	6,700	3,100	360	—	640	48	420
Trimipramine	92	34	1,050	—	—	42	—	0.1	—
Doxepin	138	24	1,000	7,100	380	720	250	0.03	160
Imipramine	186	74	3,200	38,000	610	5,000	245	16	153
Clomipramine	268	46	3,200	—	—	—	—	—	50
Nortriptyline	550	66	2,100	15,000	800	920	40	17	400
Maprotiline	590	90	9,100	—	—	—	—	—	—
Amoxapine	1,000	50	2,600	—	100	—	—	—	—
Desipramine	1,200	136	7,000	4,200	980	9,500	540	250	320

Atypical

Nomifensine	250,000	900	4,600	—	>10,000	1,400	—	—	—
Mianserin	2,400	60	53	4,400	2,200	500	—	3	67
Iprindole	6,000	6,000	8,300	21,000	6,300	>10,000	1,900	100	200
Fluoxetine	8,000	8,000	13,000	10,000	6,600	>10,000	1,300	—	—
Bupropion	47,600	50,000	>100,000	—	—	—	—	—	—
Trazodone	320,000	70	1,000	>10,000	3,000	1,700	111	460	50,000

Others

Atropine	2	—	—	—	—	—	—	—	—
Chlorpromazine	5,700	4	25	>10,000	3,500	15	28	41	300

Source: Data are summarized from a review and references therein by Baldessarini, *Biomedical Aspects of Depression and Its Treatment* (American Psychiatric Press, Inc., Washington, D.C., 1983); for muscarinic and adrenergic receptors from E. Richelson, Mayo Clinic (*Mayo Clinic Proc.* 58:40, 1983; and personal communication, 1984); and for D-2 dopaminergic receptors from B. Cohen, Harvard Medical School (personal communication, 1983).

Competition for binding of radiolabeled ligands included WB-4101 or prazosin (α_1), clonidine or rauwolscine (α_2), dihydroxyalprenolol (β), spiroperidol (D-2), serotonin (5-HT$_1$), spiroperidol (in cerebral cortex) or ketanserin (5-HT$_2$), mepyramine (or stimulation of cyclic-GMP synthesis) (H$_1$), stimulation of cyclic-AMP synthesis (H$_2$); most were evaluated with membrane preparations of rat (or human) brain tissue; muscarinic receptors (binding of quinuclidinyl benzilate, QNB) were evaluated in guinea pig ileum and rat brain tissue and the results pooled.

Note that none of these affinities correlates significantly with clinical potency, even within the tricyclic group of agents (the range of potency is limited, ranging from about 30 to 300 mg/day typical doses).

Amitriptyline and its congeners are strongly anticholinergic, while desipramine, amoxapine, and nomifensine are the least anticholinergic of the tricyclic-type and comparable agents. Amitriptyline, doxepin, and trimipramine are relatively strongly antiadrenergic and antihistaminic, as is chlorpromazine (which may correspond with sedative and autonomic side effects). Most of the atypical agents are only weakly antimuscarinic.

44). Among the tricyclic antidepressants, amitriptyline and its congeners butriptyline and protriptyline, as well as trimipramine, are relatively strongly anticholinergic, while the desmethylated products desipramine and amoxapine are among the weakest, and imipramine and others are intermediate in antimuscarinic activity. Several newer, atypical agents, such as trazodone, bupropion, fluoxetine, iprindole, and mianserin, are virtually without anticholinergic activity. Although many of the atypical agents appear to have little clinical anticholinergic toxicity, the clinical differences between typical tricyclic agents in this regard are only moderate. Since the correlation between clinical potency (not efficacy) and anticholinergic potency is weak (for example, amitriptyline and desipramine are equally effective and nearly equipotent as antidepressants but differ 35-fold in antimuscarinic potency), an anticholinergic hypothesis of antidepressant action is not supported. Nevertheless, since there is a rough correspondence between in vitro antimuscarinic actions and ability to induce atropine-like poisoning and, to some extent, cardiac toxicity in patients, screening of new agents in this way may lead to less toxic medications.

Other short-term receptor interactions of antidepressants have also failed to provide a compelling explanation for their main clinical actions or a general principle with which to guide development of new agents. Some interactions may contribute to side effects, however. For example, there is some tendency for strong anti-α_1 effects to correspond with hypotensive or sedative actions, notably of doxepin and amitriptyline (as well as chlorpromazine), which are particularly potent (see Table 44). Interactions with α_2 receptors are generally weak. Mianserin is an exception, and it has been suggested that it may facilitate release of norepinephrine from nerve terminals by blocking presynaptic α_2 receptors believed to throttle release of norepinephrine.

Interactions of antidepressants with other types of receptors are incompletely evaluated, and their significance is not always clear. Several are extraordinarily potent antihistamine agents, especially at H_1 receptors. Doxepin is one of the most potent antihistamines known, and amitriptyline and trimipramine are also very active. In addition, amitriptyline is relatively potent against H_2 histamine receptors, which are associated with gastric secretion as well as other functions, and thus shares this activity with cimetidine (Tagamet) and ranitidine (Zantac), which are effective in the treatment of peptic ulcer. This activity as well as the strongly antimuscarinic activity of amitriptyline have suggested its trial in the treatment of peptic ulcer disease, in which it has shown promising results, along with doxepin, trimipramine, and mianserin. Antihistaminic actions in the CNS may contribute to the sedative effects of these same relatively sedating antidepressants. Interactions at serotonin receptors also occur with several antidepressants, but their significance remains obscure (see Table 44).

Changes in amine receptors with repeated treatment are proposed to parallel the clinical actions of antidepressants, which are typically delayed for a week or more (aside from the more immediate sedative and hypnotic effects). Presynaptic α_2 receptors appear to become less sensitive or abundant after repeated treatment with an antidepressant, and this change may contribute to an increased release of norepinephrine per nerve impulse in cardiac and neural tissue. Simultaneously, initial decreases in the rate of production of norepinephrine and the firing of noradrenergic neurons in the brainstem diminish with repeated treatment, and these changes may also be linked with diminishing sensitivity of the α_2 receptors. Changes consistent with increased abundance and sensitivity appear at α_1 receptors, which are important postsynaptic sites of action of norepinephrine. In contrast, there are strong and consistent decreases in the abundance and stimulation of β receptors. This "down-regulation" effect has been reported after repeated treatment with many antidepressants of the typical type but also after treatment with MAO inhibitors, ECT, and a few atypical antidepressants such as iprindole. Support for this impression includes loss of stimulation of the formation of cyclic-AMP by β agonists, decreased binding of radiolabeled β antagonists, and some evidence of decreased electrophysiological response to β-active agents locally applied by micropipettes, all in preparations of mammalian brain tissue. It is not clear why α_1 and β receptors respond in an opposite manner to antidepressant treatment.

Although loss of α_2 sensitivity associated with a rise of norepinephrine production and release seems congruent with a noradrenergic hypothesis for the antidepressant action of tricyclic antidepressants, the loss of sensitivity of the β receptors seems counterintuitive. Increased alpha-adrenergic transmission through α_1 receptors is a plausible final output effect of antidepressant treatment, but since the functional, physiological consequences of altered noradrenergic receptor activity are largely unknown, it may be premature to speculate about the meaning of these changes. Indeed, such changes are most likely to represent mechanisms that tend to restore homeostasis of central neurotransmission in response to its perturbation by a drug.

Almost certainly, loss of beta-adrenergic stimulation per se is not an adequate explanation for antidepressant effects. The β antagonist propranolol is even suspected of inducing depression in some susceptible patients. Moreover, chlorpromazine and amphetamine, which are not considered antidepressants, can exert effects like those of tricyclic antidepressants on β receptors following repeated treatment.

Changes in other transmission and receptor systems are less well understood. Strongly anticholinergic antidepressants can increase the abundance of central muscarinic receptors. Changes in serotonin receptors apparently are contradictory: some binding experiments suggest a loss of receptor sites, while physiological experiments suggest an increased sensitivity to serotonin after several weeks of treatment with one of the typical antidepressants or with iprindole, which is not known to have significant acute actions on serotonin neurons. In the dopamine system, there have been suggestions that repeated treatment with an antidepressant or ECT may alter the sensitivity of presynaptic autoreceptors proposed to regulate the production and release of dopamine from nerve terminals so as to increase dopaminergic transmission. A further proposal is that such changes may come about with the passage of time following acute treatment, even without repeated daily treatment, although such a phenomenon is not known clinically.

The various alterations in neurotransmission are leading to an increasingly rich but complex picture of the effects of repeated treatment with an antidepressant. It is difficult to account for all such changes in a general theory of the actions of this class of drugs. One reasonable view is that if potentiation of the actions of norepinephrine is central to the antidepressant actions of the tricyclic antidepressants, that effect is especially likely to be mediated by α_1 receptors. Furthermore, increased availability and activity of norepinephrine, by potent blockade of its inactivation by neuronal uptake, together with weak α_1 blocking actions and eventual increase of α_1 effects may predict desirable characteristics of antidepressants similar to those now known. Desensitization of α_2 and β receptors may then follow from the increased availability of norepinephrine in the synaptic cleft. Why α_1 receptors should escape the desensitization that occurs with other adrenergic receptors is unknown, but it may reflect the mild, acute anti-alpha-adrenergic activity of many antidepressants.

A further generalization is that no single biochemical or neurophysiological hypothesis can now account for the actions of all antidepressants. Although many of the more typical agents block the uptake of norepinephrine, this action may reflect some circularity of reasoning as well as the process of developing new antidepressants by relying on such activity in initial pharmaceutical screening. Other actions, including antihistaminic and antimuscarinic effects, are more likely to account for the sedative and anticholinergic side effects of antidepressants than for their main clinical actions. A reasonable hypothesis is that the combination of high potency against the uptake-inactivation of norepinephrine, low potency to block α_1 receptors, and a tendency to down-regulate beta-adrenergic receptors is especially characteristic of antidepressants with relatively low sedative and hypotensive actions. It is not clear whether such characteristics are either necessary or sufficient to account for the mood-elevating actions of these agents, nor is it obvious that seeking more agents with similar actions will lead to drugs that are more effective or less toxic than existing antidepressants. A summary of the reported short-term and longer-term actions of typical tricyclic antidepressants is provided in Table 45.

Table 45 Actions of tricyclic antidepressants

Acute (hours)
- Block amine uptake (norepinephrine > serotonin except some atypical agents with selective effects on serotonin or no effect on amine uptake), but not dopamine (except the atypical agents nomifensine and possibly bupropion)
- Reduce firing rates of norepinephrine and serotonin neurons in brainstem
- Reduce synthesis and turnover of norepinephrine and serotonin temporarily
- Variably block muscarinic, histamine ($H_1 > H_2$), adrenergic ($\alpha_1 > \alpha_2$), and serotonin receptors

Later (weeks)
- Block of amine uptake continues
- Decreased sensitivity of presynaptic (and postsynaptic) α_2 adrenergic receptors
- Return of firing rates and turnover of monoamines to, or above, normal
- Increased release of norepinephrine
- Decreased sensitivity of beta-adrenergic receptors (mainly β_1) with possible permissive effect of serotonin
- Probably some increase in abundance of α_1 receptors as well as increased affinity for, and sensitivity to, α_1 agonists
- Uncertain effects at serotonin receptors, possibly increased sensitivity to serotonin
- Hypothesized decrease in sensitivity of dopamine autoreceptors but little change in postsynaptic dopaminergic receptors
- Variable increase in muscarinic acetylcholine receptors

Clinical Use

Treatment of depression is made difficult by the diversity of conditions subsumed under the generic term *depression* and by the inconsistency with which clinicians and investigators categorize depressions. Regardless of the scheme of categorization, it is generally agreed that depressions vary in severity. The more severe forms of major depressive illness include those referred to as *endogenous* or *vital, manic-depressive, melancholic, retarded, agitated, involutional,* or *psychotic,* depending on the clinical form of the illness and the patient's history. In contrast, the less severe forms are said to be *minor, dysthymic, reactive, neurotic, situational,* or *anxious* depressions. Although the prognosis for the less severe depressions is usually better, the efficacy of medical treatments has been better demonstrated for the more serious depressions with more pronounced "biological" symptoms, such as anorexia, insomnia, loss of energy, drive, and sexual interest, and diurnal change. Patients with the lesser depressive illnesses tend to recover more rapidly, to have spontaneous remissions, and to respond to psychotherapy, sedatives, antianxiety medications, stimulants, or nonspecific treatments including placebos nearly as well as to antidepressants.

An additional difficulty in evaluating medical treatments of depression is that spontaneous remission rates for unselected depressions of various degrees of severity are about 20–25% within the first four to six weeks and exceed 50% within a few months. Even severe depressions eventually underwent remission after many months in the era prior to ECT or antidepressant drugs. Moreover, adding a placebo increases remission rates of unselected acute depressions to about 30–50% in the first month or two.

The tricyclic antidepressants have their clearest effects in the more severe depressions, for which their performance in controlled clinical trials has been fairly consistent though not dramatic (Table 46). The best performance of these drugs has been documented in trials that attempted to exclude the less severe depressions, used adequate doses of medication (more than 100 mg of imipramine or the equivalent of another agent), and continued for at least a month. In controlled trials with a mixture of depressive syndromes of varying severity, overall improvement rates with tricyclic antidepressants have been about 65–70%, in contrast to about 30–40% with placebo; thus, only about an additional 30% of patients with significant depressive illnesses respond to the active medication. A few

Table 46   Comparison of antidepressant treatments with placebo

Agent	Number of trials	Agent superior to placebo (%)[a]
Tricyclic		
Imipramine	38	68
Amitriptyline	20	70
Maprotiline	12	75
Nortriptyline	8	62
Desipramine	6	66
Amitriptyline + Perphenazine	5	80
Protriptyline	3	100
Doxepin	1	100
Atypical		
Trazodone	12	75
MAO inhibitors		
Isocarboxazid	6	33
Phenelzine	11	55[b]
Tranylcypromine	4	75
Other treatments		
ECT	9	89
Amphetamines	3	0
Chlorpromazine	3	100

Sources: Morris and Beck, *Arch. Gen. Psychiatry* 30:667, 1974; Appleton and Davis, *Practical Clinical Psychopharmacology* (Williams and Wilkins, Baltimore, 1973 and 1980), chap. 4.

a. Summarizes controlled trials with a variety of depressive disorders in inpatient and outpatient settings where test agent produced results better than a placebo, with statistical significance at least 5%. The mean placebo response rate, by patients, averaged 34%.

b. Includes doses ranging from 30 to 90 mg per day and conditions other than major or melancholic depression, including disorders with neurotic, atypical, anxious, or pain symptoms.

who respond poorly to a tricyclic agent may respond satisfactorily to an MAO inhibitor, and about half of those who respond poorly to a tricyclic agent respond to electroconvulsive treatment (ECT). ECT has consistently outperformed MAO inhibitors or tricyclic antidepressants, but the overall gain is only on the order of 10–20%, in terms of either the proportion of patients responding or the success rates of therapeutic trials.

Selection of Agents

Among the specific antidepressants, there are more similarities than differences in overall effectiveness (Tables 46 and 47). The tricyclic antidepressants often perform better than MAO inhibitors, with the possible exception of tranylcypromine (Parnate), which has amphetamine-like properties as well as the ability to inhibit MAO and produced results about equal to those of imipramine in a small number of comparisons (see Table 46). Recent experience with doses of phenelzine adequate to produce strong inhibition of MAO activity (above 45 mg/day) has further altered this impression since results have been similar to those of standard tricyclic antidepressants in several recent trials. Among the tricyclic antidepressants, amitriptyline (Elavil) may have produced somewhat better overall results than a placebo in comparison with other tricyclic agents. Moreover, in direct comparisons of amitriptyline with imipramine, the former was somewhat more effective, but not consistently so. Desmethylimipramine (desipramine; Norpramin, Pertofrane) may be slightly less effective than the other tricyclic agents.Thus, although desipramine was better than a placebo in 66% of its controlled trials, imipramine was superior to its desmethylated congener in 18% of 11 direct comparisons of the two agents (and about equal in the other 82%; see Table 47). There is no consistent evidence that the N-desmethylated derivatives of either imipramine or amitriptyline or the newer agents such as amoxapine and maprotiline are more rapid in their onset than the older tertiary amine compounds. Nortriptyline (Aventyl, Pamelor) may be slightly more potent (or toxic) than amitriptyline in that the recommended maximum dose is only 150 mg/day. Moreover, whereas another desmethylated analogue of amitriptyline, protriptyline (Vivactil), is more potent than either amitriptyline or nortriptyline, its overall efficacy and speed of action are no greater than those of the other tricyclic antidepressants and its effectiveness may even be slightly inferior.

Amitriptyline, trazodone (Desyrel), and amoxapine (Asendin) produce more sedation (at least initially) than most other antidepressants; the desmethylated antidepressants as well as nomifensine and bupropion (Wellbutrin) generally produce less sedation, and may even have early stimulating actions. Amitriptyline has more potent anticholinergic activity than other tricyclic antidepressants, and nomifensine and desipramine the least, with other agents clustering between them (see Table 44). This consideration suggests that desipramine may be a more rational choice for elderly patients at high risk of anticholinergic delirium or of cardiac

Table 47 Efficacy of antidepressant treatments compared with a standard tricyclic antidepressant

Agent	Number of trials	Similar (%)	Inferior (%)	Superior (%)
Tricyclic				
Amitriptyline				
(vs. imipramine)	11	71	0	29
Amitriptyline + perphenazine				
(vs. imipramine)	7	57	14	29
Desipramine				
(vs. imipramine)	11	82	18	0
Doxepin	11	64	9	27
Imipramine				
(vs. amitriptyline)	11	36	45	19
Maprotiline	22	100	0	0
Nortriptyline	9	100	0	0
Protriptyline	8	75	25	0
Atypical				
Trazodone	21	100	0	0
MAO inhibitors				
Phenelzine	9	56	44	0
Isocarboxazid	5	60	40	0
Tranylcypromine	3	100	0	0
Other treatments				
ECT	7	57	0	43
Chlorpromazine	3	100	0	0
Chlorprothixine	1	100	0	0
Thioridazine	1	100	0	0

Sources: Morris and Beck, *Arch. Gen. Psychiatry* 30:667, 1976; Appleton and Davis, *Practical Clinical Psychopharmacology* (Williams and Wilkins, Baltimore, 1973 and 1980), chap. 4.

Data summarize controlled inpatient and outpatient comparisons of an index treatment against a standard antidepressant (imipramine or amitriptyline), with results reported as the proportion of trials in which the test agent was apparently similar, inferior, or superior to the standard treatment.

Note that the results among the tricyclic antidepressants are quite variable, although amitriptyline tended to be superior to imipramine in some studies. The MAO inhibitors phenelzine and isocarboxazid tended to be inferior to a standard tricyclic antidepressant (even including recent studies of phenelzine in doses up to 90 mg/day and for conditions other than major depression, with "atypical," "anxious," "neurotic," or pain symptoms for which MAO inhibitors have putative selective benefits). ECT was superior to a tricyclic antidepressant in 43% of such comparisons. The apparent "antidepressant" effects of the neuroleptic agents includes benefits in patients with agitation and psychotic features.

toxicity, although its greater safety has not been demonstrated clinically. Nomifensine and bupropion may carry a risk of excessive stimulation. Maprotiline has been associated with an excessive risk of grand mal seizures at doses above 200 mg per day. Amoxapine can induce extrapyramidal side effects at ordinary doses and has induced seizures after overdoses.

Doxepin (Sinequan) has acquired a probably undeserved reputation for having special antianxiety or mixed "antipsychotic" and antidepressant qualities; much of this impression is based on its most successful use in outpatients with mild neurotic depressions and anxiety. This agent also has an unjustified reputation for not inhibiting uptake into noradrenergic neurons. Although in vitro studies support the generalization that the tertiary-amine tricyclic antidepressants (such as imipramine and amitriptyline as well as doxepin) are less potent inhibitors of uptake into postganglionic sympathetic neurons than their desmethylated analogues (see Table 43), these distinctions do not seem to make clinically important differences, perhaps because the *di*methylated compounds are readily converted in vivo to their *des*methylated metabolites. Specifically, the idea that doxepin does not block the uptake and hence the antihypertensive actions of the postganglionic sympathetic blocking agent guanethidine (Ismelin) is not correct, although this antihypertensive agent may be less effective for the first two or three weeks of treatment with low doses of doxepin.

The main conclusion based on these various comparisons of antidepressant agents is similar to that for the antipsychotic agents: although differences in the overall efficacy of the various tricyclic antidepressants are not easy to document, subtleties based on the relative chances for various side effects or drug interactions do call for some judgment and for selection of a specific agent on the basis of sound pharmacologic principles and clinical observations.

In selecting a treatment for a specific case of depression, antipsychotic drugs must also be considered. In a few comparisons of tricyclic antidepressants and antipsychotic agents in groups of relatively unselected cases of serious depression, the overall benefits of the two types of agents have apparently been about the same (Table 47). In one of the earliest studies, thioridazine (Mellaril) was used, whereupon it acquired an exaggerated reputation as a specific agent for severe or psychotic depression. However, it is likely that any antipsychotic agent would perform about as well as any antidepressant in such unselected comparisons, although comparisons of the same agents in schizophrenic patients would yield poor results with the antidepressant. In the comparison of antipsychotic and antidepressant agents, the types of depressive syndromes specifically helped by the two classes of drugs are probably different: antipsychotic agents are most helpful in cases of psychotic or "involutional" depression with a great deal of agitation and guilty, morbid, or somatic rumination of delusional proportions; tricyclic antidepressants are often useful in such syndromes but are also particularly useful for more quiet, ruminating, anergic, psychomotorically retarded depressions, as bipolar depressions often are. Tricyclic antidepressants may even increase agitation in some cases of psychotic depression, and the addition or even the exclusive use of an antipsychotic agent or ECT in the first days or weeks of the treatment of such an illness can bring about more rapid benefits than a tricyclic antidepressant alone. The phenothiazine thioridazine has also been reported to have beneficial effects in dysthymic or "neurotic" depressions, for which tricyclic antidepressants are sometimes helpful, but for which the benzodiazepines such as chlordiazepoxide, diazepam, or alprazolam (Librium, Valium, or Xanax) are also useful and probably safer.

Generalizations that seem reasonable at the present time include the following. First, the tricyclic antidepressants are the treatment of first choice in severe, major depression, especially with melancholic features marked by striking vegetative, "medical" symptoms. There are probably not important differences in efficacy among the various agents now available, and the choice of specific agents usually requires attention to the risks of various side effects typical of the different agents. The newer agents have not been proved convincingly to have important advantages in terms of efficacy, rapidity of action, or safety over older typical tricyclic antidepressants. Some newer or experimental agents may have less risk of anticholinergic intoxication and may be less likely to be fatal after ingestion of acute overdoses, but they tend to present risks of other side effects or to have less secure efficacy in severely depressed patients. Generally, the efficacy of antidepressants in dysthymic disorder or persistent or frequently recurrent neurotic disorders with dysphoric features is less secure than their effects in major depression. There is some evidence that MAO inhibitors may be especially useful for ambulatory patients with milder illnesses marked by dysphoria but also with anxiety and "neurotic" features, as well as "atypical" symptoms such as excess sleep and increased appetite. Antidepressants also have an important role in the treatment of disorders marked mainly by symptoms of anxiety and phobias, particularly with panic attacks, as discussed in Chapter 5. Clomipramine has also been found to be superior to other medical and psychological treatments for obsessive-compulsive disorder. Antipsychotic agents may have a useful short-term adjunctive role in depressive disorders marked by profound agitation and psychotic features or acute mixed manic-depressive syndromes, but are not recommended for routine use as a primary treatment of major depression, especially for longer than six months. ECT remains more effective than medical treatments for severe melancholic and psychotic depression.

Short-Term Treatment

The clinical use of the various available antidepressant agents is similar in short-term treatment. An elaborate medical evaluation before starting treatment is usually not productive in younger and healthy individuals, but it is wise to have a good appreciation of cardiovascular, cerebrovascular, gastrointestinal, urinary, and ophthalmologic status, especially of elderly patients, who are at greater risk of toxic effects, and to have ruled out medical conditions that might be mistaken for idiopathic depression. In outpatients or elderly patients, treatment usually is begun with moderate doses of a tricyclic antidepressant agent; the equivalent of 50–75 mg/day of imipramine is typical. An initial daily dose as small as 25 or even 10 mg of imipramine or its equivalent is extremely low, but might be appropriate for an infirm, elderly depressed patient. The amount is usually increased by 25 to 50 mg every day or two, to doses of at least 100–150 mg/day of imipramine (or the equivalent of another agent; see Table 39). With inpatients it is more common to start with 75 or 100 mg and quickly reach doses of 200–250 mg/day. Daily doses above 200 mg of imipramine or its equivalent are associated with increased risks of toxic effects, including cardiovascular effects, psychotic agitation, and organic confusion or delirium, and are best reserved for carefully supervised hospitalized patients, preferably after a trial of two or three weeks at 150–200 mg per day. In severe depression and when food and oral medications are refused, an injectable form of imipramine or amitriptyline can be used (initially, 100 mg/day in divided doses, intramuscularly), although there is no compelling evidence that the efficacy or speed is increased in this way. If there is psychosis or severe agitation, it is common to add an antipsychotic agent, or a lithium salt if dysphoric mania or a mixed manic-depressive state is suspected. It is usually not necessary to add an additional hypnotic medication for sleep, and barbiturates are not used because of their interactions with the metabolism of antidepressants. If agitation, psychosis, and suicidal risk are prominent, several unilateral electroconvulsive treatments can be given while waiting for the effects of the antidepressant.

Although ECT can be given safely while antidepressants are being used, it is wise to omit the first dose of antidepressant on the morning of ECT and to use an additional anticholinergic agent to dry secretions sparingly, if at all, during ECT. Although it might seem to be a good idea, it is not usual to give a stimulant in the first few days of hospitalization while awaiting the antidepressant effects of a tricyclic agent, because the benefits of amphetamine-like agents are meager and there are added risks of inducing agitation and hypertension.

An important feature of nearly all antidepressant agents is the *delay in clinical onset* of antidepressant effect, typically at least a week, sometimes up to three weeks. The failure of objective improvement in activity, sleep, appetite, mood, or social interest within a week is an unfavorable prognostic sign and suggests that the final result will be unsatisfactory. The patient is usually the last to acknowledge subjective improvement, but if the objective response is poor after four or five weeks of adequate doses and plasma levels of a tricyclic agent, and if there is not even slight improvement in two or three weeks, there is little likelihood that changing to another agent or increasing doses above 300 mg of imipramine or its equivalent will help. At that point the main choices are to try an atypical antidepressant, an MAO inhibitor, or ECT; there is little reason not to go directly to ECT since it is more likely to have additional benefit in severe, melancholic major depression. With outpatients, a period in a hospital at that point may also provide additional benefits. If an MAO inhibitor is used, for example in a patient who refuses ECT, it is safer (although slower) to allow at least a week or, better, two weeks for the tricyclic agent to be metabolized and excreted before adding the MAO inhibitor to avoid the rare but potentially catastrophic drug interactions, including hyperpyrexia and convulsions, that may occur.

Antidepressant agents are not so stimulating and behaviorally activating as to worsen the insomnia that typically accompanies serious depressions. Indeed, antidepressants even facilitate the deeper phases of sleep that are usually decreased in adult depression. On the other hand, imipramine used in the management of childhood enuresis has been reported to be associated with a partial suppression of the deeper phases of sleep. Although it is often possible to treat the insomnia of depression with an antidepressant alone, a sedative-hypnotic benzodiazepine can be added temporarily to treat insomnia.

The half-lives of the tricyclic agents are long enough that it is reasonable to use the bulk of a day's dose at bedtime, both for convenience and to combat insomnia. Furthermore, it is best to prescribe preparations of tricyclic antidepressants with the highest unit strength (milligrams per pill), since this is usually the least expensive. For outpatients, the more slowly released pamoate salt of imipramine (Tofranil-PM) may also be used at the same daily doses as for the hydrochloride salt; however, this preparation is more expensive and does not offer a clear advantage over imipramine hydrochloride, which is available as a less expensive generic drug. When large doses of an antidepressant are used (above the equivalent of 150 mg/day of imipramine), it is safer to use divided doses to minimize anticholinergic and cardiotoxic actions of the drugs, as well as nightmares or "nocturnal terror," which occasionally follow large doses at bedtime. As with the antipsychotic agents, the "clinically equivalent doses" of antidepressant agents summarized in Table 39 have been established with the assumption that the doses are attained gradually. Thus, to avoid toxic reactions, it is best to avoid switching immediately from equivalent doses of one agent to another, and to allow several days for a gradual transition. Because of the potentially severe toxicity and limited margin of safety of most antidepressant agents, it is unwise to dispense more than a week's supply to a depressed and possibly suicidal outpatient. The risk of suicide may increase with initial improvement, since activity usually increases before mood elevation.

It has been suggested that various biological considerations or measurements might improve the efficacy or safety of antidepressants. These have had little systematic investigation in the treatment of depressed patients, except in relation to short-term use of antidepressant agents. For example, there have been repeated suggestions that an initial behavioral-activating response to a dose of d-amphetamine of 20–30 mg in one day might predict a later beneficial response to treatment with an antidepressant, perhaps especially to an agent with strong norepinephrine uptake-inhibiting action. This proposal remains experimental and insufficiently supported to be recommended for routine clinical application. There have also been repeated suggestions that metabolic features of depressed patients might help to predict responses to specific types of antidepressants. For example, "noradrenergic" versus "serotonergic" depressions have been hypothesized, the former characterized by relatively low excretion of the catecholamine metabolite MHPG in the urine, and the latter by decreased urinary or CSF concentrations of 5-HIAA, the major metabolite of serotonin (see Figures 12-15). It has been suggested that such evidence of a relative deficiency of norepinephrine output might predict selective responsiveness to an agent with potent and selective actions against the uptake of norepinephrine (such as imipramine, desipramine, or maprotiline), while the latter condition might predict a preferential response to an agent with activity against the uptake of serotonin as well as norepinephrine (such as fluoxetine, clomipramine, citalopram, or amitriptyline). Although there is some evidence suggestive of such correlations, it is not compelling, and these relatively complex and inaccessible assay methods arc not routinely used clinically.

There is also preliminary research support for several other related proposals. For example, an antidepressant can suppress the onset of REM (rapid eye movement) sleep, which is often accelerated in major depression, after one or two small test doses at bedtime (such as 50 mg of amitriptyline, the agent most extensively evaluated in this way). Such responses may predict a therapeutic response to a month of treatment with usual clinical doses. Also, initial failure to suppress the secretion of cortisol after a small dose of dexamethasone (1 mg at bedtime) during the following 24 hours ("dexamethasone suppression test") may predict a beneficial short-term response to an antidepressant of ECT, and later recovery of normal suppression during treatment may predict a favorable prognosis in the near term. Several other endocrinological features of depression are currently under investigation.

Thus far all these approaches remain largely of research interest, and none has yet been proved to predict clinical responsiveness to an antidepressant more effectively than the clinical characteristics of the syndrome treated (especially the presence of prominent melancholic, biological signs and symptoms in major depression), or the use of effective doses of any typical tricyclic antidepressant. A summary of proposed predictors of a favorable response to antidepressants is provided in Table 48. Given the present state of knowledge, none of the research proposals concerning predictors of antidepressant response would override the appropriate treatment of a depressed patient based on clinical, descriptive criteria.

Tricyclic antidepressants have also been used for conditions other than depression. The usefulness of MAO inhibitors and tricyclic antidepressant agents in treatment of panic anxiety has been mentioned and is discussed further in Chapter 5. These agents and ECT are occasionally helpful in some pain syndromes that might represent "depressive equivalents," as well as in migraine, narcolepsy, and other "psychosomatic" conditions, including eating disorders (particularly bulimia). Several disorders of children including enuresis, school phobias, and a variety of "nervous habits" have been treated with antidepressants, especially with doses of imipramine of 25–75 mg/day given an hour or more before bedtime. The success of antidepressant treatment in a growing list of such

Table 48 Predictors of favorable response to antidepressants

Relatively well established predictors
- Acute, major depressive episode with "endogenous" or melancholic features or depressive phase of bipolar disorder
- Past success of biological treatment of a similar episode
- Dose above the equivalent of 150 mg of imipramine daily
- Blood concentration of antidepressant plus major active metabolites above 100 ng/ml
- Inhibition of platelet MAO activity more than 85% by some MAO inhibitors (best established for phenelzine)

Investigational proposals
- Relatively low concentration of urinary MHPG or high concentration of 5-HIAA in the CSF may predict preferential responsiveness to imipramine, desipramine, or maprotiline, while the opposite might predict preferential responsiveness to clomipramine or amitriptyline
- Activation of behavior or mood by an oral test dose of 20–30 mg of amphetamine daily for one or two days
- Suppression of onset of REM sleep into the normal range (more than 70 minutes) by a small test dose of an antidepressant (50 mg of amitriptyline at bedtime best evaluated) may predict therapeutic benefit of usual clinical doses of the same agent given for a month
- Initial failure to suppress plasma concentrations of cortisol below 50 ng/ml within 24 hours after a bedtime dose of 1 mg dexamethasone, especially if followed by normalization of suppression on follow-up testing a week or more later

disorders is encouraging research into genetic, epidemiological, and other similarities between these conditions and major depression. Table 49 provides a summary of psychiatric, neurological, and medical disorders for which there is some experimental or clinical evidence of beneficial effects of a tricyclic antidepressant.

The role of antidepressant agents is not clearly defined in schizophrenic illnesses. There have been clinical trials of at least moderate doses of antidepressants in withdrawn or apathetic schizophrenics, usually without clear benefits, and the antidepressants have been added to the treatment of depressive phases of schizophrenic or so-called schizoaffective illnesses. These practices are not without risk, however, because stimulants, L-dopa, and MAO inhibitors as well as tricyclic antidepressants can increase or induce agitation, delusions, and hallucinations in schizophrenic and other psychotic patients, and occasionally antidepressants have been reported to be associated with the "uncovering of latent psy-

Table 49   Indications for treatment with tricyclic antidepressants

Relatively well established indications
• Acute major depression
• Prevention of relapse of major, nonbipolar depression for at least one year
• Secondary depression in psychiatric, neurological, or medical disorders, especially given melancholic features
• Panic disorder
• Enuresis (especially imipramine)
• Attention deficit disorder with hyperactivity in children (especially imipramine)
• "Pseudodementia" with depression in the elderly
• Bulimia
• Chronic pain

Investigational proposals
• Obsessive-compulsive disorder (especially clomipramine)
• Peripheral diabetic neuropathy symptoms
• Narcolepsy (especially clomipramine)
• Migraine syndrome
• Sleep apnea (especially protriptyline)
• School phobia and other separation anxiety disorders of children
• Peptic ulcer disease (especially amitriptyline, doxepin, and trimipramine)
• Some behavioral disorders marked by aggression and agitation in the mentally retarded or brain-damaged
• Anorexia nervosa (?)

chosis" in patients with schizoid, hysterical, paranoid, or "borderline" characters, as well as with the induction of manic or psychotic reactions in bipolar patients. Moreover, there is a risk of compounding psychosis with anticholinergic, toxic delirium, particularly with daily doses of antidepressants above 200 mg of imipramine or its equivalent, and with even lower doses if an antipsychotic agent and an anticholinergic antiparkinsonism agent are also being used. There have been repeated reports and clinical impressions that patients with major depressive episodes with agitation and psychotic features may respond unfavorably to a tricyclic antidepressant alone but may do better if an antipsychotic or antimanic agent or ECT is added to the regimen.

Long-Term Treatment

After appreciable clinical improvement of a severe depressive illness has been achieved with a tricyclic antidepressant agent, it is usual to continue the treatment with at least 100 – 150 mg/day of imipramine or its equivalent for several months, and perhaps up to a year for severe illness or in patients with a prior history of frequently recurrent depression. Daily doses as low as 75 mg/day in this phase of treatment are probably less effective in preventing relapses, although the point has not yet been adequately investigated. A similar regimen should be followed by patients treated initially with ECT, even if inadequate response to an antidepressant led to the use of ECT. This approach has evolved from clinical experience and many reports of relapse after partial treatment of depressions. The exact duration of the treatment depends on the individual patient's response, ability to resume normal responsibilities, premorbid history, ongoing stresses and life situation, and the duration, rate of recurrence, and response to treatment of prior depressions.

Although this practice of maintaining patients on effective doses of an antidepressant for a period of time following apparently adequate clinical recovery is usual, the information supporting this practice, based on controlled, prospective studies, is limited. It is clear that the risk of immediate relapse of major depression following adequate initial treatment is high, especially within the first six months. This period of high risk corresponds approximately to the expected duration of an untreated episode of major depression. The course of major depression in patients assigned at random under double-blind conditions to follow-up treatment with a placebo indicates that the risk of relapse is especially high within the first month of follow-up (probably as high as 50%), perhaps only half as great in the next several months, and possibly as low as 10–20% between the sixth month and the end of the first year of follow-up. Overall one-year relapse rates from many studies have averaged 60–70% of those in studies where patients were assigned to a placebo following adequate initial treatment with an antidepressant.

Table 50 gives the findings of representative studies which followed patients for three to eight months after assignment to a tricyclic antidepressant or a placebo; the risk of relapse in this early period was reduced sharply with the use of an antidepressant, from 52% to 21% or more than twofold. Table 51 summarizes additional data on the effects of antidepressants (including European studies of mianserin as well as trials of typical tricyclic antidepressants) or a lithium salt over a year of follow-up to compare the efficacy of the two forms of maintenance thymoleptic (mood-altering) treatment. Here, the relapse rate of 67% with an inactive placebo was reduced to 41% (1.7-fold) by use of an antidepressant. The sparing of relapse was similar, or slightly greater, when lithium was used alone or in combination with an antidepressant (37% or 26% relapse,

Table 50 *Antidepressant treatment and early relapse in nonbipolar major affective illness*

| Study | Year | Total N | Relapse rates (%) | | Protection ratio |
			Placebo	Antidepressant	
Seager and Bird	1962	28	69	17	4.1
Mindham et al.	1973	92	50	22	2.3
Prien et al.	1973	77	67	37	1.8
Klerman et al.	1974	99	29	12	2.4
Coppen et al.	1978	29	31	0	>30
Stein et al.	1980	55	69	28	2.5
Prien et al.	1984	73	52	28	1.9
Total or mean (7 studies)		453	52.4	20.7	2.5

Source: Review and references therein by Prien, *Schizophrenia and Affective Disorders: Biology and Drug Treatment,* ed. A. Rifkin (Wright-PSG, Boston, 1983), pp. 95–115; and six-month data of Prien et al., *Arch. Gen. Psychiatry* 41:1096, 1984. Studies involved the use of a placebo and imipramine or amitriptyline and followed patients for 3 to 8 months after recovery of an index episode of major depression. Means are weighted by the number of patients per study.

Table 51 *Treatment to prevent relapse or recurrence of nonbipolar depression for one year*

Treatment	Patients (N)	Relapse rate (%)	Protection ratio
Placebo	321	67.2	1.0
Antidepressant[a]	281	40.6	1.7
Lithium salt	226	37.3	1.8
Antidepressant plus lithium	105	25.9	2.6

Sources: Review and references therein by Schou, *Arch. Gen. Psychiatry* 36:849, 1979; and reports by Peselow et al., *Psychopharm. Bull.* 17:53, 1981 and *Am. J. Psychiatry* 138:747, 1982; Quitkin et al., *Psychopharm. Bull.* 17:142, 1981; Kane et al., *Arch. Gen. Psychiatry* 39:1065, 1982; and Prien et al., *Arch. Gen. Psychiatry* 41:1096, 1984.

a. Most studies used imipramine or amitriptyline (without systematic evaluation of the effect of dose); a few used maprotiline or mianserin.

Compare the results above with those summarized in Table 30 in Chapter 3 regarding the use of lithium alone in nonbipolar depression for 0.5 to 3.0 years, in which relapse rates on placebo and lithium treatment averaged 75.5% and 43.5%, respectively (protection ratio = 1.7).

Prien et al. also provided data at two years of follow-up, at which relapse rates are estimated to have been 75%, 45%, 62%, and 38% for the four treatment conditions, respectively. Peselow et al. reported on results at two and three years as well; at three years, the rates for the same respective treatment groups were 84%, 69%, 62%, and 64%. Thus these longer-term follow-up results suggest a waning of protective effect after the first year.

respectively). Lithium might, therefore, exert useful effects in nonbipolar affective disorders as it clearly does in bipolar disorder, as discussed in the preceding chapter and summarized there in Table 30. There is a suggestion from the data just reviewed in Table 51 that lithium may add to the preventive effect of an antidepressant on relapse of recurrent major affective disorders that appear to be nonbipolar; some of these may include cases of bipolar type II disorder (recurrent major depression and subclinical, mild hypomania) or the 5% to 10% of apparently unipolar cases that later prove to be bipolar disorder. A lithium salt is sometimes added to an antidepressant in the long-term treatment of patients with recurrent, apparently nonbipolar major affective syndromes, especially when the response to an antidepressant alone is unsatisfactory. However, it is not a sound practice to add an antidepressant to lithium routinely and continuously in the long-term maintenance treatment of bipolar affective disorders because of the suspected risk of inducing manic or psychotic reactions.

Although such relatively short-term preventive effects of antidepressants on early relapse of depression are well documented, long-term benefits are not as well evaluated. The few recent studies of antidepressants that have continued for a year or more following initial recovery from an episode of major nonbipolar depression are summarized in Table 52. They suggest that, although a prophylactic effect may persist beyond the first year, it is apparently only moderate on average, since there was only a 1.4-fold sparing of relapse in studies continued for an average of nearly two years. There is very little research involving follow-up for longer than two years of treatment with a tricyclic antidepressant or lithium salt in nonbipolar depression (see Tables 30, 51, and 52).

Further analysis of data from the studies cited in Tables 51 and 52 adds to the impression that the ability of an antidepressant or lithium salt to prevent relapse or recurrence of nonbipolar depression is especially high within the first six to twelve months after recovery from an index episode of major depression, but may diminish over time. Thus, the ratio of relapse rates of patients on placebo to those on an active tricyclic antidepressant averaged 2.4 at six months of follow-up, 1.7 at one and two years, and only 1.2 by three years. Similarly, this index of the protective effect of the combination of an antidepressant and lithium was 3.0 at six months, 2.6 at one year, 2.0 at two years, and only 1.3 by three years. The effect of a lithium salt alone appears to be consistent but more modest, with protection ratios of 1.5, 1.8, 1.2, and 1.4, respectively, at the same times of follow-up. In general, the potential power of truly prophylactic actions of

Table 52 Antidepressant treatment and late recurrence in nonbipolar major depression

Study	Year	Total N	Relapse rate (%) Placebo	Relapse rate (%) Antidepressant	Protection ratio
Peselow et al.	1981	83	84	69	1.2
Quitkin et al.	1981	12	100	83	1.2
Kane et al.	1982	24	77	55	1.4
Prien et al.	1984	73	65	33	2.0[a]
Total or mean (4 studies)		192	76.9	54.4	1.4
Annual relapse	—	—	39.8	28.6	1.4

Sources: Review and references therein by Prien, *Schizophrenia and Affective Disorders: Biology and Drug Treatment,* ed. Rifkin (Wright-PSG, Boston, 1983), pp. 95–115; and Prien et al., *Arch. Gen. Psychiatry* 41:1096, 1984, in a study in which imipramine plus lithium yielded an even lower relapse rate of 26%).

The duration of the four studies was 3.0, 0.92, 1.4, and 2.25 years, for a mean duration of 1.9 years following recovery from an index episode of major depression, and typically with at least two months of recovery prior to assignment to placebo or continued treatment with a tricyclic antidepressant (usually imipramine). Means are weighted by the number of subjects (N) per study. Note that the prophylactic effect is apparently less robust than the protection against immediate relapse within the expected duration of the natural course of untreated depression shown in Table 50.

a. $p < 0.05$.

these agents in preventing late recurrences of major depressive episodes remains inadequately evaluated. A particular methodological problem is that few studies have attempted to control for the strong effects of antidepressant agents to prevent early relapses in the first months following clinical recovery from an index episode of major depression, even though these effects undoubtedly contribute to benefits implied by cumulative risk rates reported for late times of follow-up evaluation.

MAO inhibitors have been especially poorly evaluated, even in relatively short-term studies of the prevention of relapse or recurrence of major depression. There is likewise little information on the sustained benefits of long-term treatment of patients with chronic dysthymic disorder or such chronic conditions punctuated with episodes of acute major depression (so-called double depression). Nevertheless, it is a common practice to try prolonged thymoleptic treatment in such illnesses on a case-by-case, empirical basis. There have been a few anecdotal reports of apparent tolerance to the mood-altering effects of tricyclic antidepressants or MAO inhibitors in some patients treated for more than six months; the benefits of treatment sometimes returned following an increase of dose or a switch to a dissimilar antidepressant.

The long-term risks of prolonged antidepressant treatment appear to be no greater than the risks associated with short-term treatment or continuation of treatment for several months. There is also no evidence that the toxicity of combining a lithium salt with an antidepressant in ordinary doses is greater than the sum of the toxic actions of each agent given separately, although the point is not well evaluated. Combined overdoses of these two potentially lethal types of agents are obviously very dangerous.

An important clinical impression arising from this overview of existing evidence concerning long-term benefits and potential risks of prolonged treatment with an antidepressant or other mood-stabilizing agent in recurrent nonbipolar depression is that support for indefinitely prolonged treatment is limited, particularly for times greater than one year. Accordingly, it is reasonable to evaluate the potential benefits and indications for continued treatment of this kind on a case-by-case basis. Patients with a past history of frequently recurring, severe depression or with chronic dysthymic conditions may be candidates for treatment with an antidepressant for more than one year, ideally with repeated attempts to reduce the dose of medication and to reassess the continuing need for it. Those with suggestive bipolar-like characteristics (such as subclinical hypomania, cyclothymia, and possibly an early age of onset, high attack frequency, or strong family history) may be candidates for the addition of a lithium salt.

Influence of Age on Treatment

Depression is very common but frequently overlooked in elderly patients, who can be treated with tricyclic antidepressants or, in cases marked by agitation, temporarily with antipsychotic agents. In the elderly, depression can present signs and symptoms that mimic dementia, and it may occur in addition to underlying senile changes in brain function or secondary to brain disorders such as Alzheimer's disease or stroke. It is important to treat the reversible and treatable forms of mood change in senescence in order to avoid secondary complications including malnutrition, withdrawal, and isolation. Somatic and hypochondriacal symptoms are common and occur early. Improvement in behavior and cognition and decreased hypochondriasis are useful indicators of a therapeutic response to antidepressants in elderly patients.

The tricyclic antidepressants frequently produce serious toxic effects in the elderly, particularly organic mental syndromes, postural hypotension,

and anticholinergic effects. They should be used in small, divided, and gradually increased doses. In very elderly and infirm patients, it is not unusual to start with doses as low as the equivalent of 10–25 mg of imipramine per day, and to increase doses very cautiously and slowly. Agents with strong anticholinergic and sedating properties have become less favored in the elderly; amitriptyline is probably particularly risky in this age group. Although doxepin has acquired a reputation as an appropriate choice for elderly depressed patients, it is not clear that this drug is safer than other typical tricyclic compounds in therapeutic doses. Trazodone is attractive for use in the elderly since it has little anticholinergic activity, but it may be excessively sedating in some elderly patients and is occasionally associated with confusional reactions or suspected of association with myocardial irritability. Desipramine is currently favored for its relatively weak anticholinergic effects, and nortriptyline may provide the advantage of relatively low likelihood of inducing postural hypotension. These secondary-amine antidepressants are given in relatively small, divided, and slowly increased daily doses.

MAO inhibitors have not been well evaluated for efficacy or safety in elderly depressed patients, but they can be expected to produce potentially dangerous postural hypotension and to interact in complicated ways with other medications commonly given to elderly patients. Therefore, they are not recommended for routine use in this age group. Methylphenidate, amphetamines, and other stimulants are occasionally used in elderly patients, especially for relatively minor depressive disorders that may arise secondary to a medical or neurological disorder. However, stimulants present the risk of inducing greater dysphoria, agitation, and paranoia, as well as confusion and anorexia, and thus may complicate or worsen the condition being treated. When agitation and paranoid symptoms are prominent with depression in elderly patients, low doses of high-potency neuroleptic agents can be given safely. Low-potency antipsychotic agents, such as thioridazine and chlorpromazine, should be avoided because of their excessive risk of sedation, confusion, hypotension, and anticholinergic intoxication. When psychotic symptoms are prominent in depressive disorders of the elderly, and when a tricyclic antidepressant provokes increased agitation, paranoia, or confusion, reliance on an antipsychotic agent may be a safer alternative, although ECT is also often a reasonable option when reversible organic causes of agitation or confusion due to neurological, systemic, metabolic, nutritional, or toxic conditions have been considered and excluded.

The use of antidepressants for school-age children is increasing and is a

topic of active investigation. The only "officially approved" agent for use in this age group recognized by the U.S. Food and Drug Administration is imipramine for the treatment of enuresis, and only in small doses up to 2.5 mg/kg (or 50 mg) per day. Although imipramine is effective in treating enuresis and has the support of several controlled experimental trials, it is not recommended as an ideal or sole treatment of this problem. Its effects are generally temporary, and usually nocturnal incontinence returns soon after the medication is discontinued. Behavioral techniques, including electric warning alarms placed in the bed, may be more effective, but are sometimes combined with imipramine, at least initially.

There is also substantial research support for the efficacy of tricyclic antidepressants, especially imipramine and desipramine, in the treatment of attention deficit disorder with hyperactivity ("minimum brain dysfunction" syndrome with hyperactivity). These agents have been found most effective when doses and plasma levels were gradually increased to those usual in adult patients. Thus, doses as high as 3–5 mg/kg have been used safely in school-age and young adolescent patients, at least for short periods of time. However, the efficacy of antidepressants in this syndrome is less secure than that of the stimulants; the treatment of hyperactivity is one of the few remaining indications for the stimulants. The beneficial effects of the tricyclic antidepressants in attention deficit disorder with hyperactivity may disappear with time, and there is a high risk of relapse even following very gradual withdrawal of the medication. In addition, the long-term safety of tricyclic antidepressants compared with the stimulants, especially with respect to growth and development, is not well established. MAO inhibitors have not been evaluated for this or other conditions in children and are not used routinely in this age group. It is interesting that the effects of antidepressants in enuresis and in hyperactivity are virtually immediate—an exception to the general rule in the treatment of other disorders of adults or children that the clinical benefits are typically delayed by more than a week or two.

The affective disorders of childhood are a topic of especially active clinical investigation at present. Bipolar and manic syndromes of childhood were discussed in the preceding chapter, along with the use of lithium in children. In addition, the syndrome of major depression is recognized increasingly commonly in school-age, prepubertal children. Several studies support the efficacy of tricyclic antidepressants in this syndrome; the most extensive experience has been with imipramine. In addition to the classic presentation of major depression with melancholic, biological signs and symptoms of adult depression, children may also

present symptoms of discouragement, guilty rumination, and suicidal behavior. Moreover, children believed to have an acute affective disorder may present potentially more confusing symptoms, including conduct disorders, aggression, learning disorders, or phobias. It is not surprising that clinical research increasingly indicates that some cases of conduct disorder, separation anxiety or school phobia, panic disorder, and some specific developmental disorders or learning disabilities may respond favorably to a trial of imipramine or another tricyclic antidepressant. Similar benefits of antidepressants have been reported in eating disorders, especially with bulimia in adolescence. Whether such responses suggest a biological similarity among these apparently diverse conditions as various forms of affective disorder, or simply an increased range of indications for

Table 53 Emerging indications for the use of tricyclic antidepressants in children and adolescents

---

Effective (with rapid onset)
• Enuresis (especially imipramine)
• Attention deficit disorder with hyperactivity ("miminum brain disfunction with hyperactivity")

Probably effective
• Major depression (possibly with atypical presentations)
• Panic disorder (sometimes with rapid onset)
• Bulimia

Possibly effective or investigational
• Conduct disorders (possibly in low doses)
• Specific developmental disorders (learning disabilities with normal general intelligence and especially with attention deficits or hyperactivity)
• Separation anxiety or school phobia (especially with panic syndrome)
• Anorexia nervosa (?)

Note: The only "official" FDA sanction and manufacturer's recommendations at the present time are for small doses of imipramine for enuresis, even though some research results and growing clinical experience support the other indications, approximately in the order of the groupings stated. Low doses (ca. 50 mg/day) of imipramine may be effective in enuresis and hyperactivity (and have rapid onset), but effective doses may approach those required for adults in other disorders (3–5 mg/kg), and should be attained gradually and cautiously: doses above 5 mg/kg have been associated with electrocardiographic evidence of conduction defects in children. Optimal blood levels have not been as well investigated in children as in adults. There is some evidence that blood levels of imipramine plus desipramine required for maximally effective use of imipramine in severe childhood depression may be above 200 ng/ml. There is also an impression that optimal levels of nortriptyline may parallel those suggested for adults, or about 50–150 ng/ml, and that nortriptyline may be particularly well tolerated by children.

antidepressant agents in children, is unclear. Family history and other epidemiological and follow-up studies suggest that some of these disorders share features with major affective disorders in certain families. Similarly, there is growing evidence that symptoms responsive to a stimulant or an antidepressant in adolescents or adults with antisocial or aggressive behavior may follow earlier attention deficit disorder with hyperactivity in childhood.

Despite these growing possible indications for an empirical trial of an antidepressant in children or adolescents, and their increasingly common use to treat such conditions, it must be pointed out that for most of the syndromes just discussed, these uses have only partial or tentative experimental support. Typically, except for enuresis, hyperactivity, and some cases of panic disorder, the effects of an antidepressant in these various childhood conditions are delayed for one to three weeks, and they may require doses as high as those used in adults (up to 3–5 mg/kg, or total daily doses up to 200–300 mg of imipramine or the equivalent of another agent). These emerging possible indications for tricyclic antidepressants in children and adolescents are summarized in Table 53.

Side Effects and Toxicity

Important toxic effects occur in perhaps 5–10% of patients treated with tricyclic antidepressants; of these, more than 10% represent cerebral intoxication, and the incidence of nervous system toxicity is much higher in patients over age 40. The toxic effects of tricyclic and other typical (non-MAO-inhibitor) antidepressants are summarized in Tables 54 and 55. The most common toxic side effects of the tricyclic antidepressants are extensions of their pharmacologic activities and include *anticholinergic actions* leading to dry mouth, sweating, and ophthalmologic changes. The ophthalmologic problems are variable but usually include mild mydriasis and often some degree of cycloplegia with blurred near vision because of impaired accommodation. These side effects are more annoying than dangerous and can usually be managed by simple means such as sugar-free candy or mild mouth washes to offset reduced salivation, and reading lenses to compensate for reduced near vision. Cholinergic eye drops, cholinergic mouth washes, or systemic medications have been tried for these various symptoms, but are often not helpful. Moreover, some degree of tolerance to the side effects normally develops.

These side effects can occasionally be more serious, however: the over-

Table 54 Common toxic effects of typical antidepressants

- Apparent anticholinergic or other autonomic symptoms (impaired accommodation, salivation, and function of gut and bladder and impaired erectile or orgasmic sexual functions
- Confusion, delirium
- Postural hypotension
- Weight gain
- Sleep disturbance
- Cardiac conduction impairment, arrhythmia (rare unless overdose)
- Overdose: coma, seizures and involuntary movements, anticholinergic syndrome, cardiac toxicity
- Withdrawal: nonspecific symptoms if rapid

use of candy for dry mouth can lead to monilial infections, and grossly excessive water intake secondary to dry mouth on rare occasions can lead to water intoxication with significant hyponatremia, particularly in confused patients. Water intoxication also occurs infrequently with the use of antipsychotic drugs. It is not yet clear whether this problem is caused by endocrinologic effects of antidepressant or antipsychotic agents, such as an inappropriate increase in the release of antidiuretic hormone (ADH); it is sometimes preceded by excretion of very dilute urine (specific gravity < 1.003).

Table 55 Representative rates of toxic effects of typical antidepressants

Effect	Risk rate (%)
All toxicity	15.4
CNS intoxication[a]	5.8
Anticholinergic effects (severe)	2.7
Cardiac toxicity in cardiac patients[b]	6.2
Sudden death[c]	0.4

Source: Data adapted from Boston Drug Surveillance Group, *Lancet* 1:529, 1972.

a. CNS intoxication mainly involves confusion or delirium, but some instances of psychosis or abnormal movements as well.

b. Cardiac toxicity includes conduction blocks, arrhythmia, and congestive heart failure in patients with a history of cardiac disease and treated cautiously with relatively low doses of a tricyclic antidepressant (typically, 75 mg/day of imipramine or amitriptyline); the comparable rate in a group of similar patients not given an antidepressant was 9.6% (not significantly different).

c. This rate did not differ from that in a large comparison group of medical patients not given an antidepressant (0.8%), nor was there a difference in sudden death rate in cardiac patients given or not given an antidepressant.

Among the more serious aspects of the anticholinergic actions of anti-depressants is the induction of *glaucoma,* including acute, narrow-angle glaucoma; this medical emergency was discussed in Chapter 2 regarding the antipsychotic agents. Serious *antivagal effects* of the antidepressant drugs, some of which are highly anticholinergic, include paralytic ileus and acute urinary retention; thus extra caution is required in elderly patients and men with prostatism, and urgent medical intervention is necessary when these conditions develop. Treatment entails eliminating or reducing the dose of antidepressant, and giving cholinergic smooth-muscle stimulants such as bethanechol (Urecholine), 2.5 or 5.0 mg sub-cutaneously as needed. When severe inhibition of gastrointestinal or uri-nary function occurs with even small doses of antidepressants, it may be necessary to change the treatment to ECT or an MAO inhibitor other than phenelzine (the latter may also impair the function of bowel and bladder by uncertain mechanisms). Among the tricyclic agents, desipramine has the least peripheral and CNS antimuscarinic activity in animal tissues, while amitriptyline is the most potently anticholinergic — about 35 times as potent as desipramine and 1% as potent as atropine, but given in doses more than 100 times greater than atropine. The clinical significance of differences in anticholinergic properties among typical tricyclic antide-pressants, though real, appears to be limited (Table 56; see also Table 44). Some of the newer, atypical antidepressants such as trazodone and bu-propion, however, present low risks of anticholinergic and other auto-nomic side effects.

Various *skin reactions* have been described, including hair loss and an

Table 56 Decrease in saliva flow with various antidepressants

Agent	Decrease in saliva flow (%)	
	50 mg	100 mg
Desipramine	32	48
Imipramine	47	73
Doxepin	50	65
Amitriptyline	54	69

Source: Data are adapted from Blackwell et al., *Am. J. Psychiatry* 135:722, 1978, and *Commun. Psychopharmacol.* 2:145, 1978, and represent mean effects in groups of 9 to 10 young women volunteers, before and after the stated dose of the four agents. The differences are not striking, but generally parallel the in vitro differences in antimuscarinic potency of these agents as summarized earlier in Table 44.

allergic-obstructive type of *jaundice* that occurs early in the course of treatment (both conditions are rare). *Purpura* has been reported in a few cases. *Agranulocytosis* is rare. There is a tendency for some patients to *gain weight,* and there are occasional *hypoglycemic effects* of the tricyclic agents. *Sexual dysfunction,* such as altered orgasmic function, may occur, and trazodone has been associated rarely with sustained penile erection (priapism), which has required surgery in some cases.

A serious consequence of the anticholinergic and direct quinidine-like properties of the tricyclic antidepressants is their potential *cardiac toxicity.* Palpitations and mild tachycardia are not rare, and cardiac conduction defects or arrhythmias are to be expected in cases of acute overdosage. Accordingly, the tricyclic antidepressants should be used in lower doses and with great caution in elderly patients at risk for myocardial infarction and stroke, and should be avoided altogether within several months after myocardial infarction. Amitriptyline may be particularly cardiotoxic, although this impression derives from studies in animals; there is no convincing clinical evidence that any typical tricyclic-type antidepressant is consistently more or less cardiotoxic than the others. Moreover, the hope that newer, and especially the more atypical, antidepressants might be less toxic is not securely established. The atypical agents such as trazodone and bupropion are less anticholinergic and may be less likely to induce lethal toxicity on acute overdose, but their effects on the cardiovascular system are less certain. Evidence of cardiac irritability or conduction defects has been reported with the use of trazodone and maprotiline. Amoxapine has been associated with atrial arrhythmias.

Generally, the likelihood is low that a tricyclic antidepressant, given in usual therapeutic doses, will be associated with a cardiac arrhythmia. This impression is supported by experience in depressed patients without evidence of cardiovascular disease (Table 57) but also in some with known cardiac disorders (Table 58). The most probable effects are mild atrial tachycardia (probably in part an anticholinergic effect) and mild decreases in cardiac conduction (probably a direct, quinidine-like cardiac depressant effect). It has been found recently that tricyclic antidepressants can actually have *anti*arrhythmic actions; the best evaluated are the quinidine-like effects of imipramine to reduce the rate of premature ventricular contractions (see Table 58). It is, accordingly, considered a dangerous practice to add an antidepressant with such effects to the regimen of a patient already receiving a cardiac depressant, antiarrhythmic agent such as quinidine, procaineamide, or disopyramide (Norpace). Similarly, it is extremely dangerous to give a tricyclic antidepressant to a patient with a

Table 57 Effects of antidepressants on cardiac function in medically healthy patients

Measurement	On drug (day 20)	Off drug (day 50)	On drug (13 months)
Pulse rate (min⁻¹)	82 ± 2	77 ± 2	84 ± 3
QRS width (msec)	86 ± 2	80 ± 2	82 ± 3
PR interval (msec)	161 ± 4	157 ± 3	154 ± 5
QT_c (msec)	397 ± 3	390 ± 3	403 ± 5
T amplitude in ECG lead V_5 (mV)	275 ± 10	325 ± 12	310 ± 40
Systolic BP: supine/standing	130/120	135/130	130/125
BP drop on standing (mm Hg)	10	5	5

Source: Data are adapted from Burckhardt et al., *J.A.M.A.* 239:213, 1978, concerning 66 random depressed patients (mean age 43 years) treated for three weeks with the following mean daily doses: amitriptyline (118 mg), imipramine (188 mg), trimipramine (169 mg), maprotiline (81 mg), or mianserin (40 mg); 19 patients were followed for 13 months, and all were evaluated after three weeks on, and one month off treatment. The effects were generally minor and reversible. All data are means ± S.E.M. The various ECG measurements are stated, including the QT interval corrected for pulse rate (QT_c); blood pressure (BP) changes are stated for measurements in the supine and standing position and the decrease on standing.

Table 58 Cardiovascular effects of imipramine in depressed cardiac patients

Measurement	Baseline	With medication	Percent change
ECG changes (msec)			
Rate (min⁻¹)	78.2 ± 3.7	83.1 ± 2.3	+ 6
PR interval	106.0 ± 25.1	190.0 ± 8.8	+79
QRS width	98.1 ± 15.8	124.6 ± 15.4	+27
QT_c interval	256.4 ± 54.8	432.1 ± 51.6	+21
Blood pressure (mm Hg)			
Supine	130/81	124/83	−5/+2
Standing	124/83	106/72	−15/−13

Source: Data adapted from Kantor et al., *Am. J. Psychiatry* 135:534, 1978, concerning 7 cardiac patients with major depression (aged 35–71 years) given imipramine (175–400 mg/day, mean = 275 mg/day) for five weeks with blood levels of imipramine plus desipramine averaging 280 ng/ml. In two cases, spontaneous PVCs were markedly *suppressed* by treatment with this quinidine-like agent.

known cardiac conduction defect, such as bundle-branch block, because of the risk of worsening the conduction defect and increasing the risk of a malignant ventricular arrhythmia.

Although clinically important cardiac changes are not usual with ordinary doses of antidepressants, they are commonly encountered following acute overdoses. The most common electrocardiographic effects are summarized in Table 59. These toxic effects following an overdose have a complex and poorly understood pathophysiology, but antivagal, antiadrenergic, and direct cardiotoxic effects probably play a role, as do hypotensive effects and interference with the membrane transport of potassium ion. Tricyclic antidepressants accumulate in muscle to higher levels than are found in plasma, and accumulations in cardiac tissue may be especially high. The presence of drug molecules in such tissue may be particularly prolonged following an overdose, contributing to the risk of cardiac arrhythmias for a week or more after initial treatment of the acute intoxication. The optimal medical treatment of the cardiac aspects of acute intoxication with a tricyclic antidepressant is a specialized and complex matter requiring the attention of experts in emergency medicine and cardiology. Some general principles that are currently widely accepted by such experts are provided in Table 60.

There has been some tendency to feel that tricyclic antidepressants are generally too dangerous to be employed in the treatment of depressed cardiac or stroke patients. Although it is reasonable to be cautious in the treatment of such patients, it is necessary in evaluating a patient for treatment to consider the risk of untreated major depression as well as that of possible toxicity of the treatment. For example, the risk of worsening or complicating a medical illness by the morbidity due to severe depression

Table 59 Characteristic electrocardiographic effects of typical tricyclic antidepressants at toxic doses

- Prolonged atrioventricular or intraventricular conduction (prolonged PR, QRS, QT intervals; QRS greater than 100 msec)
- Bundle-branch and other serious atrioventricular conduction blocks
- Mild atrial tachycardia, fibrillation, or flutter (less often, bradycardia)
- Ventricular tachycardia, fibrillation, or arrest
- Depressed T and ST segments
- Large U waves

Note: Similar changes can occur with overdoses of low potency neuroleptic agents, especially thioridazine.

Table 60 Suggested guidelines for management of acute cardiac toxicity with overdose of a tricyclic antidepressant

- Expect to find classic signs: altered consciousness or coma, seizures, hypotension, arrhythmia, mydriasis, and antivagal effects
- Obtain blood for confirmatory assay of drug level
- Monitor patient for at least several days in a cardiac intensive care unit following stabilization of acute intoxication
- Support airway, blood pressure, plasma potassium and pH (patient may require infusion of bicarbonate, which may have antiarrhythmic effects even without evidence of acidosis)
- Avoid blood volume expansion (risk of acute congestive failure); treat hypotension conservatively or with a pure alpha-adrenergic agonist such as *l*-norepinephrine
- Dialysis and diuresis are useless
- Repeated gastric lavage with 20–30 g of activated charcoal may help to bind residual unabsorbed drug in gut
- Avoid use of quinidine, procaineamide, or disopyramide; lidocaine or phenytoin is probably safer against ventricular irritability
- The role of propranolol and physostigmine is still uncertain and controversial
- Electrical cardioversion can be used for ventricular arrhythmias
- Consider early transvenous pacing
- Simultaneous grand mal seizures are likely to complicate cardiovascular management; phenytoin is unlikely to be adequate treatment, but diazepam may help (avoid barbiturates or rapid infusion of physostigmine)

is often serious. A further consideration in analyzing the risk : benefit ratio of these agents is that there is evidence that the risk of suicide falls with increased vigor of antidepressant treatment (Table 61), even though suicide by acute overdose of an antidepressant agent does occur. Suggestions to consider in the clinical management of patients with known cardiac disease and major depression are provided in Table 62. An important consideration in choosing a treatment for serious depression in elderly or infirm patients is that ECT, with its modern modifications, is probably as safe as the antidepressant drugs if not safer. Mortality rates with the tricyclic agents and ECT are both low, but the incidence of serious morbidity and mortality with the drugs may be higher than with ECT if overdoses are included. Certainly the total morbidity rate with the drugs is considerable, especially if minor as well as more serious toxic effects and overdosages are taken into account.

Although there is much concern about the possible induction of cardiac

Table 61   Suicidal behavior and level of antidepressant treatment

Daily dose (mg)	Prevalence of suicidal behavior (%)
0–74	30.4
75–149	10.1
150–249	5.1
250 or more	0.5

Source: Keller et al., *J.A.M.A.* 248:1851, 1982, based on a study of 217 patients with major depression who were given no treatment or various daily doses of an antidepressant (given as equivalent to imipramine). The behaviors included suicide attempts as well as successful suicides.

conduction defects or arrhythmias, the most common, but underrecognized, cardiovascular complication of the use of antidepressants is hypotension, and especially *postural hypotension.* This effect can be dangerous, especially in those at risk of myocardial infarction or stroke, and falls or faints can lead to head trauma or orthopedic injuries such as hip fractures. The risk of mild postural hypotension may be in excess of 20% overall, but there is evidence that the risk of severe hypotension is even

Table 62   Suggestions for the clinical management of depressed cardiac patients

- Evaluate the risk : benefit ratio (including morbidity due to depression and suicide risk)
- Be especially cautious with elderly cardiac patients
- Collaborate closely with an internist or cardiologist
- Treatment is most safely started in hospital
- Avoid use of amitriptyline, imipramine, trimipramine (may be relatively cardiotoxic) or protriptyline (long-acting)
- Low doses of nortriptyline, desipramine, or atypical antidepressants may be safest (status of doxepin, maprotiline, and trazodone uncertain in this situation versus other agents)
- Start with very small doses; always divide doses; avoid blood levels over 200 ng/ml or dispensing more than a week's supply at one time
- Avoid cardiac depressants (especially those with quinidine-like actions), low-potency neuroleptics, antiparkinsonism agents, MAO inhibitors
- Diuretics and moderate doses of propranolol may be relatively safe for hypertension, but watch closely for orthostatic hypotension when antidepressant is added
- Untoward interactions with digitalis are not proved
- Consider ECT (can be used even with a pacemaker)

Table 63 Incidence of postural hypotension with tricyclic antidepressants

Patient group	Incidence of hypotension (%)		
	Mild	Moderate	Severe
Cardiac	37	14	24
Medically well	28	7	0

Source: Miller et al., Clin. Pharmacol. and Ther. 2:300, 1961, based on a study of 82 patients, half of whom had identified cardiac disease. Definitions of severity were as follows: mild, less than 20 mm decrease in blood pressure on standing, no symptoms; moderate, 10–20 mm decrease with mild symptoms of dizziness or faintness; severe, more than 20 mm decrease in pressure with fainting. The risk tended to decrease with repeated exposure to the antidepressant.

greater, and the consequences correspondingly more serious, in patients known to have cardiac disease (Table 63). For most cardiovascular and other toxic effects of antidepressants, the elderly and young children are at high risk, especially when doses greater than 2.5–3.0 mg/kg of imipramine or its equivalent are given daily, or blood levels are above 300 ng/ml. With hypotension, however, recent clinical reviews indicate that these associations are not strong, and that postural hypotension tends to be idiosyncratic and not easily predicted by age, dose, or type of agent. Patients with preexisting postural hypotension appear to be at higher risk, and in general elderly and cardiac patients should be monitored especially carefully to avoid complications arising from this common and potentially very dangerous reaction. Evidence of the hypotensive actions of antidepressants was also provided in Tables 57 and 58.

The management and treatment of postural hypotension remain unsatisfactory. The usual measures are reducing the daily dose, giving smaller doses at one time, or changing to a different agent, as well as considering ECT if the problem or risk is severe. There is a clinical impression that nortriptyline may be less likely to induce postural hypotension than other tricyclic antidepressants. MAO inhibitors also produce this effect commonly, as do the more recently introduced tricyclic antidepressants in use in the United States; the status of atypical or experimental antidepressants in this regard is not well established. There have been occasional reports that steroids, such as cortisone, as well as dihydroergotamine (at a dose of about 10 mg/day) may be useful in reducing this reaction, but these treatments are not widely accepted and their utility and safety are not well established.

The untoward effects of tricyclic antidepressants on the *central nervous system* include mild dizziness and light-headedness, insomnia and restlessness, or fatigue and somnolence. Fine and occasionally gross resting tremors are common and may respond to diazepam (Valium), but extrapyramidal syndromes are rare except after an acute overdose. The powerful anticholinergic action of these drugs is often sufficient to produce antiparkinsonism effects, which are occasionally encountered when antidepressants are combined with neuroleptic agents or when they are given to depressed patients with Parkinson's disease. Tricyclic antidepressants should be used with caution in the treatment of patients receiving antiparkinsonism medications, because of the risk of combined anticholinergic toxicity. These agents would be expected to worsen choreas, including tardive dyskinesia, as antiparkinsonism drugs can. There is also some risk of provoking or worsening agitation and psychosis in patients with psychoses or unstable characterological conditions in addition to depression, and large doses or acute overdoses of the tricyclic antidepressants can induce a toxic psychosis.

Confusion and delirium are not infrequent complications of treatment with antidepressants; they may or may not be accompanied by signs suggesting anticholinergic intoxication. There is a clear increase in risk of such cerebral intoxication with increasing age, and the risk may exceed 30% in patients above age 60 (Table 64). An additional side effect is the possible induction of *grand mal seizures* with tricyclic antidepressant treatment. Although this association has been noted infrequently with older antidepressants, there is a growing suspicion that maprotiline may

Table 64 Effect of increasing age on risk of confusional states with tricyclic antidepressants

Age (years)	Risk rate (%)
10–19	0
20–29	0
30–39	4
40–49	25
50–59	43
60–69	33
70–79	50
Overall risk	13

Source: Davies et al., *Am. J. Psychiatry* 128:95, 1971, from a review of 150 patients. About half of these patients also received a neuroleptic agent alone or with an antiparkinsonism agent, which would be expected to inflate the risk due to a tricyclic antidepressant alone.

Table 65 Apparent relative risk of epileptic seizures with antidepressants of the tricyclic type

Agent	Frequency of use (%)	Seizures reported (N)
Maprotiline	3.6	112
Amitriptyline	34.2	35
Imipramine	13.5	15
Nortriptyline	2.2	11

Source: Rothblatt, *Drug Intell. and Clin. Pharmacy* 16:749, 1982. The data on frequency of use represent estimates of contemporary "market share" as a percentage of total antidepressant prescriptions. The cases of seizure are those reported in the literature or to the manufacturer or the U.S. Food and Drug Administration and thus may be unreliable as absolute indexes of risk, although they may suggest relative risks, especially when compared to the frequency of their use.

carry a higher risk of seizures than other tricyclic-type antidepressants (Table 65). This risk appears to be dose-related and more common at daily doses of maprotiline above 200 mg. Past history of epileptic seizures is probably also a risk factor. The relative risk of seizures with other newer or atypical antidepressants is not clear. Usually, a depressed epileptic patient can be safely treated with an antidepressant provided that adequate anticonvulsant therapy is continued or, if necessary, increased in dose.

Other CNS effects of tricyclic antidepressants include *disturbances of sleep* (large doses at bedtime may produce nightmares) and *withdrawal reactions.* These latter reactions have been reported to follow the abrupt discontinuation of high doses of tricyclic antidepressants (more likely if doses exceed 300 mg/day of imipramine or its equivalent); they include restlessness, anxiety, and akathisia but almost never seizures. Thus it is best to discontinue unusually high doses slowly. Nomifensine has occasionally been associated with fever, presumably on a central basis.

Severe CNS depression and *coma* (rarely lasting more than 24 hours) can result from large, acute overdoses of tricyclic-type antidepressants, but it is common to see signs of *anticholinergic poisoning* early or with milder confusional or delirious states associated with therapeutic doses. The latter syndrome includes restless agitation; confusion; disorientation; perhaps seizures and hyperthermia; dry, sometimes flushed skin; tachycardia; sluggish and at least moderately dilated pupils; decreased bowel sounds; and often acute urinary retention (Table 66). These effects are probably a result of CNS and systemic anticholinergic and antivagal actions of these potent muscarinic blocking agents (see Table 44). Sys-

Table 66 *Anticholinergic and cholinergic excess syndromes*

Anticholinergic Syndrome

Causes

Acute overdose or excessive prescription of medications with antimuscarinic properties, especially in combination: tricyclic antidepressants, most antiparkinson agents, some antipsychotics (especially thioridazine), many proprietary sedative-hypnotics, many antispasmodic preparations, several plants (e.g., Jimson weed, some mushrooms).

Neuropsychiatric signs

Anxiety, agitation; restless, purposeless overactivity; delirium, disorientation; impairment of immediate and recent memory; dysarthria; hallucinations; myoclonus; seizures.

Systemic signs

Tachycardia and arrhythmias; large, sluggish pupils; scleral injection; flushed, warm, dry skin; increased temperature; decreased mucosal secretions; urinary retention; reduced bowel motility.

Treatment

Adults: initial or test dose: 1–2 mg physostigmine salicylate, intramuscularly, or *slowly* intravenously; repeat as needed after at least 15–30 minutes.

Children: 0.5–1.0 mg physostigmine salicylate, as for adults. (Neostigmine, pyridostigmine, etc., do not enter the CNS.)

Physostigmine-Induced Cholinergic Excess

Neuropsychiatric signs

Confusion, seizures, nausea and vomiting, myoclonus, hallucinations, often after a period of initial CNS improvement when physostigmine is given to treat the anticholinergic syndrome.

Systemic signs

Bradycardia, miosis, increased mucosal secretions, copious bronchial secretions, dyspnea, tears, sweating, diarrhea, abdominal colic, biliary colic, urinary frequency or urgency.

Treatment or prevention

Atropine sulfate (CNS + systemic actions): 0.5 mg per mg of physostigmine, intramuscularly or subcutaneously.

Methscopolamine bromide (Pamine) (no CNS action): 0.5 mg per mg of physostigmine, intramuscularly (methscopolamine and methylatropine, a similar agent, may not be readily available).

Glycopyrrolate (Robinul) (no CNS action): 0.1 to 0.2 mg per mg of physostigmine, intramuscularly.

Note: In cases of severe (and especially mixed) overdoses with coma, and unstable vital functions, the first responsibility is to support respiratory and cardiovascular function; the role of physostigmine is not clear and may even make such situations worse.

temic, including cardiac, toxic effects of acute overdoses of various agents with anticholinergic activity have been treated effectively and safely with reversible anticholinesterase agents, including neostigmine (Prostigmin) and pyridostigmine (Mestinon). However, only physostigmine (eserine, Antilirium) lacks the charged, quaternary ammonium moiety of this group of anticholinesterase agents and is able to penetrate the blood-brain diffusion barrier to exert central as well as peripheral cholinomimetic actions. There are also experimental agents with central anticholinesterase activity (such as tetrahydroaminoacridine and galanthamine), but only physostigmine is in common clinical use. Suggestions for the use of physostigmine are provided in Table 66, along with potential complications of excessive treatment with this cholinomimetic agent.

The possible clinical utility of including physostigmine in the management of intoxications caused by tricyclic antidepressants or other agents with antimuscarinic activity is currently a matter of uncertainty and controversy, and the basis of the central actions of this agent are increasingly uncertain. It is clear that there are risks of serious toxic effects from the overly aggressive or inappropriate use of physostigmine, including the precipitation of acute asthma in susceptible patients and the routine induction of grand mal epileptic seizures by rapid intravenous injection, especially in doses above 1.0 mg. Other signs of a state of cholinergic excess are summarized in Table 66. Moreover, it is crucial to realize that physostigmine is not a highly specific antidote for poisoning with a tricyclic antidepressant. These drugs exert complex toxicologic actions, only a portion of which can be ascribed to their antimuscarinic effects. Several recent clinical reports on the use of physostigmine in the management of patients acutely poisoned with an overdose of an antidepressant have led to mixed and sometimes highly unsatisfactory results. In part, this outcome probably reflects excessive expectations of physostigmine as well as its early and rapid administration in excessively aggressive doses, while deferring more critical life-supporting measures such as maintenance of adequate ventilation and blood pressure. The principles of attending to the cardiovascular aspects of acute antidepressant poisoning outlined in Table 60 apply more broadly to the overall management of such life-threatening and dangerous intoxications. If physostigmine has a place in this overall management, it is secondary to the support of vital functions, and a step to be considered carefully and applied cautiously by an expert in the management of overdoses of this type.

Another possible use for physostigmine is in the diagnosis and management of lesser degrees of intoxication that are often encountered in psychiatric settings, especially reactions marked by confusion or mild delirium in association with the classic signs of atropinic intoxication as outlined in Table 66. Small intramuscular or slowly infused intravenous injections of physostigmine in such circumstances, especially with an otherwise healthy patient, can be safe and effective. The primary approach, however, should be immediate discontinuation of the suspected intoxicating agent or agents. This recommendation is especially important because recent clinical experience has suggested that the antidelirium actions of physostigmine may not be limited to anticholinergic agents; for example, physostigmine has been found to diminish the central depressant effects of sedatives, antianxiety agents (such as benzodiazepines), and even general anesthetics — none of which has important antimuscarinic activity. Thus, a favorable response of a confusional state to a small dose of physostigmine may not necessarily prove the diagnosis of central anticholinergic intoxication, since the actions of physostigmine on the CNS remain incompletely understood.

Other aspects of the pharmacology of the tricyclic antidepressants should also be appreciated in the management of overdoses. For example, the ability of these compounds to potentiate directly sympathomimetic amines such as norepinephrine complicates the use of such pressor substances in managing the hypotension and shock of tricyclic poisoning. Furthermore, the tricyclic antidepressants potentiate and prolong the actions of barbiturates, probably through competition for hepatic microsomal enzymes, which are particularly important in inactivating the shorter-acting barbiturates. Although small doses of very short-acting barbiturates have been advocated for the control of seizures associated with tricyclic antidepressant poisoning, diazepam (Valium) is probably a safer anticonvulsant in this situation and is less likely to induce respiratory depression. After an acute overdose, it is impossible to remove the tricyclic agents by dialysis; forced diuresis adds little, and rapid volume expansion may contribute to cardiac failure. Although attempts to increase the dialysis of antidepressants by the use of oils, resins, or charcoal have not been successful, activated charcoal is sometimes introduced into the gut during gastric lavage in an attempt to bind and inactivate any remaining unabsorbed drug. Several of these points are summarized in Table 67 (see also Table 60).

The agents used in the treatment of mood disorders (tricyclic antidepressants, MAO inhibitors, and lithium salts) are much more toxic in acute overdosage than the antipsychotic agents and, unfortunately, must be given to patients at increased risk of attempting suicide. The tricyclic

Table 67 Relationship of aspects of the clinical pharmacology of tricyclic antidepressants to management of their acute intoxication

Pharmacologic characteristic	Treatment consideration
1. Rapidly absorbed	1. Rapid intoxication
2. Bound to lipid and protein	2. Dialysis ineffective
3. Tissue (especially cardiac) levels greatly exceed plasma concentration and fall slowly	3. Plasma levels may be misleading; risk of cardiac intoxication may persist for more than a week
4. Several active metabolites arise	4. Conventional plasma level assays may be misleading
5. Less than 5% of active agent and by-products excreted by kidney	5. Diuresis ineffective and may risk heart failure
6. Some (ca. 5%) enterohepatic recycling occurs; concretions form in gut	6. Delayed uptake and fluctuating course common; charcoal may reduce the effect
7. Strongly antimuscarinic	7. Variable delirium, mydriasis, and anti-vagal signs, seizures, tachycardia
8. Directly cardiac depressant; block vascular reflexes, unpredictable effects at adrenergic receptors	8. Hypotension, cardiac conduction defects and arrhythmias common
9. Complex, obscure CNS effects	9. Delirium and seizures, myoclonus and choreoathetosis as well as coma
10. Respiratory depression	10. Apnea (may be delayed) and complication of course by atelectasis and pneumonitis
11. Actions of indirect sympathomimetic pressor amines blocked; beta-adrenergic agents may increase splanchnic pooling of blood; direct alpha-adrenergic agents potentiated	11. Hypotension common (but blood pressure often fluctuates unpredictably); can manage mild hypotension by elevating feet; avoid indirect and beta-adrenergic pressors; can use intravenous *l*-norepinephrine cautiously
12. Hypoxia and acidosis common	12. Ventilation crucial; may need infusions of supplemental potassium and bicarbonate

antidepressants are a common choice in suicide attempts by increasingly younger persons. Acute doses above 1,000 mg are almost always very toxic, but doses as low as a few hundred milligrams, especially of amitriptyline, have been severely toxic in adults as well as children. Acute doses in excess of 2,000 mg can be fatal. The average fatality rate after an acute overdose of a tricyclic antidepressant is at least 1% in adults, and more than 10% in children. The monomethylated (desmethylated) derivatives may be slightly less toxic than the tertiary amine parent compounds. Because of the relatively low margin of safety of all tricyclic antidepressants, it is unwise to dispense more than a week's supply, and certainly never more than 1,000 mg of imipramine or the equivalent of another agent. Realistically, however, since patients may hoard pills for potential later use in a suicidal overdose or may have accumulated similar or other potentially toxic agents from other sources, it is well to maintain a high index of suspicion and to inquire about access to potentially lethal collections of medicines.

Tricyclic antidepressant agents have many *interactions with other drugs* (Table 68). Tricyclic antidepressants increase the CNS depression caused by alcohol, antihistamines, barbiturates, and other sedatives as well as antipsychotic agents and anticonvulsants. The barbiturates and glutethimide (Doriden) much more than the benzodiazepines also induce hepatic microsomal enzymes required for the metabolism of the tricyclic antidepressant agents, and thus may decrease the efficacy of the tricyclics. Since the seizure threshold may be lowered, increased doses of anticonvulsants may be required. The effect of any anticholinergic agent (including antiparkinsonism drugs) is additively increased by the antimuscarinic activity of the tricyclic antidepressants, and this combination creates a risk of toxic confusional brain syndrome, agitation, and sometimes fever. Antipsychotic agents are contraindicated in cases of toxic agitation produced by overdoses of tricyclic antidepressants because of the moderate anticholinergic and other autonomic actions of the former drugs.

A difficult combination to manage satisfactorily is *depression and hypertension.* Antihypertensive agents, possibly because of their central antiadrenergic properties, are sometimes associated with depression of mood. This association may occur unpredictably at any time in the treatment of hypertension; it is most common in patients with a prior history of depression, and has most frequently been reported with reserpine and other *Rauwolfia* alkaloids, and occasionally with alpha-methyldopa (Aldomet). Guanethidine is one of the few antihypertensive agents that has little CNS activity and is not likely to induce or worsen depression, although, surprisingly, anecdotal reports of its sporadic association with depression exist. Because the tricyclics exert a blockade of guanethidine uptake into postganglionic sympathetic nerve fibers (Table 68), the treatment of hypertension with guanethidine in patients who are also depressed is usually rendered unsuccessful by the addition of any of the typical tricyclic-type antidepressants (and to some extent the phenothi-

Table 68 Interactions of various agents with tricyclic antidepressants (TCAs)

Agent	Interactions
Alcohol, antihistamines, barbiturates, and nonbarbiturate sedatives (e.g., ethchlorvynol, glutethimide)	More sedation; may induce TCA metabolism and lower blood levels
Anesthetics	Possibly increased risk of cardiac arrhythmias
Narcotics	Some potentiation and risk of respiratory depression; some increase in TCA metabolism and decrease of plasma levels
Anticonvulsants (especially phenytoin)	Less effective control of seizures, may increase blood levels of TCA; carbamazepine induces hepatic metabolism and lowers plasma TCA levels
Disulfiram (Antabuse)	May increase TCA levels
Anticholinergic agents (antiparkinsonism agents, antispasmotics)	Potentiate each other; more anticholinergic effect
L-dopa	Absorption of dopa may decrease; unpredictable effects on BP, ECG, mood
Stimulants, anorexics (e.g., methylphenidate, fenfluramine)	May potentiate each other, may induce hypertension; compete for hepatic metabolism and thus increase plasma TCA levels
Reserpine	Risk of hypertension if reserpine added acutely, later some loss of hypotensive effect; may worsen depression
Alpha-methyldopa (Aldomet)	May reduce hypotensive effect; some risk of paradoxical excitement; may increase depression
Postganglionic sympathetic antagonists (e.g., guanethidine, bethanidine, debisoquine)	Hypotensive action antagonized; may have severe hypotension when TCA removed; small increase in TCA plasma levels
Any agent with MAO inhibitory properties (e.g., Eutonyl, Furoxone, Matulane as well as antidepressant MAO inhibitors)	May increase TCA plasma levels; rare but potentially catastrophic CNS reaction with hyperpyrexia and seizures
Alpha-adrenergic agonists (e.g., norepinephrine, methoxamine, phenylephrine)	Potentiate by blocking neuronal uptake

Table 68 (continued)

Agent	Interactions
Clonidine (Catapres)	Hypotensive action lost due to CNS interaction with TCAs, but not bupropion
Indirect sympathomimetic amines (e.g., tyramine in foods)	Antagonize pressor effects
Alpha-adrenergic antagonists (e.g., phentolamine, phenoxybenzamine)	May diminish hypotensive effects
Beta-adrenergic agonists (e.g., epinephrine, isoproterenol)	May potentiate epinephrine; less effect on isoproterenol, which is not taken up by sympathetic terminals
Beta-adrenergic antagonists (e.g., propranolol, atenolol, metoprolol, pindolol)	May antagonize hypotensive effects; may increase cardiac depressant effects of TCA; plasma levels of both may rise slightly
Anticoagulants (e.g., coumarins, indanediones)	Small increase in blood levels of coumarin; slight increase in anticoagulant effect
Cardiac agents (e.g., quinidine, digitalis)	Dangerously potentiate class I cardiac depressants such as quinidine; safe with digitalis for congestive failure but may increase risk of cardiac depression and irritability; phenytoin and lidocaine are relatively safe antiarrhythmics with TCAs; can substitute imipramine for quinidine
Thyroid hormones and thyroid-stimulating hormone	May increase risk of cardiac toxicity; may increase plasma levels of TCAs
Steroids (including contraceptives)	Unpredictable; may increase TCA levels, with uncertain clinical effect
Insulin and oral hypoglycemics	Unpredictable, may potentiate hypoglycemia; tolbutamide may increase TCA levels
Oral alkalis (e.g., Amphojel) and resins (e.g., Questran)	Absorption of TCAs decreased
Aspirin	May decrease plasma binding of TCAs and potentiate their actions

Other reported interactions include the effects of cigarette smoking and exposure to insecticides to increase hepatic metabolism, and decrease plasma levels of TCAs.

azines as well, but less so with haloperidol or molindone). Although doxepin (Sinequan) has been claimed to have this effect much less than the other antidepressants, the claim is at best only partially valid for relatively small doses of the antidepressant (less than 150 mg/day) given for brief periods of time (less than two or three weeks). The antihypertensive effects of several other agents, including reserpine and the *Veratrum* alkaloids, can also be diminished by the tricyclic antidepressants. It is safe to use diuretics with tricyclic antidepressants for the management of hypertension in depressed patients, although moderate degrees of hyponatremia may have mood-depressing effects. It is also possible to treat hypertension with large doses of a beta-adrenergic blocking agent such as propranolol (Inderal) alone, or combined with the vascular smooth-muscle relaxant hydralazine (Apresoline); however, high doses of the former can produce central sedative effects and may induce depression, and hydralazine has occasionally induced toxic psychoses. Moreover, this combination of antihypertensive agents with tricyclic antidepressants has not yet been evaluated, although propranolol can be used safely with tricyclic antidepressants.

The safety of antidepressant drugs in *pregnancy and lactation* is not established. They pass the placental barrier and can be secreted at low levels in human milk. In severe prepartum and postpartum depression, ECT can be used safely. There have been rare reports of neonatal distress in infants born to mothers given antidepressants; these reactions included muscle spasms, myoclonus, tachycardia, congestive heart failure, and respiratory distress.

MAO Inhibitors

Inhibitors of the enzyme *monoamine oxidase* (MAO) are historically important because they had a major impact on the medical treatment of depression and on the biological theories that attempt to relate brain metabolism to psychiatric illness. In the early 1950s the first useful antidepressant, iproniazid (Marsilid), was introduced and its inhibitory effects on MAO were described. A few years later, the ability of reserpine to deplete serotonin and norepinephrine in the mammalian brain while inducing behavioral "depression" was noted by Bernard Brodie and Parkhurst Shore at the U.S. National Institutes of Health. Speculation then began that a functional deficiency of brain amines may underlie depression and that MAO inhibitors and other antidepressants as well as

ECT may act by reversing this deficiency. This view was formulated very early by Nathan Kline, who, simultaneously with several other American investigators, demonstrated the usefulness of iproniazid in serious depression. After that time, the MAO inhibitors fell into a position of limited use. The tricyclic agents were found to be somewhat superior as antidepressants (see Tables 46 and 47), and the MAO inhibitors acquired a reputation for pharmacologic complexity and toxicity as well as limited efficacy in major depression. Several MAO inhibitors, including iproniazid, were removed from the market because of severe hepatocellular toxicity, limited efficacy, or hypotensive effects. Moreover, these agents are severely toxic on acute overdosage and can also induce dangerous interactions with other drugs, chemicals, hormones, or metabolic conditions. Although the likelihood of inducing serious drug reactions with an MAO inhibitor is small, and overall morbidity is probably not greater than that due to ECT or the tricyclic antidepressants, some reactions to MAO inhibitors are serious and potentially fatal (in about 0.001% of cases). Thus the dangers of toxicity, the inconvenience of restrictions required for the safe use of MAO inhibitors, and the impression of limited efficacy of these agents in serious depression resulted in their near abandonment in this country until recently.

The situation has changed in recent years as dosage requirements and the range of indications for the MAO inhibitors have been clarified. At present, although these agents are generally considered drugs of second choice for major depression, they can be of use to some patients who fail to respond to other antidepressants, and also to some patients with chronic disorders marked by anxiety, phobias, or panic as well as dysphoria, especially if doses are increased sufficiently to induce strong inhibition of MAO in tissues such as blood platelets. Moreover, there is much experimental interest in developing new MAO inhibitors with selective actions on a type of enzyme characteristic of many monoamine-containing nerve endings (so-called "type A" MAO) as well as another type ("type B" MAO) that has been tentatively associated with dopaminergic neurons in the human brain. At the present time, three MAO inhibitors are available in the United States for clinical use in the treatment of depression: phenelzine (Nardil), tranylcypromine (Parnate), and isocarboxazid (Marplan, which is not actively marketed). Figure 16 shows the chemical structures of these three agents. There are also several agents used for other medical indications that have MAO-inhibitory properties, as well as experimental MAO inhibitors, as discussed.

The development of the antidepressant MAO inhibitors can be traced

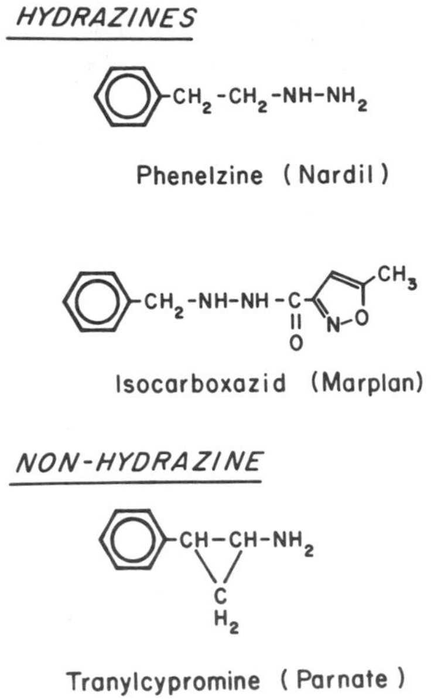

HYDRAZINES

Phenelzine (Nardil)

Isocarboxazid (Marplan)

NON-HYDRAZINE

Tranylcypromine (Parnate)

Figure 16   Chemical structures of monoamine oxidase inhibitors.

to the introduction of isoniazid and its isopropyl analogue iproniazid in 1951 as antibacterial agents, especially for the treatment of tuberculosis. It was noted that iproniazid had mood-elevating properties in tuberculous patients and suggested that it be tried as an antidepressant. Although iproniazid (Marsilid) can be considered the first successful modern antidepressant, based on trials in the United States and Europe in 1952–1957, its association with severe parenchymal damage to the liver led to its abandonment in the 1960s. This agent (as well as phenelzine and isocarboxazid, which are in current clinical use) are derivatives (hydrazides) of hydrazine, a highly hepatotoxic substance. It was found later that other compounds unrelated to hydrazine have potent MAO-inhibiting properties. Some are analogues of amphetamine and were developed to take advantage of combined stimulant-like and MAO-inhibiting properties; the sole representative of this type of MAO inhibitor in clinical use in the United States is tranylcypromine, a reversible inhibitor of MAO with a cyclized side chain. Other agents contain the propargyl moiety, a reactive group that binds to the flavin cofactor component of the MAO enzyme system to produce irreversible inhibition after initial association as a "pseudo-substrate" or so-called "suicide inhibitor" which is acted upon by the enzyme to initiate covalent attachment. Examples of this type of

Table 69   Dosage forms and doses of antidepressant MAO inhibitors

Agent	Trade name	Dosage form	Dose range (mg/day)
Phenelzine sulfate	Nardil	(T) 15 mg	15–90
Tranylcypromine sulfate	Parnate	(T) 10 mg	10–30
Isocarboxazid	Marplan	(T) 10 mg	10–30

All are supplied only as tablets (T).

Because of the prolonged biological effective half-life of the MAO inhibitors (especially the irreversible MAO inhibitors phenelzine and isocarboxazid), it is often possible to use small doses less often than daily once initial strong inhibition of MAO has been achieved. The efficacy of phenelzine in major depression at doses below 45 mg/day is not secure. Tranylcypromine has stimulant properties and is not recommended for routine use in the elderly or for cardiac patients. It is occasionally used in doses up to 60 mg/day if lower doses are ineffective but well tolerated. Other MAO inhibitors have been used but are no longer marketed (Catron, Marsilid, Monase, Niamid), or are not used in psychiatric practice (*furazolidone:* Furoxone, an antimicrobial agent; *pargyline* hydrochloride: Eutonyl, Eutron, an antihypertensive; and *procarbazine:* Matulane, a cancer chemotherapy agent).

The therapeutic index (ratio of toxic or lethal dose to therapeutic dose) is equivalent to about a week's supply of all three of the above MAO inhibitors, indicating the need for careful dispensing of small amounts to unreliable or potentially suicidal patients.

MAO inhibitor are the antihypertensive agent pargyline (Eutonyl), the selective MAO inhibitor clorgyline (against type A MAO) and (−)deprenyl (against type B MAO), and several additional experimental agents. The clinically available antidepressant MAO inhibitors and their doses are given in Table 69.

Pharmacology

These agents inhibit the enzyme monoamine oxidase (MAO), which is located in monoamine-containing nerve terminals, including the sympathetic nervous system and the CNS, but also in liver and other tissues. MAO is crucial in inactivating exogenous monoamines arising from foods or the action of bacteria in the gut, including the indirect sympathomimetic pressor amine tyramine. The MAO inhibitors also interact with other enzymes, including hepatic enzymes required for the metabolism of many drugs. Accordingly, they can interfere with the inactivation of many other agents. In addition, it remains uncertain whether their antidepressant effects can be ascribed solely to the MAO-inhibiting properties; for example, tranylcypromine also has amphetamine-like actions to inhibit the uptake of monoamines, similar to the tricyclic antidepressants and stimulants.

MAO is a flavin-containing enzyme located mainly in mitochondrial membranes within cells; it is biochemically dissimilar to a nonspecific amine oxidase found in soluble form in plasma. MAO occurs in close functional association with an aldehyde reductase, the activity of which determines whether the final deaminated product is an alcohol (such as MHPG) or a carboxylic acid (such as VMA, HVA, or 5-HIAA; see Figures 12–15 earlier in this chapter). It is now believed that MAO occurs in biological materials in two major forms, types A and B, the tissue distribution of which varies among species. In man, types A and B are both found in liver and brain; type A is characteristic of gut mucosa and skin fibroblasts; type B is found in blood platelets, which are a convenient tissue with which to assay the degree of MAO inhibition induced by most MAO-inhibitor antidepressants. All three of the currently available agents are more or less nonspecific with respect to types A and B and thus inhibit MAO in all tissues to an approximately similar degree. Although generally nonselective, phenelzine has shown a slight preference for type A substrates of MAO (approximately 6 : 1) in vivo, while tranylcypromine has shown a slight preference (2 : 1) for type B substrates and isocarboxazid has virtually identical affinity for A and B substrates. The salient characteristics of types A and B MAO activity are listed in Table 70.

Table 70   Characteristics of MAO subtypes in human tissues

	Type of MAO activity		
Characteristic	*A*	*A + B*	*B*
Preferred substrates	Norepinephrine, serotonin, octopamine	Dopamine, tyramine, tryptamine	Phenethylamine, benzylamine, N-methylhistamine
Tissues	Nerve terminals, gut mucosa, skin fibroblasts	Liver, CNS	Blood platelets
Preferred inhibitors	Clorgyline, KY-1349, LY-51641[a]	Phenelzine, tranylcypromine, isocarboxazid	(−)deprenyl, AGN-1133, AGN-1135, U-1424 pargyline, norpargyline[a]

Source: Baldessarini, *Psychopharmacol. Bull.* 20:230, 1984, and references therein.
Note: The distribution of types A and B activity varies in other species. The clinically available MAO inhibitors are not specific and inhibit both types of MAO activity in all tissues.
   a. The numbered compounds are experimental agents as yet unnamed.

The three antidepressant MAO inhibitors in current clinical use in the United States are readily absorbed after oral administration and exert maximal inhibition of MAO in animal tissues or in human blood platelets within a few days, although their mood-elevating actions are usually delayed for one to three weeks, as with tricyclic antidepressants. The reversible inhibitor tranylcypromine is more rapidly removed from the enzyme system than the irreversible hydrazide MAO inhibitors, and substantial return of tissue MAO activity can be expected within a week or ten days after tranylcypromine treatment is discontinued. The irreversible inhibitors exert "hit and run" effects in which the drug molecules attach to the enzyme system and exert a persistent inhibition long after the drug itself is no longer detectable in plasma by sensitive assays. Return of MAO activity, accordingly, requires production of new enzyme or cofactor molecules—a process that occurs gradually over a period of about two weeks. Thus, the risk of a drug interaction may persist long after such irreversible inhibitors have been discontinued. A slow return of MAO activity is also characteristic of the irreversible propargyl MAO inhibitors such as pargyline, clorgyline, and deprenyl.

Assays of plasma levels of MAO inhibitors have not been evaluated extensively for their possible clinical correlations, and one would not expect a close relationship given the slow offset of the irreversible inhibitors. On the other hand, the biological actions of MAO inhibitors have been found to provide a useful indication of adequate dosing, at least with phenelzine. Recent studies have found that inhibition of human platelet MAO (B) activity by more than 85% is predictive of a high probability of antidepressant effect with this agent. This degree of inhibition usually requires doses of phenelzine of 45 mg/day or more, and thus the currently recommended upper limit of an effective dose of phenelzine has been increased to 90 mg/day (see Table 69), at least for initial treatment. It is possible to maintain strong inhibition later with smaller doses, or even with intermittent treatment, although precise guidelines concerning such maintenance treatment have not been established and must be determined empirically on a case-by-case basis. If aggressive dosing is employed and treatment is guided by clinical response, it is not necessary to follow MAO activity by routine laboratory testing. On the other hand, increasingly available clinical assays of platelet MAO-B activity can be useful if poor response is found after the use of high doses of phenelzine for several weeks, or if marked intolerance of small doses is encountered. It is not established that platelet MAO assays are helpful in guiding treatment with MAO inhibitors other than phenelzine and perhaps deprenyl, which is selective for the type of MAO activity found in human blood platelets (type B). There is some anecdotal experience to suggest that such assays may be useful in evaluating treatment with isocarboxazid and instances of poor responses to apparently adequate doses of tranylcypromine, although the latter agent may produce strong inhibition of platelet MAO activity in relatively low doses that may not be clinically effective.

The pharmacokinetics and metabolism of MAO inhibitors are not well evaluated. The hydrazide compounds are believed to be cleaved at the hydrazine moiety to liberate pharmacologically active products, which are secondarily modified metabolically, largely by acetylation. About half of the American and European populations are relatively inefficient in carrying out the last step ("slow acetylators"), and even higher proportions of Eskimo and certain Oriental populations are inefficient in acetylating hydrazine derivatives, including phenelzine. Such pharmacogenetic metabolic differences among individuals and races may contribute to exaggerated effects of MAO inhibitors in some patients, although routine laboratory assessment of acetylation capacity has not been proved to be a clinically powerful technique and is not recommended except as a research measurement.

Clinical Use

In controlled trials of the currently available MAO inhibitors, their efficacy generally has been inferior to that of ECT and the tricyclic antidepressants. They produced results significantly better than a placebo in only about 60% of published trials of nialamide and tranylcypromine (see Table 46). Moreover, imipramine or amitriptyline proved to be superior in 40 to 44% of comparisons with MAO inhibitors other than tranylcypromine (Table 47). An exception to these less than compelling results in a mixture of major depressive and dysthymic disorders has been the amphetamine-like nonhydrazine MAO inhibitor tranylcypromine (Parnate), which outperformed a placebo in three of four studies and was found equal to imipramine in antidepressant efficacy in all of three studies (see Tables 46 and 47). In addition, whereas most antidepressants and MAO inhibitors require one to three weeks to produce beneficial effects, tranylcypromine usually acts within a few days, possibly because of its amphetamine-like stimulant actions. The only other MAO inhibitor presently in common use as an antidepressant in this country is phenelzine (Nardil), and in recent trials it has performed about as well as the tricyclics when given at doses above 45 mg/day. Although the MAO inhibitors have not always yielded strong and consistent antidepressant effects, it should also be realized that the tricyclic antidepressants have produced results better than a placebo in only 71% of 93 controlled clinical trials, while ECT has been effective in nearly 90% of its controlled trials (see Table 46).

At present, given their uneven clinical performance and toxicologic complexity, the main indication for the use of MAO inhibitors in major depression is as a second choice of medication when a vigorous trial of a tricyclic or atypical antidepressant has been unsatisfactory or if ECT is not possible or acceptable. This step requires a *delay of at least 7-10 days after stopping the tricyclic agent* to permit its metabolism and excretion in order to avoid the rare but potentially severe interactions with MAO inhibitors. It is often better to hospitalize patients and to add ECT for cases of serious depression responding poorly after several weeks of an adequate dose of a tricyclic agent.

If an MAO inhibitor is to be used, at present tranylcypromine is the most consistently effective antidepressant; it is the most rapid in onset of its clinical effects and termination of its chemical effect. However, it may also be especially toxic on acute overdosage. An additional reason to consider tranylcypromine as an initial therapy for severe depression is that it lacks the severe anticholinergic and potentially cardiotoxic effects of the tricyclic agents; thus it offers a theoretical advantage in elderly patients with heart disease, provided that contact with sympathomimetic agents can be scrupulously avoided and that hypotension does not complicate the treatment. Phenelzine (Nardil) is a reasonable alternative to other antidepressants or ECT in depressed adult patients if it is used in doses of 45 mg/day or more.

Some psychiatrists have claimed, and an increasing number of controlled trials indicate, that there may be special effects of the MAO inhibitors in certain conditions that are not necessarily depressions and are marked by neurotic anxiety and phobia in adults or children, although tricyclic antidepressants may produce similar results. This use of MAO inhibitors in adults is particularly well thought of in England, where MAO inhibitors and tricyclic antidepressants are also sometimes combined. Nevertheless, the routine combination of MAO inhibitors or stimulants with tricyclic antidepressants cannot be recommended as sound practice unless further experimental data become available to support the additional benefits of this approach. The safety of such combinations has been debated repeatedly; the impression remains that the CNS intoxication reactions associated with combinations of a tricyclic antidepressant and

Table 71   Possible indications for antidepressant MAO inhibitors

---

* Acute, primary, major depression (high doses)
* Prevention of early relapse of major depression (long-term use to prevent recurrences is not adequately evaluated, and some tolerance may occur)
* Panic disorder (probably similar in efficacy to imipramine)
* Secondary depressions with other psychiatric or medical disorders (given freedom of risk of interactions with other medications)
* Neurotic dysthymic disorders with anxiety, atypical features, and hysteroid traits that are usually chronic (may be more effective than other agents)
* Posttraumatic neurosis
* Bulimia
* Obsessive-compulsive disorder

The MAO inhibitors may also have beneficial effects in disorders of childhood, including attention deficit disorder with hyperactivity, panic disorder, and other phobic states and also in eating disorders, but are not recommended for routine use in school-age children. For most of the possible indications listed above, the research evidence remains incomplete or fragmentary.

an MAO inhibitor, while rare, can be catastrophic. Similar reactions may also occur when different MAO inhibitors (presumably including those used in general medicine) are combined. A summary of suggested possible indications for antidepressant MAO inhibitors is provided in Table 71.

Toxic Effects

When MAO inhibitors are used clinically, both minor and serious toxic effects may be encountered. Hypotensive effects, usually *orthostatic hypotension,* are sometimes a troublesome problem; they may result from gradual accumulation in sympathetic nerve endings of amines lacking direct sympathomimetic activity, at the expense of the normal synaptic transmitter, norepinephrine ("false transmitter" hypothesis). The hypotensive effects of MAO inhibitors have been applied to the treatment of moderate hypertension, for example with pargyline (Eutonyl), although the main effect is to induce orthostatic hypotension rather than sustained reduction of diastolic pressure. Hypotension is the most common potentially serious side effect of MAO inhibitors and may be worrisome in patients at high risk of heart attack, stroke, or fractures. The diminution of sympathetically regulated arteriolar tone may also contribute to the reported antianginal effects of some MAO inhibitors. The orthostatic hypotension associated with these agents can sometimes be minimized by increasing dosage slowly. Although various steroid compounds have been proposed to counteract these hypotensive effects, as with the tricyclic antidepressants, they are not commonly used and are not recommended.

In general, MAO inhibitors have little anticholinergic activity in laboratory test systems. This also appears to be the case clinically with tranylcypromine. Curiously, there have been frequent instances (> 20%) of *apparently "anticholinergic" effects* of phenelzine (especially when given at high doses), such as dry mouth, constipation, urinary retention, and sexual dysfunction (impotence and orgasmic dysfunction). Since all of these functions represent a physiological balance between cholinergic and sympathetic autonomic functions, similar symptoms may result either from a deficiency of vagal, pelvic, and other muscarinic parasympathetic functions or from an excess of adrenergic, sympathetic function.

Severe *parenchymal hepatotoxic reactions* occur infrequently and are usually much more serious than the biliary stasis associated with antipsychotic and tricyclic antidepressant agents. This toxicity is serious enough to justify frequent (perhaps weekly initially) determinations of serum bilirubin and transaminase activities and to contraindicate the use of MAO inhibitors in patients with chronic liver disease. For such patients, small doses of a tricyclic antidepressant can be given cautiously, or ECT can be considered.

Manifestations of *CNS toxicity* include agitation, insomnia, and toxic psychoses, as well as provocation of previously quiescent functional psychoses. Severe CNS intoxication with excitement and seizures is a regular feature of acute overdoses of MAO inhibitors, which can be lethal in acute overdoses equivalent to about a week's supply. Rapid discontinuation of high doses of an MAO inhibitor has been associated with withdrawal reactions, including acute psychosis. Severe CNS reactions can also occur as part of several drug interactions with MAO inhibitors, described later in this section.

The most serious toxic effect of the MAO inhibitors (perhaps especially with tranylcypromine) is their ability to provoke *acute hypertensive crises,* typically associated with severe, throbbing headache and sometimes with intracranial bleeding and collapse. These severe and potentially damaging or fatal reactions are fortunately infrequent, and can largely be prevented by scrupulous avoidance of medications, foods, and beverages containing appreciable quantities of sympathomimetic amines and other pressor agents. This reaction has been associated classically with *tyramine,* a natural pressor amine by-product of bacterial fermentation found in many foods, such as well-ripened cheeses ("cheese reaction"). A list of

Table 72 Foods and beverages containing tyramine or other pressor agents potentiated by MAO inhibitors

Source	Content	Source	Content
Cheeses and dairy products		*Meat or yeast products*	
Liederkranz	+++++	Yeast products (Bovril, Oxo, Marmite, dietary supplements containing brewer's yeast)	++++
Argenti	++++		
Blue	++++		
Boursault	++++	Fermented sausages (bologna, pepperoni, salami, summer sausage)	++++
Brick	++++		
Brie	++++	Caviar	++++
Camembert	++++	Pickled herring	++++
Cheddars	++++	Liver, meat, or fish products if unrefrigerated, preserved, or spoiled	++++
D'Oka	++++		
Edam	++++	Snails (preserved)	++
Gruyère	++++		
Romano	++++	*Fruits and vegetables*	
Stilton	++++	Avocado (esp. overripe; guacamole)	++
Swiss	++++	Fava (broad) bean pods	++
Tulum	++++	Figs (overripe, canned, spoiled)	++
Gouda	+++	Raisins	+
Limberger	+++	Banana peel (less in pulp)	+
Mozzarella	+++	New Zealand spinach	+
Parmesan	+++	Sauerkraut	+
American processed	++		
Sour cream	+	*Beverages*	
Yogurt	+	Chianti wine	++
Cottage cheese	+/0	Red wines (variable)	+
Cream cheese	+/0	Sherries, liqueurs (variable)	+
		White wines	0/+
Miscellaneous		Distilled spirits	0
Chocolate (large amounts)	+	Caffeinated beverages (coffee, tea, cola, cocoa, in large amounts)	+
Soy sauce	+		
Cyclamate sweeteners	+		

The crucial active agent in most of the above sources is tyramine, a product of bacterial fermentation, or other related sympathomimetic amines. Broad bean pods contain dopa or dopamine; chocolate contains traces of phenethylamine. Rare reactions have been associated with soy sauces, possibly due to sodium glutamate, and with the use of cyclamate-containing artificial sweeteners. The ratings from 0 to 5+ indicate approximate levels of pressor, although these vary markedly among samples so that effects are unpredictable, as patients tempted to cheat on their diets should be warned. Sources with low concentrations do not present a high risk of hypertensive crisis if taken in small amounts. Hypertensive reactions can be expected if 10 mg of tyramine or more is ingested in the presence of an MAO inhibitor. Liederkranz cheese, an unusually rich source of tyramine, is reported to contain 1.5 mg/g; other cheeses have levels of about 0.2 mg/g. Thus, an ounce of cheese (28.4 g) may contain about 6 mg of tyramine, so as little as 2 ounces could be dangerous. The most likely sources of pressor substances are the highly ripened, veined, or triple-cream cheeses and foods prepared from them (such as fondue or pizza). Patients receiving an MAO inhibitor should be given a list such as this one, as well as a list of medications to avoid.

food products to be avoided by patients taking an agent with MAO-inhibiting activity is provided in Table 72. Other aromatic amines can induce a similar response as a result of their ability to release norepinephrine from sympathetic nerve terminals. These indirectly sympathomimetic amines are usually cleared from the portal blood by the liver, but they are not inactivated by deamination when MAO is inhibited and thus are more available to act systemically. Possibly an even more important mechanism is the buildup of norepinephrine in sympathetic nerve terminals following inhibition of MAO, especially of type A. Accordingly, inhibitors of type B (such as deprenyl) are less likely to potentiate tyramine since they have much less effect on the metabolism of norepinephrine than of tyramine.

In addition to foods containing tyramine-like pressor amines, a large number of prescription drugs and over-the-counter proprietary medications contain *sympathomimetic agents* or other compounds that can induce hypertensive and other reactions in the presence of an MAO inhibitor. Medications to be avoided or used cautiously include the amphetamines and other sympathomimetic phenylalkylamines: Benzedrine, Dexedrine, methamphetamine (Desoxyn), ephedrine, pseudoephedrine, norephedrine, oxymetazoline (Afrin), and phenylephrine (Neo-synephrine), some of which occur in proprietary cold and sinus medications and decongestant inhalers. Because L-dopa and alpha-methyldopa (Aldomet) are converted metabolically to sympathomimetic amines, they should also be avoided. Patients with pheochromocytoma (catecholamines in excess) or carcinoid syndrome (excessive production of serotonin) should not receive an MAO inhibitor (and toxic reactions have been encountered in patients with hyperthyroidism as well). Moreover, the combination of an MAO inhibitor with reserpine, guanethidine, or other agents with acute amine-releasing effects can also induce paradoxical hypertensive reactions and CNS excitation. If such a hypertensive reaction is encountered, the specific treatment is immediate, but slow, intravenous injection of a potent alpha-adrenergic blocking agent, such as *phentolamine* (Regitine) in doses of 5 mg, as needed. In an emergency, if a specific adrenergic blocking agent is not at hand, parenteral injections of chlorpromazine (Thorazine), 50 to 100 mg intramuscularly, can be used while appropriate medical treatment is arranged.

MAO inhibitors also produce unwanted *interactions with other medications* (Table 73). They potentiate many central depressants, including the barbiturates, benzodiazepines and other sedatives, phenothiazines, antihistamines, opioid analgesics, and alcohol. Meperidine (Demerol) in

Table 73 Partial list of drugs that may interact with MAO inhibitors

Agent	Effect
Sympathomimetics	
d- and d,l-amphetamine, methamphetamine, ephedrine, pseudoephedrine, norephedrine, oxymetazoline, phenylephrine, tranylcypromine, all catecholamines (including epinephrine or other vasoconstrictors added to procaine), L-dopa, foods or beverages containing pressor substances (see Table 72), and possibly serotonin and its precursor amino acids	Potentiation, excess CNS stimulation or intoxication, hypertension with organ damage or intracranial hemorrhage
Central depressants	
General anesthetics, alcohol, antihistamines, barbiturates, nonbarbiturate sedatives, benzodiazepines, neuroleptics, anticonvulsants, narcotics (except meperidine)	Potentiation, excessive CNS depression or intoxication; may also diminish MAO inhibition by hepatic induction
Analgesics	
Meperidine	Hyperpyrexia, seizures, coma.
Aspirin	May induce hypertension(?)
Antiparkinsonism agents and anticholinergics	
All anticholinergic antiparkinsonism agents, atropine, scopolamine	Potentiate, atropinic intoxication syndrome; may decrease metabolism of MAO inhibitor (?)
L-dopa	Potentiate; unpredictable changes in blood pressure; may induce CNS excitation or intoxication
Antihypertensive agents	
Reserpine (and congeners), alpha-methyldopa, guanethidine	When added to an MAO inhibitor can induce acute paradoxical hypertension and CNS excitation; unpredictable
Bethanidine, debrisoquin	Potentiate (not known to have acute pressor response as with guanethidine)
Clonidine	May potentiate
Hydralazine	Potentiate
Salt-losing diuretics	Hypotension

Table 73 (continued)

Agent	Effect
Other antidepressants and MAO inhibitors	
Imipramine and all typical tricyclic antide-pressants (and possibly carbamazepine and cyclobenzaprine); all antidepressant MAO inhibitors, pargyline, nitrofuran antibiotics, and procarbazine (or other agents with MAO inhibitory activity)	Additive toxicity; unpredictable hypertension or hypotension; may induce rare but cata-strophic CNS excitation, seizures, hyper-pyrexia of unknown cause (not due to pres-sor amines)
Sympathetic receptor-blocking agents	
Alpha-antagonists	May potentiate
Beta-blockers	Unpredictable: may antagonize early and po-tentiate later
Antidiabetic agents	
Insulin, oral hypoglycemics	Potentiate
Anticoagulants	
Coumarins and indanediones	May potentiate (?)

Source: Baldessarini, in *Goodman and Gilman's The Pharmacological Basis of Therapeutics,* 7th ed., ed. A. G. Gilman, L. Goodman, and A. Gilman (New York, Macmillan, 1985), and references therein.

particular has been associated with severe reactions that are not well understood pharmacologically; these include states characterized by ex-treme excitement, seizures, and fever, as well as reactions resembling overdoses of a narcotic, and even coma. Narcotics should never be used for headache in patients taking an MAO inhibitor, and the headache requires immediate evaluation of blood pressure.

The use of MAO inhibitors requires particular caution in the manage-ment of surgical anesthesia, since complex and unpredictable changes in cardiovascular function and interactions with other agents present un-wanted risks. An MAO inhibitor should be discontinued for at least several days prior to elective surgery or ECT. Even in minor surgery or dental procedures, local anesthetic preparations (for example, procaine; Novocaine) often contain epinephrine to provide local vasoconstriction, but are capable of inducing excessive systemic sympathomimetic actions when given with an MAO inhibitor.

The combination of an *MAO inhibitor and a tricyclic antidepressant* can, as mentioned earlier, rarely induce severe reactions of unknown cause, including central excitation, seizures, hyperpyrexia, variable

changes in blood pressure, and sometimes death, especially when parenteral or high doses of the tricyclic agents are used. This reaction has been
reported most frequently in association with tranylcypromine, but any
MAO inhibitor combined with any tricyclic-type antidepressant should
be suspect. The infrequency of such reactions (less than 0.1%) makes it
difficult to assess risks of specific combinations of agents. Although the
cause of this potentially catastrophic reaction is not known, it is almost
certainly *not* similar to the hypertensive reaction to sympathomimetic
agents during treatment with an MAO inhibitor. Indeed, there is good
evidence that tricyclic antidepressants with potent blocking effects on the
uptake of amines into sympathetic nerve terminals can actually *reduce*
the pressor effects of tyramine infusions in man (Table 74). Reactions
similar to those between an MAO inhibitor and a tricyclic antidepressant
may also occur between different MAO inhibitors, so it is good practice to
wait two weeks between discontinuing an MAO inhibitor and adding any
other agent with MAO-inhibiting activity (including those used in general
medicine; see Table 69) or any typical tricyclic-type antidepressant. The
risk of such interactions with newer, atypical antidepressants such as
trazodone, alprazolam, and others is unknown. Since bupropion and
nomifensine or their metabolites may block uptake of catecholamines,
they should be used with extra caution in combination with an MAO
inhibitor. Tricyclic agents with high potency and selectivity against the
uptake of norepinephrine may also present a risk of inducing hypertensive reactions when combined with an MAO inhibitor.

Potentiation of anticholinergic or antiparkinsonism agents, oral hy-

*Table 74 Effects of tricyclic antidepressants and MAO inhibitors on pressor
responses to tyramine infusion*

Subjects	Tyramine pressor dose (mg)
Normal controls	3.6
Untreated major depression	3.4
MAO inhibitor alone	0.3
Amitriptyline + MAO inhibitor	3.0
Trimipramine + MAO inhibitor	0.8

Source: Klein et al., *J. Clin. Psychopharmacol.* 2:434, 1982. Data are for 3 to 5 human
subjects per condition, given sufficient tyramine intravenously to elevate systolic blood
pressure by 30 mm. MAO inhibitors were phenelzine or tranylcypromine given to depressed
patients in clinical doses. Compare these results with the potency of amitriptyline vs. trimipramine against the uptake of norepinephrine in Table 43 ($IC_{50} = 50$ vs. 1,875 nM), which
documents the relatively weak action of trimipramine.

poglycemics, thyroid hormones, and insulin by MAO inhibitors can also be anticipated. MAO inhibitors in combination with salt-losing diuretic agents have induced severe hypotension. These varied and complex interactions of drugs with MAO inhibitors are summarized in Table 73. Because of the potentially severe reactions that may be encountered, it is good practice to provide patients not only with lists of foods and drugs to avoid while taking an MAO inhibitor, but also with some means of identification, such as a card or bracelet, indicating their use of an MAO inhibitor in case they should require emergency medical or surgical treatment or be found in an unconscious state.

CNS Stimulants

Stimulant drugs, and especially the amphetamines, were formerly used in the attempt to treat depression, often in combination with a barbiturate for anxiety and agitation. They are still occasionally employed for the short-term management of mild depression but are not recommended for routine use in the treatment of major depression because of their limited efficacy and the risk of increasing agitation and somatic symptoms of major depression, including insomnia and anorexia. Small doses of amphetamines or methylphenidate are sometimes given cautiously to elderly or demented patients in an effort to combat withdrawal and apathy, but again, risks of excessive stimulation, insomnia, and anorexia have discouraged this practice. A possibly related group of agents have also been used in elderly, withdrawn, and mildly demented patients in an effort to improve their functioning. These include agents with smooth muscle relaxing effects (such as papaverine), as well as ergolines such as Hydergine (with possible stimulant-like effects), and experimental peptides (such as fragments of ACTH). While there is much interest in such "anti-dementia" agents in Europe and other areas, they do not have an important place in current neuropsychiatric practice in the United States, although they are of research interest. These agents are discussed further in Chapter 6.

Stimulant agents continue to have a role in the treatment of *narcolepsy* and related disorders of the sleep-waking cycle and are still occasionally used in weight loss programs, for which their efficacy is doubtful. They do have anorexic and mood-elevating effects that may be useful temporarily in the management of obesity, but these effects typically are lost rapidly with tolerance.

The most important role of stimulants at the present time in the United

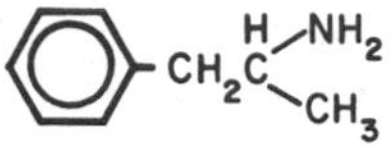

Amphetamine (Benzedrine, Dexedrine)

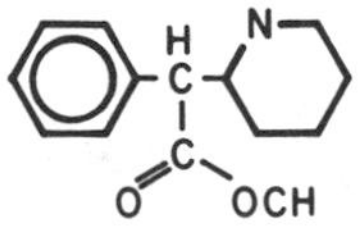

Methylphenidate (Ritalin)

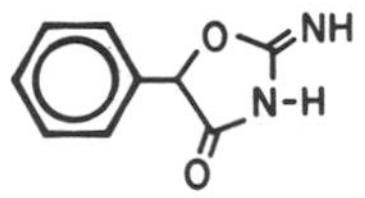

Pemoline (Cylert)

Figure 17   Chemical structures of stimulants.

States is in the treatment of *attention deficit disorder with hyperactivity* in children (hyperactivity syndrome, "minimal brain dysfunction" syndrome). The possible utility of imipramine and other tricyclic antidepressants for this disorder was discussed earlier in this chapter. Of the stimulants used in this pediatric syndrome, d-amphetamine, methylphenidate, and pemoline are most commonly employed (Figure 17; Table 75).

Table 75   Stimulants: Preparations and doses

Agent	Trade name	Dosage form	Dose range (mg/day)	
			Usual	Extreme
d-Amphetamine	Dexedrine (and generic)	(T) 5 mg (SR-T) 5, 10, 15 mg (S) 5 mg/5 ml	10–30	2.5–60
Methylphenidate	Ritalin	(T) 5, 10, 20 mg (SR-T) 20 mg	20–30	10–60
Pemoline	Cylert	(T) 18.75, 37.5, 75 mg	56.25–75	37.5–112.5

Dosage forms: tablets (T), sustained release tablets (SR-T), and soluble elixir (S).

The stimulant agents are rapidly absorbed after oral administration and are not given parenterally. They have relatively short half-lives of elimination, of about 8 to 12 hours, and so are given two or three times per day (with attention given to minimizing their anorexic and sleep-reducing effects). Typical clinically attained plasma levels of amphetamine have been reported to be about 10–20 ng/ml, but are not used to guide treatment. The amphetamines are converted to products oxidized and conjugated by hepatic enzymes but partially excreted unchanged by a process dependent on urinary acidity (acid urine increases excretion). Methylphenidate is converted mainly to the carboxylic acid derivative of its side-chain, again by hepatic microsomal mechanisms. Pemoline is about 60% converted to inactive conjugates, oxidized (dione) products, and mandelic acid, and 40% excreted in unchanged form. The ability of stimulants to compete for hepatic enzymes can reduce the metabolism of antidepressants, neuroleptics, and many other drugs.

The actions of the commonly used stimulants include activation of the brainstem reticular activating system to induce cerebral stimulation and arousal. These effects are due in part to the ability of stimulants to diminish the inactivation of norepinephrine by neuronal uptake—a property shared with the typical tricyclic antidepressants. In addition, however, the stimulants block uptake of dopamine and may thus increase arousal through forebrain mechanisms that include stimulation of dopaminergic circuits between midbrain and the subcortical and cortical portions of the limbic system. Similar noradrenergic and dopaminergic mechanisms may contribute to the effects of stimulants on sleep, while potentiation of catecholamine activity in the hypothalamus may contribute to their appetite-suppressing effects. It has been suggested that the effects of stimulants in the hyperactivity syndrome of children may represent a paradoxical form of sedation or behavioral inhibition, possibly uniquely in persons with an underlying brain dysfunction. This view is currently in great doubt, however, partly because of observations of similar, if milder, actions in children who are neurologically and behaviorally normal, as well as actions that include increased arousal, attention, and selective inhibition of irrelevant behaviors rather than sedation. It is a plausible hypothesis that stimulants may act by exerting maximal function from cortical and other higher centers of the brain, and that these effects may be most noticeable clinically in persons with an immature or mildly dysfunctional central nervous system.

Many of the effects of stimulants are relatively short-lived, including euphoria and decreased sleep and appetite. Children sometimes experience dysphoria with stimulants. Although physiological dependence on the stimulants similar to that of other habituating substances has not been demonstrated, they have been popular substances of abuse and are produced in quantities that far exceed their legitimate medical uses. (Methylphenidate and pemoline are evidently less commonly abused than amphetamines.) In the abuse state, tolerance to euphoriant effects develops rapidly and tolerance to many of the sympathomimetic and other effects of these agents is common, permitting consumption of high doses that might otherwise be highly toxic or lethal. Rapid withdrawal, especially of high doses and after severe abuse, can lead to profound inertia and depression of mood ("crashing"). In this sense a state of physiological dependence is apparent, although agitation, nausea, pain, seizures, and delirium typical of withdrawal from opioids or sedatives do not occur. Psychosis may occur after severe abuse, or in some susceptible persons after clinical doses. Effects that can be ascribed to extrapyramidal dopaminergic stimulation, including tics and behaviors similar to those in Gilles de la Tourette's syndrome, have been reported infrequently among children given stimulants for hyperactivity.

Acute overdoses of 10 days' supply of most stimulants are likely to be very toxic and possibly lethal, particularly in children. Acute intoxication includes profound overstimulation of the sympathetic and central nervous systems, which is usually short-lasting. The management of acute intoxication sometimes includes use of a neuroleptic or benzodiazepine. Theoretically, acidification of the urine as well as dialysis should be effective, but these measures have not been evaluated systematically.

A remarkable feature of the clinical actions of the stimulants is that their beneficial effects in attention deficit disorder with hyperactivity not only appear almost immediately, but are usually sustained with little evidence of tolerance over months or even years of continued treatment. There is some risk of inducing insomnia in children, and there has been much concern that the anorexic effects of stimulants might retard growth and development. Minor, and usually temporary, slowing of development can occur and requires monitoring, but clinically significant changes are unlikely. The use of amphetamines and other stimulants for children has been controversial, however, partly because of the notoriety surrounding the amphetamines as common drugs of abuse as well as concern about the side effects of stimulants. The evidence and clinical experience concerning the efficacy of pemoline for treating hyperactivity in children are somewhat less secure than with d-amphetamine and methylphenidate.

The use of stimulants is considered only one part of the comprehensive clinical management of children with attention deficit disorder. There is currently much interest in knowing the long-term outcome of cases of attention deficit disorder, and in considering the possible utility of stimulant or antidepressant agents in adults who had this disorder as children. There is an emerging impression that some such persons continue to manifest attention deficits as adults or may show antisocial or dysthymic characteristics that sometimes respond to treatment with a stimulant or an antidepressant.

Alternative and Experimental Treatments
Problems in the Development of Improved Antidepressant Treatments

The existing antidepressants have serious limitations in terms of both efficacy and safety, as well as a slow onset of action. Even given classic cases of major depression with melancholic features and adequate doses of an effective antidepressant for more than one month, as many as 20–30% of patients respond unsatisfactorily. The problem of clinical management of treatment-refractory patients in psychiatric referral settings is becoming even greater as a higher proportion of poorly responsive, relapsing, or chronically ill patients is encountered. One recent survey found that between one-quarter and one-third of patients with major depression treated in university-affiliated general hospital psychiatric services in the United States went on to a course of chronic illness, usually incompletely responsive to medical treatment (Keller et al., 1984). In part, this pattern may reflect the partial success of antidepressants since many relatively straightforward, medically responsive cases of major depression are treated adequately in general medical settings by physicians without specialized training in psychiatry. At the same time, medically treatable major depression continues to be underdiagnosed and often not treated or undertreated, partly because of inadequate psychiatric training of many physicians and surgeons, and partly because of widespread professional and public misconceptions and prejudices concerning psychiatric disorders.

Another feature of the partial success of existing antidepressant treatments is that the existence of even an imperfect treatment makes it difficult to develop and test potentially improved new treatments. This problem is especially noticeable in the evaluation of new treatments for severely depressed, and especially hospitalized, patients; ethical issues arise in proposals such as withholding an available treatment for the purposes of evaluation, or assigning a patient to an inactive placebo or a novel treatment. These issues remain unresolved, much to the consternation of clinicians, investigators, regulatory agencies, and the pharmaceutical industry. As the requirements to demonstrate the efficacy and safety of new pharmacologic treatments have been increasing in the past decades, the availability of appropriate patients for experimental therapeutic studies has been falling. The result is that many studies rely on patient populations that contain many persons with atypical, chronic, or even relatively mild illnesses, who are sometimes acquired through advertising and often treated in ambulatory settings.

Partly in response to these ethical issues, experimental protocols now often do not include a placebo condition, but typically compare a standard treatment with a novel agent or method. Unless the test population is well characterized and the prognosis clearly defined in advance, such protocols risk producing results indicating that the old and new treatments seem similar in efficacy, even though "not different from" is not equivalent statistically to "as good as." Rarely do studies reveal that a new agent provides clearly superior results to a standard agent. Given the relatively high probability of spontaneous or placebo-associated remission in major depression and allied conditions, and the past history of uneven performance of standard agents against a placebo (see Tables 46 and 47), it does not seem reasonable to rely heavily on "treatment A versus treatment B" designs unless a placebo condition is also included.

It has been argued by some biostatisticians that the total morbidity present in an experimental therapeutic trial lacking a placebo condition is often much greater than when a placebo condition is included. This conclusion follows from considerations of the power of the experimental protocol to detect changes or differences. Increasing the contrast between the test and control groups or conditions (such as new agent versus placebo) generally *reduces* the number of subjects required as well as the length of time of assessment — both of which tend to minimize the total morbidity to be endured by the test population, as well as yielding the least ambiguous results. As a result of these problems, the efficacy of newer antidepressants tends to be less secure than that of older agents, especially regarding treatment of severely depressed hospitalized patients.

An additional problem is that the sketchy knowledge of the pathophysiology of major depression and the lack of a coherent theory of its etiology, or of the necessary and sufficient actions of antidepressants, have fostered remarkable conservatism in the development of new treatments. Most of the agents recently introduced into medical practice in the United States, following a long period of little innovation, are already well known in other countries or are remarkably similar pharmacologically to older agents. Most have exploited catecholamine-potentiating screening tests as a prerequisite for consideration and thus have led to a growing list of "me-too" agents. Important gains have been made, however, especially in regard to the toxicity of antidepressants. Some of the newer, atypical antidepressants, many of which remain experimental in this country, lack the sympathomimetic and anticholinergic toxicity of older drugs as well as their high risk of lethality on acute overdose. Nevertheless, their efficacy, especially in severe, classic, major melancholic depression, is generally less well supported than that of the older agents, and they often present trade-offs of lesser toxicity of one type for more of another.

Use of Adjunctive Medications in Treatment-Refractory Depression

When a well-established antidepressant has been tried in adequate doses for more than a month, perhaps with confirmatory blood assays to ensure an approximately adequate dose and adherence with the treatment program, it is not highly likely that trials of additional agents will bring success, although it is reasonable to try several dissimilar agents serially and with increasing doses based on individual tolerance. Given a continued poor outcome, and especially with severe melancholic depression, a trial of ECT is often a reasonable next choice. However, ECT is not always readily acceptable to patients or physicians, despite its proven superiority to all other medical treatments of major melancholic depression and its relative ease and safety with modern improvements.

Because of these difficulties in treating a substantial minority of depressed patients, a number of innovative or experimental proposals have been made to try to improve the rate of success. Many of these newer approaches include adding other agents to an antidepressant. One such proposal was to add a stimulant, such as *methylphenidate,* for early and additional stimulant effects, and to increase plasma levels of the antidepressant by competition for hepatic microsomal enzymes. This tactic has not been widely accepted, and it is doubtful that it is more effective than simply increasing the dose of the primary antidepressant. It may also increase the risk of hypertensive and other toxic reactions.

Thyroid status may alter responses to antidepressants, and it is usual practice to evaluate thyroid function as part of an initial comprehensive evaluation of a patient with major depression (in part to test for rare cases of hypothyroidism that may present with some resemblance to clinical depression), or at least if treatment response has been inadequate after a month or more of apparently adequate treatment. There have been repeated suggestions that adding small doses of thyroid hormones (such as 25–50 μg of *l-triiodothyronine* [Cytomel] daily) may increase the efficacy or speed of onset of effects of imipramine or other typical antidepressants, even in a patient who is physiologically euthyroid. The evidence for this phenomenon is uneven and appears to be best supported with respect to the rate of onset of clinical benefit in middle-aged female patients, although there is also some evidence that adding thyroid hormone can increase efficacy later in an unsuccessful course of antidepressant treatment. There is probably some risk in aggressive use of thyroid supplements, especially with respect to cardiovascular toxicity in patients at high risk, such as the elderly or those with cardiac disease. Evidence that thyroid-stimulating hormone (TSH) or thyrotropin-releasing hormone (TRH) given by intravenous infusion may have mood-elevating effects is suggestive and intriguing, but tentative.

Other endocrine strategies are only beginning to be considered. It is unclear whether the evident overactivity of the hypothalamic-pituitary-adrenal axis and the high output of corticosteroids in major depression are merely manifestations of pathophysiology or an indication of attempts to restore homeostasis that might be exploited pharmacologically. For example, the effect of exogenous steroid molecules in depression is unclear, especially since the treatment of medical illnesses with cortisone or prednisone, as well as the use of antifertility steroids, has led, unpredictably, to depression as well as euphoria. There is some evidence that fragments of the ACTH molecule may have central neuropharmacologic effects that might be worthy of further exploration, and some years ago there were reports that very high doses of estrogen steroids might have antidepressant effects in some otherwise treatment-unresponsive women.

Another tactic has been to combine dissimilar antidepressants. Most commonly, an *MAO inhibitor and a typical tricyclic agent* have been combined—a practice that is common in some countries, but generally regarded with skepticism in the United States. A usual pattern of treatment is to try a typical tricyclic agent first for at least a month or six weeks, with increasing doses according to the patient's clinical tolerance, and possibly with confirmatory plasma assays of drug concentration. If the response remains unsatisfactory, one can discontinue the tricyclic antidepressant in diminishing doses over several days, and then wait for at least a week or ten days before introducing an MAO inhibitor. The cycle is then repeated with gradually increasing doses of the MAO inhibitor, perhaps with a confirmatory assay of platelet MAO activity before and during treatment to assess the degree of enzyme inhibition. If this treatment is unsuccessful after another month, the dose of MAO inhibitor can be reduced somewhat and a tricyclic antidepressant added cautiously, starting with very *small, divided doses.* The dose can then be increased every two or three days, with careful monitoring of the patient's cardiovascular and mental status, ideally at first in an inpatient setting. Although it is reasonably certain at present that such combinations are rarely severely toxic, it is not clear that this treatment results consistently in substantial gains over aggressive use of either agent alone, including doses above those usually recommended. There are anecdotal reports of gains with such combination therapy, but these, like many uncontrolled experiences with innovative treatments of affective disorders, are difficult to interpret: some may represent more aggressive use of the medications, the nonspecific benefits of embarking on an unusual and potentially dangerous course or of added psychological support or hospitalization, or the mere passage of time in which spontaneous remission is more probable. Since the evidence of therapeutic gain is limited and the risks small but potentially catastrophic, this treatment approach cannot be recommended unless other more conventional alternatives have been exhausted. There is no rationale for combining like agents, such as two tricyclic antidepressants or two MAO inhibitors, and the latter may present risks similar to those of combinations across classes of drugs. Additional investigation of the efficacy and safety of combining an *atypical* antidepressant with a tricyclic agent or an MAO inhibitor may be in order.

One combination of mood-altering or thymoleptic substances that is worth considering is that of an antidepressant of any type with a *lithium salt.* The possible beneficial effects of lithium on nonbipolar as well as bipolar depression were discussed in Chapter 3. There is growing evidence that some treatment-refractory cases of major depression have benefited from the addition of lithium, especially when combined with a typical tricyclic antidepressant. Again, questions concerning nonspecific factors and the passage of time in these results remain to be addressed in appropriate prospective, controlled trials.

A final combination therapy that has been investigated for years in Europe is the addition of an *aromatic amino acid* in high doses to another agent, usually an MAO inhibitor. There is also some experience with the use of such compounds alone, although the evidence for a clear antidepressant effect of L-tryptophan, L-5-hydroxytryptophan (5-HTP), L-dihydroxyphenylalanine (dopa), or L-tyrosine alone is weak. This approach has been strongly stimulated by the success of L-dopa as a precursor of dopamine in the treatment of Parkinson's disease. L-dopa itself is probably ineffective in major depression, although it has been reported to have some stimulant-like effects and may induce mania or psychosis in high doses. Although it has been believed that tyrosine hydroxylase is normally saturated with its substrate, L-tyrosine, some recent findings suggest that large amounts of tyrosine might increase the rate of production or turnover of catecholamines in mammalian brain, especially under conditions of increased demand or turnover. To date, however, results of attempts to employ large doses of tyrosine as an antidepressant remain highly preliminary and uncertain.

A larger number of studies have involved the use of L-tryptophan, and a few have evaluated 5-hydroxytryptophan, either alone or in combination with an MAO inhibitor or tricyclic antidepressant to treat depression. A recent review of these efforts with tryptophan is representative; a summary of its results is provided in Table 76. Doses of tryptophan were typically 3 – 10 grams/day. The trials are highly variable in scientific quality; most lacked a placebo control condition and, as one might predict, led to many results "no worse than" an alternative treatment, but not necessarily better. For example, tryptophan was reported to be similar in apparent efficacy to a standard tricyclic antidepressant in 9/11 trials (82%) and apparently to potentiate a tricyclic or MAO inhibitor antidepressant in only 8/14 studies (57%). As has been found with most pharmacologic therapies of major depression, tryptophan was not better than ECT in any of 6 trials. A critical analysis, however, is not supportive of an antidepressant effect of tryptophan. Thus, when the amino acid was used alone it was claimed to be effective in only 4/12 trials (33%) and among only 48/146 patients (35%), or at rates similar to those expected with an inactive placebo. Worse yet, none of only five available placebo-controlled trials found tryptophan better than a placebo. The doses of tryptophan employed were apparently sufficient to alter indoleamine metabolism, since CSF levels of 5-HIAA were increased when it was measured. The results of combining tryptophan with an MAO inhibitor emerge as the most encouraging, in that 4/5 (80%) of such trials found added benefits from the combination over those of the MAO inhibitor alone. The apparent safety of this combination is also encouraging; toxic effects in the reported studies have been few and usually mild. Mild gastrointestinal symptoms, nausea, headache, and some sedation were the most common problems. In contrast, side effects common to traditional antidepressant

Table 76 Effects of tryptophan in depression

Clinical effect	Studies (N)
Antidepressant effect of tryptophan alone	
Efficacy claimed	4
Not effective	8
Potentiation of MAO inhibitor	
Combination claimed superior	4
Results similar to MAO inhibitor alone	1
Tryptophan vs. ECT	
Similar to ECT	4
ECT superior	2
Tryptophan vs. tricyclic antidepressant	
Similar to tricyclic antidepressant	9
Tricyclic antidepressant superior	2
Potentiation of tricyclic antidepressant	
Combination claimed superior	4
Results similar to antidepressant alone	5

Source: Baldessarini, *Psychopharmacol. Bull.* 20:224, 1984, and references therein.
Note: Only 5/12 of the studies of the amino acid alone included a placebo control, and none found the experimental agent more effective. Most studies of tricyclic antidepressants employed imipramine, amitriptyline, or clomipramine. The most encouraging results were with the combination of tryptophan with an MAO inhibitor.

therapy, such as postural hypotension, anticholinergic effects, confusion, and impaired cardiac conduction, were rare. High doses of tryptophan have occasionally been associated with tremor or myoclonic seizures. It is not clear whether there is commercial interest in exploring such combinations further, since tryptophan is an inexpensive and readily available natural product.

An increasing number of studies have investigated 5-hydroxytryptophan as an alternative to tryptophan as a precursor of serotonin. The results are mixed, since only 5/12 studies (58%) found favorable results in 289/547 (53%) of patients with 5-hydroxytryptophan as a primary treatment of major depression (Baldessarini, 1984). These results are tantalizing, but not striking. Several reports of combinations of 5-hydroxytryptophan with an MAO inhibitor or clomipramine, a selective inhibitor of the uptake of serotonin, are also encouraging. Doses of the indoleamino acid have usually ranged from 50 to 500 mg/day; the lower doses were made possible by the addition of an inhibitor of peripheral decarboxylation outside the central nervous system (such as carbidopa or benserazide, which have also been combined with L-dopa to reduce the total daily dose for patients with Parkinson's disease). While 5-HIAA levels in the CSF were increased by such doses of 5-hydroxytryptophan, there have also been metabolic findings that suggest catecholamines may be released by this treatment. The side effects and toxicity of such treatment appear to be more frequent and severe than those reported with tryptophan, especially signs of cerebral intoxication with nausea, tremor, ataxia, dysarthria, and confusion. Hypotension has been infrequent. Some of these side effects may result from local gastrointestinal or other peripheral reactions and might be minimized by use of a peripheral decarboxylase inhibitor, the more soluble methyl ester of the amino acid, or with alternative pharmaceutical preparations of the large amounts of amino acid required. There are also anecdotal reports that the indoleamino acids are unlikely to induce mania (the "switch process"), and suggestions that they may have mood-stabilizing effects in patients with bipolar affective disorders. These results are intriguing and deserve further study, but all such combinations of amino acids with other antidepressants, or their use alone to treat depression, are considered experimental even though they involve use of natural or dietary products.

Experimental Antidepressant Treatments

It has been mentioned that the U.S. Food and Drug Administration and American pharmaceutical manufacturers have been slow to accept new antidepressant agents in common use in other countries. While many of these agents are similar pharmacologically to typical tricyclic-type antidepressants, some have unique or interesting features and several are under active clinical investigation in the United States. *Clomipramine* (Anafranil) has been in common clinical use for years in many countries, including Mexico and Canada. Although it has many features of imipramine-like agents, its reported special efficacy in obsessive-compulsive disorder is potentially important since the treatment of this sometimes severely disabling and baffling disorder remains unsatisfactory. Clomipramine is also unusual in having a strong preference to block the uptake of serotonin rather than norepinephrine (see Table 43). Other agents with similar pharmacologic properties have been developed more recently. These include *fluoxetine* and its congeners as well as *citalopram* and *zimelidine,* which are relatively potent and selective inhibitors of the uptake of serotonin by nerve terminals. Fluoxetine and citalopram are under clinical investigation, with some encouraging results in depressed patients. Zimelidine, while possibly an effective antidepressant, has been associated with a small number of cases of ascending paralysis of the Guillain-Barré type, and its trials have been discontinued. *Mianserin*, an antidepressant of uncertain mechanism of action, has been in clinical use in Europe for several years, typically in daily doses of 40–60 mg. Curiously, it has *anti*serotonergic actions. Although it is a relatively weak inhibitor of the uptake of monoamines, it may potentiate the release of norepinephrine by a moderate antagonistic effect at presynaptic α_2-adrenergic receptors. *Nomifensine* (Merital) is also in clinical use in Europe in daily doses of 50–200 mg. It has potent effects against the uptake of norepinephrine, but also against that of dopamine; it also has stimulant-like properties, possibly reflecting its dopaminergic actions.

Among truly atypical agents, *iprindole* has no effect on monoamine uptake and lacks anticholinergic activity. However, experimental trials testing its efficacy have led to inconclusive results, and its future is uncertain. Yet another curious agent is the natural metabolic product *S-adenosyl-L-methionine* (SAMe). This compound is the major donor of methyl groups in biological transmethylation reactions in the liver and other mammalian tissues. Its pharmacology is obscure, but it may play a role in modifying the structure and functions of biological membranes by altering the synthesis and distribution of methylated lipids, and so possibly modifying the function of receptors or transport systems. It is used clinically as an antidepressant in Europe and is available only for intravenous injection. Several trials, mainly involving comparisons with a standard tricyclic antidepressant, support its possible efficacy and striking lack of side effects or toxicity, and at least one trial indicates its superiority to a placebo. There are a few instances of its association with switches of mood from depression to mania in patients with bipolar disorder.

Yet another example of an interesting agent without a known mechanism of action in depression is *alprazolam* (Xanax), a triazolo-benzodiazepine. This agent is already in clinical use in small doses as an antianxiety agent, and there is also good evidence that it exerts anti-panic effects (similar to imipramine), possibly more so than other benzodiazepines. It has also been reported in a few trials to exert apparent antidepressant actions, especially in relatively mildly depressed and usually anxious outpatients. It is thus not clear whether these effects are unique and clearly different from those of other sedatives and antianxiety compounds in neurotic, dysthymic patients, or whether they may apply also to patients

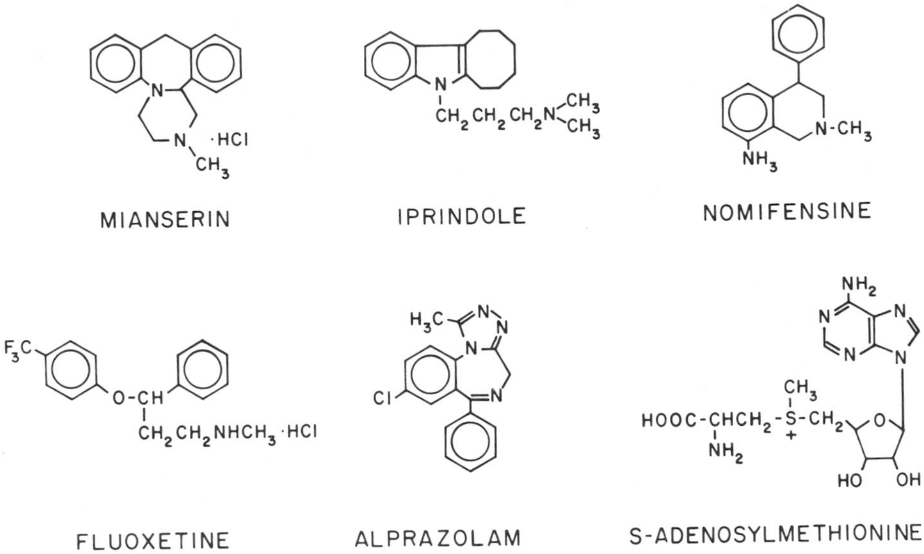

Figure 18 Chemical structures of atypical antidepressants.

with major melancholic depression, for whom this agent is not as well evaluated. Doses associated with apparent antidepressant effects (up to 10 mg/day) have sometimes been higher than those recommended for antianxiety effects. Potential problems associated with alprazolam are its sedative effects and questions about its risk of tolerance and dependence — questions also raised about other benzodiazepine agents of high potency and relatively short duration of action in the following chapter. Since the risks of other side effects or of fatal overdoses, typical of older antidepressants, are low with the benzodiazepines, this type of agent could be very attractive clinically, even if its efficacy were limited to patients with milder depressive disorders associated with anxiety symptoms, or as an alternative for treating elderly, cardiac, or otherwise medically infirm depressed patients. Several congeners of alprazolam are also under development at the present time.

Examples of new, atypical, or experimental antidepressant agents are provided in Figure 18. Although the future of many of these and other experimental antidepressants is uncertain, their development is encouraging because it indicates renewed interest in finding novel antidepressants that not only are effective, and possibly safer than the tricyclic and MAO-inhibitor types of antidepressants, but also that act by obscure mechanisms which may offer ways to escape the repetitious rediscovery of agents similar to those known since the 1950s.

Other experimental approaches to the treatment of depression are also emerging. There is preliminary work with *beta-adrenergic agonists* with central neuropharmacologic activity, and at least theoretical consideration of centrally active alpha-1 agonists. Most direct sympathomimetic agonists developed in the past have been catecholamine analogues, usually excessively polar to penetrate the blood-brain diffusion barrier. There is also interest in the possibility of developing derivatives or precursors ("prodrugs") of polar active molecules that might penetrate the brain. Similar drug distribution problems, as well as rapid metabolism, have limited explorations of *peptides* as potentially active neuropharmacologic drug substances, although such materials are currently the subject of intense investigation. Finally, there are intriguing reports of apparent mood-elevating or antidepressant effects of deliberate alterations of the circadian light-dark cycle and the sleep-waking cycle. For example, sleep deprivation, interference with rapid-eye-movement (REM) sleep, and altered timing of sleep and waking cycles, as well as exposure to strong illumination during the night or early morning, have all been reported to have interesting beneficial effects on mood in depressed patients and are the subject of continued investigation.

The study of the role of psychotherapy in depression is one of the most active and encouraging facets of psychotherapy research. There is now good evidence of the efficacy of psychodynamic insight-oriented, cognitive, and supportive psychotherapeutic techniques in depressive disorders, especially when combined with adequate chemotherapy. The best evidence exists for relatively mild or moderate cases that may or may not meet current research criteria for "major depression"; they are usually ambulatory patients and rarely suffer from severe melancholia. Nevertheless, even without complete research support, psychotherapeutic methods continue to have an important place in the overall treatment of patients with major mood disorders as well as dysthymic neuroses, particularly in patients with chronic or frequently relapsing illnesses that respond inadequately to thymoleptic treatment.

Selective MAO Inhibitors

The recent development and preliminary clinical testing of agents selective for the two major biological forms of monoamine oxidase have stimulated increased interest in MAO inhibitors for depression and other psychiatric disorders. The two most extensively investigated, representative, and selective MAO inhibitors are the propargyl compounds: clorgyline, for type A MAO, and (−)deprenyl, for type B MAO. In addition, the

PROPARGYLAMINE MAO INHIBITORS

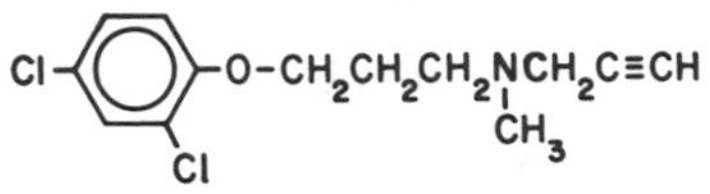

Cl—⟨◯⟩—O–CH₂CH₂CH₂NCH₂C≡CH
                            |
                           CH₃

Cl (on ring)

Clorgyline (A)

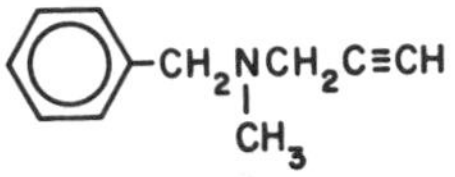

⟨◯⟩—CH₂NCH₂C≡CH
           |
          CH₃

Pargyline (B)

                CH₃
                |
⟨◯⟩—CH₂CHNCH₂C≡CH
                 |
                CH₃

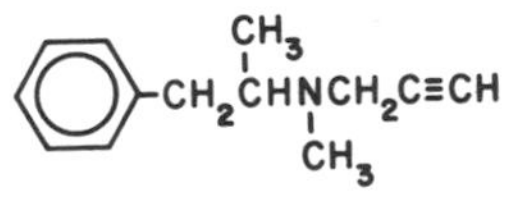

Deprenyl (B)

Figure 19 Chemical structures of selective MAO inhibitors. The properties of inhibitors selective for MAO types A and B are summarized in Table 70.

antihypertensive agent pargyline (Eutonyl) is relatively selective for type B MAO. The structures of these agents are shown in Figure 19. Clorgyline and (−)deprenyl are extraordinarily selective for types A and B substrates (see Table 70), by a factor of more than 1,000:1 in vitro. In vivo, this selectivity is lower, about 10:1. Deprenyl has a complex pharmacology. The levo (−) enantiomer is a selective MAO-B inhibitor, but some selectivity may be lost after repeated high doses in vivo. The dextro (+) isomer is reported to have amphetamine-like stimulant properties, and the structural analogy to amphetamine is apparent in the structures of these agents (see Figures 17 and 19). It is also suspected that deprenyl may be partly converted to amphetamine or methamphetamine in vivo, but the possible pharmacologic contribution of such minor metabolites is unclear. If this effect were important, one would expect deprenyl to block the pressor effects of the indirect sympathomimetic agent tyramine, which is taken up in sympathetic nerve endings to release norepinephrine, but it does not. Also, any loss of selectivity of deprenyl for MAO-B must be small in that this MAO inhibitor fails to potentiate the pressor effects of tyramine after repeated, as well as acute, administration.

In contrast, inhibitors of MAO-A are generally strong potentiators of the pressor effect of tyramine (a nonspecific substrate for MAO-A or B), probably by increasing the availability of norepinephrine for release rather than by preventing the breakdown of tyramine itself. Clorgyline strongly potentiates the pressor effect of tyramine. It was hoped that the development of selective MAO inhibitors might help in avoiding the hypertensive interactions between MAO inhibitors and various pressor amines, such as the "cheese reaction" in response to tyramine in foods, while retaining antidepressant efficacy. This hope has not been fully realized, however; although deprenyl avoids the hypertensive effects of other MAO inhibitors that interact with tyramine, it does not appear to be consistently effective for the treatment of major depression. In contrast, clorgyline almost certainly has antidepressant activity, but is also a strong potentiator of tyramine (and of norepinephrine). Nevertheless, the clinical evaluation of these and other experimental selective MAO inhibitors is still at a preliminary stage, and further investigation is required. A summary of current understanding of the actions of clorgyline and (−)deprenyl as representative selective inhibitors of types A and B MAO activity is provided in Table 77.

In addition to possible antidepressant or "antineurotic" actions, the selective MAO inhibitors may have additional properties worthy of further investigation. For example, clorgyline, in addition to yielding results similar to those of imipramine or amitriptyline in major depression, has been reported to have little tendency to induce mania while exerting useful mood-elevating and stabilizing effects in a small number of rapidly cycling bipolar manic-depressive patients, in contrast to other antidepressants or MAO inhibitors in unselected bipolar patients. Thus, it is hypothesized that clorgyline or similar agents may be especially useful in the treatment of bipolar major affective disorders, as lithium has been proved to be, and as carbamazepine may be (see Chapter 3).

Exploration of the potential of MAO-B inhibitors is even less well developed than that of clorgyline and several other MAO-A inhibitors. The evidence that (−)deprenyl is effective in major depression is mixed and generally unconvincing, although it may have utility in neurotic dysthymic disorders marked by atypical biological symptoms (increased sleep or appetite), anxiety, and a chronic course. Moreover, there are suggestions that deprenyl might be useful in the treatment of Parkinson's

Table 77 Reported actions of selective MAO inhibitors

Clorgyline and other MAO-A inhibitors
• Increase levels and actions of norepinephrine and serotonin
• Potentiate pressor effects of tyramine even if tyramine is given intravenously to avoid the liver (probably mediated by increased availability of norepinephrine)
• Probably have clinical efficacy in major depression comparable to tricyclic antidepressants
• Similar to typical tricyclic antidepressants, can downregulate α_2- and β-adrenergic receptors

(−)Deprenyl, an MAO-B inhibitor
• Potentiates L-dopa and dopamine, and thus may be useful in treating Parkinson's disease
• Spares potentiation of the pressor effect of tyramine but does not prevent the action of tyramine
• Is probably an inferior or ineffective antidepressant in major depression but may have utility in atypical or neurotic dysphorias or dysthymic disorders

disease, possibly by potentiation of dopamine, and there is some evidence that it can decrease the requirement of L-dopa in such patients; it may even slow the progress of Parkinson's disease, possibly by preventing formation of toxic metabolic products of dopamine, although this hypothesis is still highly tentative. In addition, the lack of tyramine-potentiating actions of (−)deprenyl, in contrast to the MAO-A inhibitors, is an attractive property that might increase the safety of MAO inhibitor therapy provided that MAO-B inhibitors are proved to be clinically effective in psychiatric disorders. Unlike the antihypertensive MAO-B inhibitor pargyline, deprenyl has not been reported to have marked hypotensive actions.

Finally, an imaginative new approach to the design of antidepressant agents is a proposal to combine the anti-MAO-A effects of a propargyl substituent with the amine-uptake-inhibiting properties of a tricyclic antidepressant—all in the same molecule. Such a drug might avoid the hypertensive effects of indirect sympathomimetic amines such as tyramine by preventing their uptake into sympathetic nerve endings, even while increasing the availability of norepinephrine by preventing its metabolic breakdown as well as its inactivation by neuronal uptake. Such an agent, an analogue of imipramine (KY-1349), is now under investigation.

Summary and Conclusions

The modern chemotherapy of depression arose from the use of structural analogues of the phenothiazines. In contrast to the largely antidopaminergic effects of antipsychotic agents, these "tricyclic" antidepressants potentiate the actions of norepinephrine; most also have strong antimuscarinic effects. The latter actions contribute to their annoying and more serious atropine-like effects on the eye, salivary glands, heart, gut, bladder, and central nervous system. In addition to blocking the uptake of norepinephrine, the tricyclic-type antidepressants exert complex effects on the metabolism, receptors, and functions of monoamines in the brain. It is unfortunate that the drugs used to treat patients at increased risk of suicide are so toxic and potentially lethal.

Although antidepressant effects of the tricyclic antidepressants have been demonstrated in controlled clinical trials among outpatients as well as inpatients, their efficacy is more impressive in the more severe forms of major depression with melancholic features. For milder forms of the syndrome, their effects are not much better than those of antianxiety agents, a placebo, or other nonspecific treatments, nor are they impressively better than psychotherapy. Even in serious depressions, the antidepressant drugs are usually not effective for a week or more after treatment is begun, and the rate of relapse is high unless patients are maintained on the medications for at least several months. In very severe cases of depression, more consistent and more rapid effects are obtained with ECT, which is still used in the treatment of some severe depressions, with acutely suicidal patients, and also when the tricyclic antidepressants fail to work within a month or so, as happens in as many as 30% of severe depressions. The antipsychotic agents are also useful in the short-term treatment of agitated and psychotic forms of depression.

The MAO inhibitors are now undergoing a resurgence of interest. With the exception of tranylcypromine, and possibly also phenelzine in high doses, they are inferior antidepressants and their use is complicated by many restrictions resulting from their toxic interactions with other agents. Stimulants have little if any place in the treatment of serious depressive illnesses.

Because of the limited efficacy, slowness, and toxicity of the currently available agents, the search for better antidepressants must be pursued. There has been remarkably little that is fundamentally new in the treatment of major depression since the introduction of ECT in the 1930s and the MAO inhibitors and imipramine in the 1950s. Several newer "atypical" antidepressants lack many of the pharmacologic and toxic effects of older tricyclic-type agents and challenge the need to potentiate norepinephrine to obtain an antidepressant effect. Several experimental chemotherapies for depression are being investigated, including a number of hormones and precursors of biogenic amines, as well as manipulation of sleep or light cycles.

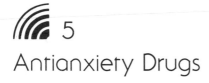

5
Antianxiety Drugs

There is no ideal generic term for the class of agents known as antianxiety drugs. Use of the synonyms "antianxiety," "anxiolytic," or "tranquilizer" to some degree represents wishful thinking based on a long search for drugs that are specific for anxiety and distinctly different from the sedatives, hypnotics, and general anesthetics. Antianxiety agents have been of interest to physicians throughout the history of medicine. A hundred years ago, the main antianxiety agents were the bromide salts, and ethanol administered as self-medication, in patent remedies, or by prescription. With the development of pharmaceutical technology in the late nineteenth and early twentieth centuries, several compounds similar to alcohol were added, including paraldehyde and chloral hydrate. Then the barbiturates, of which at least fifty came into clinical use, became the standard sedatives and hypnotics.

More recently the use of propanediols was initiated by the description in 1946 of the muscle-relaxant and sedative properties of the impractically short-acting agent mephenesin. In 1951, Bernard Ludwig and Edward Piech produced *meprobamate* (Miltown, Equanil), a structural analogue of mephenesin with more prolonged muscle-relaxant and sedative actions; these actions were demonstrated clinically by Frank Berger in 1954. Meprobamate was shown to be useful in anxious patients by Noah Dixon in 1957. Since then other propanediols, including tybamate (Solacen, Tybatran), have been developed.

The search for safer antianxiety agents lacking the addictive and potentially lethal properties (CNS and respiratory depression) of all the previously mentioned sedative-hypnotic tranquilizing agents led to the development of the *benzodiazepines*. Although this latter class of chemicals had been known at least since the 1930s, their reinvestigation during the ferment in psychopharmacology in the 1950s led to the synthesis and study by Leo Sternbach of *chlordiazepoxide* (Librium), which was introduced into clinical use in 1960. It was found to have potent taming effects in animals and anticonvulsant, skeletal-muscle relaxant, and sedative-antianxiety effects in man. Since then a large number of structural variants of chlordiazepoxide have been introduced. The enormous popularity of the benzodiazepines, which derives from their significant antianxiety effects and their relative safety, is illustrated by the fact that they have been among the most prescribed drugs of *all* kinds, at rates approaching 100 million prescriptions per year and a cost of about 500 million dollars in the United States alone. Benzodiazepines are also the standard hypnotic agents.

Despite their popularity, the sedative-tranquilizing agents in general have been severely criticized in recent years. Too often they are used in an apparent allopathic compulsion to give something to ease the patient's distress, and as a substitute for the time required to assist an anxious or unhappy patient to discover and modify the sources of psychic pain.

A limiting factor in the discovery and development of new antianxiety agents is the same as with preclinical pharmacologic identification of potential antipsychotic agents by their neuroleptic effects and antidepressants by their adrenergic potentiating effects. With the anxiolytic sedatives, animal tests that have been commonly used are those developed through experience with the barbiturates and include decreases in spontaneous and conditioned behavioral responses, elevated seizure threshold, production of ataxia, and the prolongation and potentiation of sedative effects of a standard agent such as a barbiturate. Innovative biochemical methods are also available to identify new agents that share with the benzodiazepines their recently discovered high-affinity binding sites and interactions with membrane components of gamma-aminobutyric acid (GABA) receptors and chloride ion transport systems. It is not clear whether these newer methods will lead to additional, novel agents or merely to more benzodiazepine-like compounds in addition to the large number of similar agents already available.

Pharmacology
Preparations, Dosing, and Types of Agents

Since the benzodiazepines have come to dominate clinical practice as well as recent research on antianxiety agents, they are emphasized in the following discussion. Most of those with useful antianxiety and sedative properties that are currently available for clinical use in the United States are shown in Figure 20, which also provides the structure of the new, atypical non-benzodiazepine buspirone. The preparations and doses of both anxiolytic and sedative-hypnotic benzodiazepines are provided in Table 78. Several other sedative-hypnotic benzodiazepines are known, including nitrazepam (Mogodon), a common hypnotic agent in other countries; flunitrazepam is a very potent sedative benzodiazepine and has often been used in radiolabeled form to label benzodiazepine receptor sites in brain tissue.

Older compounds that are still in use as sedatives or antianxiety agents include several barbiturates, a group of structural analogues of the barbiturates (including glutethimide, methaqualone, and methyprylon), several compounds that share structural and pharmacologic properties with alcohol (including ethchlorvynol, chloral hydrate, paraldehyde, meprobamate, and tybamate), and sedative antihistamines (including diphenhydramine, hydroxyzine, and promethazine). Most of these agents are used infrequently, and many of them are not recommended for further use because of inferior, complex, or potentially dangerous pharmacologic and toxicologic properties, as discussed in the section on clinical use. Older sedatives that are still available are listed in Table 79.

Absorption, Metabolism, and Elimination

The benzodiazepines differ from one another in pharmacokinetics and metabolism. Diazepam is one of the most rapidly absorbed benzodiazepines, reaching peak plasma levels in less than an hour after oral administration; clorazepate is also more rapidly absorbed than most other benzodiazepines. Intravenously administered, diazepam has an almost immediate effect, but—with the possible exception of lorazepam—diazepam and other benzodiazepines are absorbed unpredictably after intramuscular injection, which is not used routinely. The high potency and rapid action of diazepam may contribute to its occasional abuse to induce intoxication. Most benzodiazepines are absorbed at an intermediate rate, with peak plasma levels typically appearing in 1 to 3 hours. A particularly slowly absorbed (and slowly eliminated) compound is prazepam, peak levels of which may be delayed for 6 hours or longer. The relative rates of absorption, the approximate half-time of elimination, and the presence of active metabolites of the benzodiazepines in clinical use in the United States are summarized along with dosages in Table 78.

Most benzodiazepines are lipophilic and highly bound to plasma

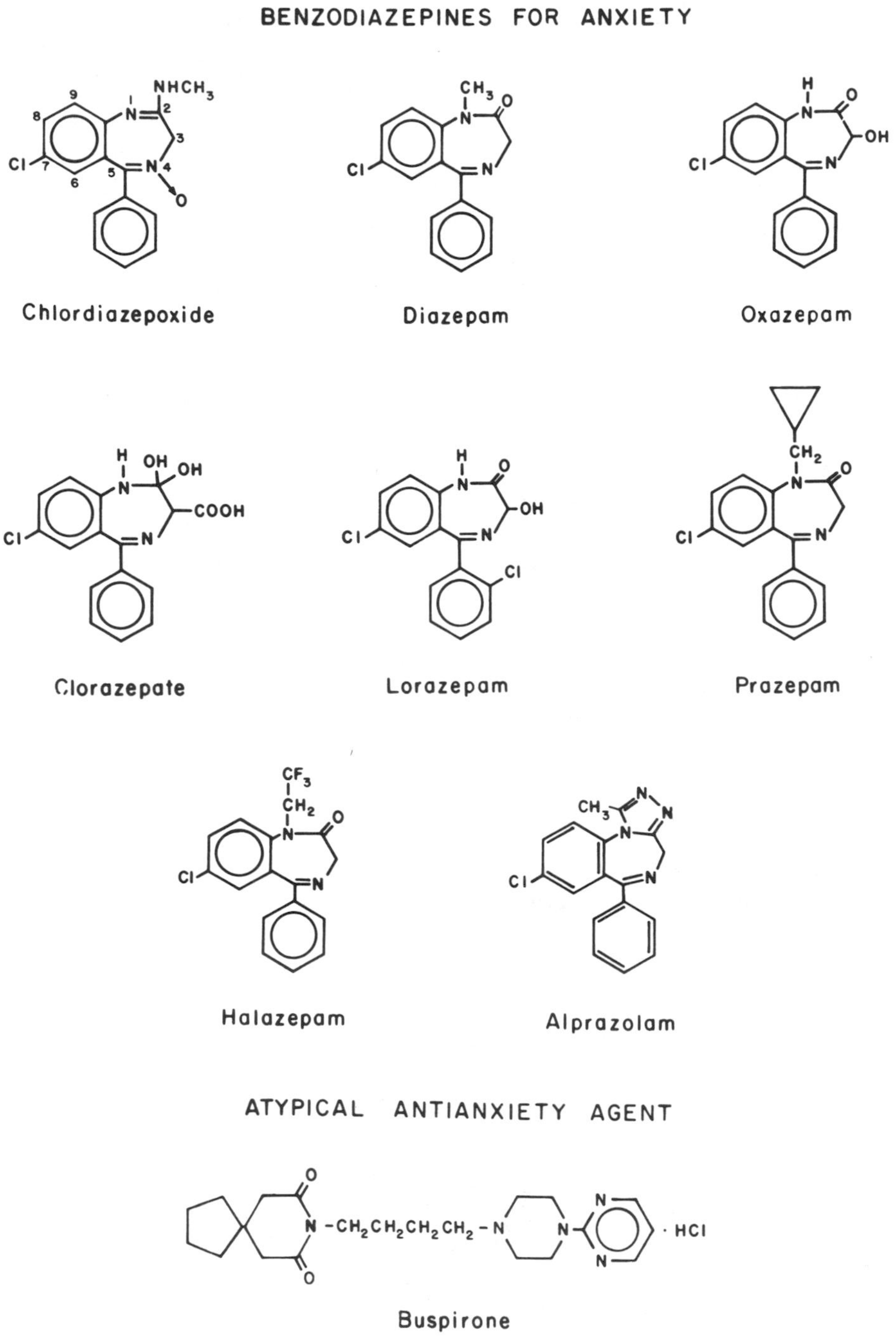
BENZODIAZEPINES FOR ANXIETY
Chlordiazepoxide
Diazepam
Oxazepam
Clorazepate
Lorazepam
Prazepam
Halazepam
Alprazolam
ATYPICAL ANTIANXIETY AGENT
Buspirone

Figure 20 Chemical structures of benzodiazepines and an atypical new agent used in the treatment of anxiety.

membranes (85 – 90%), although their apparent volumes of distribution (typically, 1 – 3 liters/kg) are not as high as those of the antipsychotic or tricyclic-type antidepressant agents. Secondary peaks in the plasma concentration of several benzodiazepines have been described (for example, after 6 to 12 hours following an oral dose of diazepam), and these may reflect enterohepatic recirculation (biliary secretion with secondary intestinal absorption). Such fluctuations in plasma levels may be associated with unstable or unpredictable clinical effects and with a fluctuating course following acute overdoses.

The pharmacokinetics of the benzodiazepines are often complex, particularly since many of these agents have active metabolites that dominate their course of activity. For example, desmethyldiazepam (nordiazepam) is a common, active metabolite of diazepam and other benzodiazepines (chlordiazepoxide, clorazepate, halazepam, and possibly prazepam) that has a remarkably prolonged half-life of elimination (as long as 100 hours). Flurazepam has an analogous, long-acting, N-dealkylated metabolite. All of the agents with such slowly eliminated active metabolites have prolonged clinical actions, and an elimination half-life from plasma in excess of two days (see Table 78). The actual pharmacokinetics of some benzodiazepines are complex and not easily analyzed by simple mathematical models. The stated values for approximate half-life are averages for active substances that are eliminated at dissimilar rates. Moreover, the stated elimination half-life does not reflect the distribution half-life, which may be of critical importance clinically and represent a key determinant of the dosing schedule. Thus, for example, diazepam has a distribution (alpha) half-life of about 2.5 hours, while the elimination (beta) half-life is about 1.5 days initially and even longer after prolonged administration (the nominal, overall estimated elimination half-life is about 60 hours). The prolonged elimination of desmethyldiazepam and other active products of the metabolism of diazepam may suggest that infrequent dosing might be a reasonable tactic. However, plasma levels only about twice those considered to be effective and safe may be associated with undesirable degrees of sedation or mild intoxication. For this reason, long-acting benzodiazepines can be given safely in two to four single daily doses if these are *small;* shorter-acting agents are also best given in two to four small portions for the treatment of daytime anxiety with a minimum risk of oversedation.

Most of the products of metabolism of the benzodiazepines are derived through the actions of hepatic microsomal and other enzymes to form N-dealkylated, ring-hydroxylated, or other oxidized products, and appear

Table 78 Benzodiazepines: Preparations, dosage forms, doses, and characteristics

Nonproprietary name	Trade names	Dosage forms[a] (mg)	Usual daily dose (mg)[b]	Extreme daily dose (mg)	Rapidity of absorption[c]	Half-life (hr)[d]	Active metabolites[e]
Anxiolytic benzodiazepines							
Alprazolam	Xanax	(T) 0.25, 0.5, 1	0.75–4	0.5–10	+++	12	Minor
Chlordiazepoxide	Libritabs	(T) 5, 10, 25	15–60	10–100	+++	18	Yes
Chlordiazepoxide hydrochloride[f]	Librium A-poxide SK-lygen (and generic)	(T) 5, 10, 25 (C) 5, 10, 25 (A) 100/2 ml	15–60 50–100 (IV per dose)	10–100 300 (IV)	+++	18	Yes
Clorazepate dipotassium[g]	Tranxene	(C) 3.75, 7.5 (T) 3.75, 7.5, 15	30	7.5–90	++++	100	Yes
Diazepam[g,h]	Valium	(T) 2, 5, 10 (A) 10/2 ml (V) 50/10 ml (S) 10/2 ml	4–40 2–20 (IV per dose)	2–60	+++++	60	Yes
Halazepam	Paxipam	(T) 20, 40	60–160	20–160	+++	50	Yes
Lorazepam[h]	Ativan	(T) 0.5, 1, 2 (V) 20 or 40/10 ml (S) 2 or 4/ml	2–6 2–4 (IM or IV per dose)	1–10	+++	15	No

Oxazepam	Serax	(C) 10, 15, 30 (T) 15	30–60	10–120	++	8	No
Prazepam	Centrax	(C) 5, 10 (T) 10	20–40	5–60	+	100	Yes
Hypnotic benzodiazepines							
Flurazepam hydrochloride[i]	Dalmane	(C) 15, 30	15–30	15–30	++++	2 + 72	Yes
Temazepam	Restoril	(C) 15, 30	15–30	15–30	++	11	No
Triazolam[j]	Halcion	(T) 0.25, 0.5	0.25–0.5	0.125–0.5	+++	2	No
Anticonvulsant benzodiazepine							
Clonazepam[k]	Clonopin	(T) 0.5, 1, 2	1.5–10	0.5–20	++	34	Yes

a. T = tablet; C = capsule; A = ampule; V = vial; S = syringe.

b. The daily doses are given as total milligrams per day, assuming doses are divided into two to four portions per day. All doses are for adults or adolescents. For children 6 to 12 years of age, chlordiazepoxide may be given in divided daily doses of 10 to 30 mg. Diazepam may be given in divided daily doses of 1 to 10 mg to children over 6 months of age. For younger children, consult the manufacturer's instructions.

c. Ranked from 5+ (fastest: diazepam, <1 hour) to 1+ (slowest: prazepam, ca. 6 hours).

d. Elimination half-life is an estimated average, including active metabolites.

e. Most include desmethylated products, notably the long-acting nordiazepam; alprazolam has some active desmethylated and hydroxylated products that do not greatly prolong elimination.

f. Chlordiazepoxide is also available in combination with clidinium bromide (Librax and Clipoxide) or amitriptyline (Limbitrol).

g. Clorazepate dipotassium is also available as slow-release tablets (Tranxene-sd) containing either 11.25 or 22.5 mg to be taken once daily. Diazepam is also available as slow-release capsules (Valrelease) containing 15 mg.

h. Parenteral preparations are available only for chlordiazepoxide hydrochloride, diazepam, and lorazepam; intramuscular administration is not advisable, except with lorazepam (which is also very active sublingually); for details concerning intravenous use, see the manufacturer's instructions.

i. Flurazepam has active metabolites (mainly norflurazepam) with a long half-life and thus a risk of inducing "hangover" or prolonged sedation, making it a less than ideal hypnotic.

j. The extraordinarily short half-life of triazolam can lead to an insufficiently sustained hypnotic effect.

k. Clonazepam, while used primarily as an anticonvulsant for petit mal epilepsy and other non–grand mal seizure disorders, has been reported to have antimanic and antipanic activity as well.

Table 79   Older sedatives

Agent	Trade name	Comments
Alcohols, aldehydes, and propanediols		
Ethanol	Generic	Not recommended[a]
Ethchlorvynol	Placidyl	Not recommended[a]
Chloral hydrate	Generic	1–2 gm for sleep
Paraldehyde	Generic	Not recommended[a]
Meprobamate	Equanil, Miltown, generic	Not recommended[a]
Tybamate	Tybatran, Solacen, generic	Not recommended[a]
Barbiturates		
Amobarbital	Amytal, generic	100–800 mg/hr, intravenously in diagnosis, or parenterally for emergency sedation
Methohexital	Brevital	10 mg/5 sec intravenously for ECT only
Pentobarbital	Nembutal, generic	Can be used for withdrawal in most sedative addictions[b,c]
Phenobarbital	Luminal, generic	30–90 mg/day[b,c]
Secobarbital	Seconal, generic	Not recommended[b]
Structural relatives of barbiturates (nonbarbiturates)		
Glutethimide	Doriden	Not recommended[a]
Methyprylon	Noludar	Not recommended[a]
Methaqualone	Quaalude, Sopor, generic	Not recommended[a]
Antihistamines		
Diphenhydramine	Benadryl	25–50 mg parenterally for dystonia[d]
Hydroxyzine	Atarax, Vistaril	Not recommended[a]
Promethazine	Phenergan, generic	Not recommended[a]

a. Some agents are not recommended for routine use as sedatives.

b. Sometimes short-acting barbiturates, though not generally recommended, are used for sleep because of their low cost; phenobarbital is a very inexpensive sedative and not often abused.

c. Pentobarbital and phenobarbital are often used to treat addiction to this entire class of agents; see Table 80.

d. Diphenhydramine and other antihistamines are sometimes used as sedatives in pediatric practice.

finally in the urine in the form of N-dealkylated, oxidized, and conjugated metabolites. Clorazepate, which itself is probably inactive pharmacologically, is rapidly converted nonenzymatically in gastric acid to the active product desmethyldiazepam, the long-acting derivative of several other benzodiazepines already discussed. Lorazepam, oxazepam, and possibly alprazolam are exceptional benzodiazepines in that they have virtually no important pharmacologically active metabolites, but all three agents rely mainly on conjugation with glucuronic acid to form inactive metabolites.

Because of heavy reliance on hepatic mechanisms to alter and inactivate the benzodiazepines, these agents should be used cautiously and sparingly in patients with liver disease, whose ability to eliminate them may be reduced by a factor of 2 to 5. Since formation of glucuronides is not limited to hepatic microsomes, oxazepam, lorazepam, and possibly alprazolam may be relatively safe agents for patients with inefficient or impaired hepatic function if given in small, divided doses. Oxazepam may be especially useful because of its unusually rapid nominal half-life of only about 8 hours. In addition to patients with hepatic dysfunction, the premature neonate and elderly persons may also have less ability to metabolize and inactivate benzodiazepines compared with healthy adults and older children, or even full-term infants. The former groups are at increased risk of intoxication by ordinary doses of benzodiazepines; their rate of elimination may be three or four times less than in other age groups, requiring proportionate decreases in daily doses to one-third or one-fourth of the usual dose.

As a class, the benzodiazepines tend to have minimal pharmacokinetic interactions with most other drugs, with the possible exception of MAO inhibitors, which can potentiate the sedative effects of the benzodiazepines. In ordinary clinical doses, benzodiazepines are unlikely to interfere with, or to induce the hepatic metabolism of, other agents (such as anticoagulants or other psychotropic agents), in contrast to the strong hepatic enzyme-inducing actions of many older sedatives.

Most benzodiazepines have relatively minor ability to induce their own hepatic metabolism. This factor is probably not a major contributor to the limited development of tolerance to these agents, in contrast to barbiturates and most other older sedatives; that is, steadily increasing doses usually are not required to obtain sustained antianxiety or hypnotic effects in clinical applications. However, a degree of tolerance to the sedative effects of these agents when employed for daytime antianxiety effects is usual and can be advantageous. Habituation can develop, but high doses of benzodiazepines usually must be given for long periods and then discontinued abruptly before marked withdrawal symptoms, occasionally including seizures, are observed. There is a clinical impression that some of the newer benzodiazepines of high potency and relatively short duration of action may present an increased risk of habituation and of symptomatic reaction to rapid withdrawal, but this risk can be minimized by slow tapering of doses. Such risks may be less with the long-acting benzodiazepines, or at least delayed. For example, withdrawal reactions to the rapid removal of prolonged, high doses of diazepam may be delayed for a week or more. Moreover, propranolol has been reported to counteract some of the autonomic symptoms of such withdrawal reactions. Nevertheless, a safe and rational practice is to use such agents in the smallest possible effective doses for the shortest practical periods, and to withdraw them slowly and gradually.

The barbiturates (see Table 79) are less and less used by physicians for the management of anxiety and dysphoria. Phenobarbital is now only occasionally used for such purposes. It is a long-acting barbiturate and is to a considerable degree excreted by the kidney (20–30%) independent of its hepatic metabolism; in contrast, the shorter-acting barbiturates are more rapidly metabolized, almost entirely by hepatic enzymatic activity. Thus, phenobarbital was formerly used cautiously in small doses even in patients with liver disease; it can be used in those with renal failure as well, although its actions are prolonged in both circumstances. The difficulty of obtaining a quick subjective "high" by intoxication with phenobarbital limits its potential for abuse, and its prolonged duration of action limits its ability to produce severe withdrawal reactions. On the other hand, the drug's persistence complicates the management of potentially lethal acute overdoses. Phenobarbital can induce synthesis and activity of hepatic microsomal enzymes, and thus its own rate of metabolism, although this effect is not believed to be an important factor in the production of tolerance to the barbiturates. However, it can have important consequences for the actions of other drugs, hormones, and metabolic products, including increased inactivation of dihydroxycoumarin and steroids and increased production or porphyrins.

The propanediols (see Table 79) are metabolized mainly by hepatic microsomal oxidases, and meprobamate shares with the barbiturates their ability to induce these enzymes. Because meprobamate is more rapidly excreted than phenobarbital (half-life is about 12 hours for meprobamate versus more than 24 hours for phenobarbital), an increased rate of oxidation probably contributes to tolerance of this drug. Tybamate is even more rapidly metabolized and excreted than meprobamate, and its useful duration of action is about 50% less. The probability of physiological habituation to tybamate is probably also reduced because much less drug accumulates in tissue. Physiological addiction to meprobamate is well known and can occur after prolonged use of doses not much greater than the upper limits of recommended doses.

Mechanisms of Action

Since the 1970s, the benzodiazepines have been the dominant antianxiety, sedative, and hypnotic agents in the United States and worldwide. Initially they were thought to be pharmacologically highly dissimilar to other sedatives, but now it is known that this class of agents shares many properties, including behavioral, neurophysiological, and biochemical actions, with older sedatives such as barbiturates and the propanediols. Thus, the benzodiazepines have widespread, diffuse inhibitory effects in the central nervous system and important anticonvulsant activity as well as muscle-relaxant activity, partly mediated by inhibitory effects on reflex activity, especially on polysynaptic reflexes at the spinal cord and higher levels. Like nearly all of the sedatives, the benzodiazepines produce slow wave and low-voltage, fast (beta) activity in the electroencephalogram (EEG). Some benzodiazepines, in common with the barbiturates, have been reported to block EEG arousal induced by direct stimulation of the brainstem reticular formation. Like meprobamate and the barbiturates, benzodiazepines depress the after-discharges following stimulation of the limbic system, including the septal region, amygdala, hippocampus, and hypothalamus. Such effects appear at lower doses than are required to produce more generalized depression of the cerebral cortex and the reticular activating system, and thus have been linked theoretically with the antianxiety effects of these agents. These responses appear to correlate with taming effects in animals and the suppression of conditioned (especially "avoidance") behaviors more than unconditioned responses in animals. In conflict-inducing procedures, benzodiazepines greatly reduce the behavior-suppressing effects of punishment. Positive effects are not found in this laboratory model with antidepressant and antipsychotic agents. It is theorized that in man, selective limbic neuropharmacologic actions of the benzodiazepines are manifested by antianxiety effects relatively separate from the sedation and mental clouding typical of older sedatives.

Evaluating or modeling the clinical therapeutic effects of antianxiety agents is particularly difficult, especially because of the contribution of nonpharmacologic factors to the treatment of anxiety. As in the case of other psychotropic agents already discussed, there is a degree of circularity in the methods of detecting possible new antianxiety agents. Although the discovery of the benzodiazepines represents a major advance in pharmacology, especially in eliminating or reducing many of the complexities and risks associated with older sedative agents, and even though their actions are increasingly better detailed, a coherent theory of the biological aspects of anxiety and methods to predict truly novel agents that are not variants on known drugs continue to be elusive. It is hoped that recent research findings, such as a relationship between increased anxiety and overactivity of the norepinephrine-containing locus ceruleus of the brainstem, the triggering of panic by infusion of lactate in susceptible subjects, and the discovery of anxiety-producing benzodiazepine antagonists, may lead to greater insights into the biology of anxiety disorders.

Actions of the benzodiazepines and other antianxiety agents on the limbic system and central components of the autonomic nervous system are the focus of particular theoretical interest at the present time, as are observations of selective potentiation of the effects of gamma (γ)-aminobutyric acid (GABA), a key inhibitory neurotransmitter amino acid in the brain, and of selective interactions with the transport of chloride ion. This area of interest has been stimulated by the discovery of selective binding sites with high affinity (nanomolar) for benzodiazepines in the mammalian brain, especially in limbic and cortical tissue of forebrain. Endogenous substances that may be physiological ligands for such binding sites have been hypothesized; candidates include nicotinamide, purines, and β-carbolines. Benzodiazepines appear to interact at macromolecular complexes in neuronal membranes that include GABA receptors and chloride ion channels, as well as binding sites for barbiturates. Such binding sites can be demonstrated with highly radioactive labeling agents, such as ^{3}H-flunitrazepam. These interactions with a molecular complex that appears to inhibit neurophysiological activity of many neurons may provide insights into important actions of the benzodiazepines as well as of barbiturates and other antianxiety-sedative agents, but the detailed account of these interactions is still emerging from very active research on this topic.

In contrast to the antipsychotic agents, the sedative-antianxiety agents have relatively little effect on autonomic functions, including blood pressure; little ability to antagonize catecholamines or acetylcholine; and little effect on the extrapyramidal motor system. Exceptions are the more "antiautonomic" sedatives, including the antihistaminic compounds such as diphenhydramine (Benadryl) and hydroxyzine (Atarax, Vistaril), as well as the new atypical antianxiety agent buspirone (Buspar), which has some antidopaminergic actions. Although sedatives lack useful long-term antipsychotic actions, they can be helpful in the practical management of acutely psychotic or manic patients, as discussed in sections of earlier chapters concerning the clinical use of antipsychotic and antimanic agents.

Most of the sedative tranquilizers (except the antihistamines and buspirone) exhibit *cross-tolerance,* the ability of one to induce tolerance to the effects of the others, as well as some degree of tolerance to their main and side effects. This observation supports the impression that the actions of these agents are similar. A practical consequence of cross-tolerance is that withdrawal of addicting doses of most of these agents can be accomplished by the use of gradually diminishing doses of any one of them; a barbiturate can be used, although it is more common to use the agent of habituation itself. The benzodiazepines appear to be less likely than older sedative agents to be limited by the development of tolerance to their main or desired antianxiety effect as well as to the degree of sedation or hypnotic effect they produce. Tolerance to their actions can limit the length of time they are clinically useful and contributes to the potential abuse of all sedatives. In addition to tolerance, almost all of the drugs employed to treat anxiety (barbiturates, propanediols, and other nonbarbiturate sedatives, as well as benzodiazepines, but not the less frequently used antihistamines and possibly not buspirone) produce physiological dependence and significant withdrawal syndromes on abrupt discontinuation of high doses. However, the benzodiazepines are less likely to produce dangerous withdrawal syndromes, and are unlikely to produce even mild withdrawal after less than two months of use. The danger of severe coma, respiratory depression, and death following an acute overdose of a benzodiazepine is also less than after a comparable multiple of the average daily dose of a barbiturate, propanediol, or other sedative. One way of summarizing the unique characteristics of the benzodiazepines is to point out that their dose-response relationships are much "flatter" than those of the barbiturates or the nonbarbiturate sedatives (but less gradual than those of the antipsychotic agents), so that doubling the dose produces proportionally less sedation than occurs with the other sedatives.

Clinical Use

Anxiety is a cardinal symptom of many psychiatric disorders, as well as an almost inevitable component of many medical and surgical conditions. Indeed, it is a universal human emotion, closely allied with appropriate fear, and often serving biologically adaptive purposes. It is infrequently a "disease" in itself. Among psychiatric disorders for which antianxiety agents may be useful, anxiety as a prominent symptom is associated with acute, chronic, or recurrent disorders formerly categorized as the "psychoneuroses" or "neuroses," in which the symptoms of anxiety are rarely satisfactorily explained by medical or psychological evaluation of the patient. In addition, symptoms of anxiety are commonly associated with depression, especially in dysthymic disorder ("neurotic depression") and many personality disorders. Sometimes, despite thoughtful and thorough medical and psychiatric evaluation of a patient, no treatable primary illness is found; and even if a specific disorder is diagnosed and appropriately treated, it may be reasonable to deal directly with the symptoms of anxiety themselves.

The antianxiety or sedative agents are rarely used as a primary therapeutic agent in severe psychiatric illness, although their occasional use for short-term sedation in acutely manic or psychotic patients can be helpful, as discussed in earlier chapters. Benzodiazepines have also been claimed to have some immediate euphoriant and antianxiety effects, as well as hypnotic actions, which may be useful in the treatment of moderately severe, anxious, "neurotic" depression or dysthymic disorder, and may be of some short-term benefit while awaiting the actions of an antidepressant in major depressive disorders. The main usefulness of antianxiety agents, however, is in the treatment of relatively transient forms of anxiety, fear, and tension. They are also widely employed in general medicine to treat anxiety associated with other disorders, as preoperative sedatives, in the management of short-lived painful syndromes, and in "psychosomatic" and other disorders with unexplained physical manifestations. They also have extraordinary popularity for relatively nonspecific indications when other medical or surgical treatment is not indicated or a specific medical disorder is not found. Consequently, these agents are much more often used in general medicine (85% of all their prescriptions) than in psychiatric practice.

Many psychiatrists believe that prolonged nonpsychotic disorders involving anxiety or dysphoria are better treated with psychotherapy, and thus limit antianxiety agents to relatively brief use in the management of less common, more acute, short-lived, and sometimes "reactive" neurotic conditions. Their prolonged use in personality disorders is often unsuccessful and may lead to misuse or abuse of the agents. The usefulness of the sedative-antianxiety agents is optimized by careful attention to subtleties of their actions and of the doctor-patient relationship. Many psychotherapists are particularly disinclined to rely on the antianxiety agents because the descriptive characteristics of patients who respond well to these agents differ from those of patients usually considered good candidates for the rational, verbal psychotherapies. Thus, a favorable response has been associated with relatively lower socioeconomic class, lack of psychological sophistication, and inability to express unhappiness verbally in terms of intrapsychic or interpersonal conflict. A more favorable response also occurs in patients with a passive attitude and almost magical expectations of the physician. An enthusiastic, charismatic presentation of the medication and its effects by the physician seems to be helpful. Patients who are active, vigorous, and extraverted tend to dislike the sedative effects of antianxiety agents, and may even be made more uncomfortable by taking them.

An important recent advance that should help to improve the specificity of use of agents with antianxiety properties is the separation of various types of anxiety disorders, including those with panic and phobic features as well as those with more generalized anxiety. Features that help to distinguish anxiety syndromes are apparently preferential responses of panic disorder and some complex phobias such as agoraphobia to tricyclic or MAO inhibitor antidepressants. Often, however, features of these putatively distinct syndromes are admixed in individual patients, especially over time, and partial or incomplete responses to any unidimensional therapy in the disorders marked by anxiety are common.

The broad and loosely defined applications of antianxiety agents severely complicate the interpretation of data based on even well-designed, controlled clinical trials. The rate of favorable responses to a placebo in many of these trials has ranged from 20 or 30% to as much as 60%, depending on the group of patients, although the placebo response rate in panic disorder is less than 10%. This variability of patient selection and the strong placebo effect in many anxiety disorders make it difficult to demonstrate significant benefits of an active antianxiety drug. In a review of 78 controlled trials, benzodiazepines proved more effective than a placebo in only 56% of the studies (Solomon and Hart, 1978). The benefits of medication are often particularly difficult to demonstrate in short-lived, reactive forms of anxiety that improve even without chemical intervention. The main conclusions based on several extensive reviews of clinical drug trials are that sedative-tranquilizing agents do have appreciable and fairly consistent antianxiety effects beyond those of a placebo, and that it is extremely difficult to demonstrate the superiority of one agent or class of agents over another. A specific agent, then, must be selected on the basis of considerations other than its demonstrated superiority in a given condition.

Drug Selection and Short-Term Treatment

The benzodiazepines (see Table 78) have become the standard sedative-antianxiety agents worldwide because their effects in anxiety are usually superior to a placebo and because they are relatively safe agents; also, it is difficult to become addicted to them or to commit suicide with them. They are relatively expensive. For reasons that are not entirely clear, diazepam (Valium) became the most commonly prescribed medicine in the United States for several years in the 1970s. The benzodiazepines continue to be among the most commonly used agents in medicine.

Unfortunately, the rapid activity of diazepam and its tendency to induce euphoria have made it a popular drug of abuse. Its prolonged duration of action and affinity for lipid and protein suggest that overdoses of diazepam may be somewhat more dangerous than those of other benzodiazepines. Oxazepam (Serax) is the most rapidly metabolized and cleared benzodiazepine commonly used to treat anxiety; this drug and lorazepam have no active metabolites or tendency to accumulate in tissue, and alprazolam has only minor amounts of active metabolites. These short-acting benzodiazepines, then, are safer for use in elderly patients or those with impaired hepatic function. Oxazepam is also a particularly potent anticonvulsant. Lorazepam is uniquely well absorbed after intramuscular injection, and very rapidly acting if given sublingually. The potential of the short-acting benzodiazepines for tolerance, habituation, and abuse requires further evaluation. Longer-acting agents may be preferable where prolonged use for more than a few days is considered. No anxiolytic has been proven superior to chlordiazepoxide, which is relatively inexpensive compared to newer benzodiazepines.

Flurazepam (Dalmane), temazepam (Restoril), triazolam (Halcion), and nitrazepam (Mogodon; not available in the United States) are more potent in their sedative effects than the other benzodiazepines and are recommended only for nighttime sedation and sleep (see Table 78). They also seem to have less tendency to induce tolerance than other hypnotics.

It appears, although it is not yet clearly established, that their lethality on overdosage and their potential for abuse and addiction appear to be no greater than for other benzodiazepines and much less than for the short-acting barbiturates and nonbarbiturate hypnotic-sedatives. Flurazepam, although the first benzodiazepine introduced into American medicine as a hypnotic agent, is actually ill-suited for this purpose because of its production of long-acting metabolites and associated risk of "hangover" or protracted daytime sedating effects. The newer, shorter-acting benzodiazepine hypnotics are probably better suited for this indication and are growing in popularity, although triazolam is so short-lived that it may not always provide an adequately prolonged hypnotic effect to last all night. Their effects appear not to undergo rapid tolerance, as was common with barbiturates and many other, older hypnotics, at least during several weeks of use for their hypnotic effects. The ability of any hypnotic agent to produce sustained decreases in the time of onset of sleep has been questioned in several research studies, and some deeper phases of sleep may even be reduced by benzodiazepines. Nevertheless, subjective and some objective data concerning the improved quality of sleep and reduced awakenings encourage the widespread use of such hypnotics. One hopes that growing research on specific sleep disorders and on the differential diagnosis of insomnia will have a growing impact on medical practice and the selection of more specific treatments.

A specialized use of benzodiazepines is to control acute toxic psychoses brought on by hallucinogenic agents, such as lysergic acid diethylamide (LSD), methylated aromatic amines, or phencyclidine, since the use of antipsychotic agents in such cases may occasionally produce unwanted drug interactions, including hypotension. Many milder cases, especially those involving LSD or mescaline, can be managed even more conservatively by protection and reassurance of the patient until the effects of the psychotogen wear off. A notable exception to this rule is the paranoid psychosis induced by large or prolonged doses of amphetamines; it responds quickly, specifically, and safely to antipsychotic agents, and is unnecessarily prolonged without such treatment. Another specialized use of benzodiazepines is for their anticonvulsant effects: intravenous diazepam is a frequent choice in status epilepticus, and clonazepam (Clonopin) is effective in petit mal epilepsy (and may have useful antianxiety effects). The long-acting benzodiazepines are also agents of choice in the management of withdrawal from alcohol.

For routine use in psychiatric patients, and indeed most patients, the short-acting barbiturates and nonbarbiturate sedatives should *not* be used for prolonged daytime sedation and antianxiety effects because of their potential for excessive sedation, their high potential for tolerance, habituation, and dependence, and their lethality on overdose. However, it is well to remember that the long-acting barbiturate phenobarbital has done about as well as the more "modern" antianxiety agents in most drug comparisons, and it is far less expensive. Although there is little reason to recommend short-acting barbiturates as antianxiety agents, they still have specialized uses in psychiatry. For example, they are occasionally used (but now less often than diazepam, lorazepam, or other benzodiazepines) in emergencies to produce rapid sedation in psychotic, manic, or enraged patients, usually in conjunction with an antipsychotic agent. Short-acting barbiturates, most commonly amobarbital, given intravenously are sometimes used to facilitate the differential diagnosis of catatonic behavior or in attempts to uncover highly defended thoughts or feelings in diagnostic examinations or abreactive therapeutic interviews, although their unique efficacy for such uses has not been proved.

The propanediols, which seemed promising in the 1950s, are no better than the barbiturates for treating anxiety disorders, and meprobamate carries an unacceptable risk of addiction and fatality on overdosage. The habituating dose of meprobamate overlaps the therapeutic range: physical signs of withdrawal can follow the rapid discontinuation of doses as low as 1,200 mg/day, and severe withdrawal and seizures can be expected at doses above 3,200 mg/day, while the therapeutic range is 1,200 to 2,400 mg/day. A newer propanediol, tybamate, is less likely to produce addiction, but comparisons with barbiturates and the benzodiazepines have shown it to be an inferior antianxiety agent.

Other agents have been employed in the treatment of anxiety disorders; some of these are considered experimental and are discussed later in the chapter. *Antipsychotic agents* are generally inferior antianxiety agents, and their toxic risks are usually considered to be excessive for short-term use and to contraindicate prolonged use. Paradoxically, some side effects, notably motor restlessness (akathisia), probably contribute to the impression that anxiety symptoms may be worsened in some patients by neuroleptics. Although some clinicians prefer to use small doses of an antipsychotic agent for prolonged periods in patients who appear to benefit from such treatment, or patients who have highly unstable personalities with symptoms suggestive of psychosis or a history of abuse or addiction to sedatives, alcohol, or opioids, such uses are to be considered nonroutine and should be carefully supported and documented on a case-by-case basis.

The utility of *antidepressants* of the tricyclic or MAO inhibitor types for the treatment of some syndromes marked by anxiety was discussed in the preceding chapter. Such agents appear to be especially useful (sometimes in relatively small doses, less than half of those used in major depression) against the manifestations of *panic* (severe, sudden, overwhelming anxiety; a sense of impending doom or catastrophe; and marked autonomic discharge with palpitations, sweating, and rapid respiration or hyperventilation). This syndrome is often associated with phobias, especially severe *agoraphobia,* as well as with more generalized and *anticipatory anxiety* leading to growing restriction of the range of activities or risks undertaken. There may also be an association of panic disorder with the mitral valve prolapse syndrome, of uncertain significance. The phobic aspects of anxiety disorders respond less consistently to antidepressants or benzodiazepines, and may show additional benefit from behavioral and psychotherapies in a comprehensive program of treatment, whereas a drug alone is seldom adequate. There is probably some overlap between the spectrums of efficacy of antidepressants and benzodiazepines. For example, several recent studies indicate that alprazolam or other benzodiazepines may be of benefit in panic and phobic disorders as well as mild or moderate depression — conditions in which antidepressants are also effective.

Some of the anguish of *obsessive-compulsive disorder* may also be benefited by a benzodiazepine as well as, or in combination with, an antidepressant; there is current interest in alprazolam for this purpose. Benzodiazepines as well as antidepressants of either the MAO-inhibitor or tricyclic types may be of benefit in *dysthymic disorders* or in forms of depression or allied conditions associated with marked anxiety or phobic features. Although the antidepressants are the agents of first choice in the treatment of major depression, especially with prominent melancholic features, benzodiazepines are, in fact, commonly employed clinically for mild, "neurotic" dysthymia, in part because of their relative safety and easy acceptability by patients and many general physicians.

A final point about the acceptability of antianxiety agents is that there are strong prejudices regarding their use by the medical profession, by psychiatrists in particular, and by the general public. Since anxiety symptoms that reasonably indicate medical treatment are so similar to "normal" everyday tensions and dysphorias, many individuals are reluctant to give or to accept medication for such disorders, even when they are severe and disabling. Such attitudes appear to arise partly from societal values about individual responsibility and partly from a general association of sedative agents with problems of overuse, abuse, habituation, and acute overdoses. Although such attitudes are understandable, there is a risk that undertreatment may result. Recent studies indicate that some physicians use benzodiazepines very conservatively and may even undertreat patients with clinically significant anxiety; they may either withhold medication unless symptoms or dysfunction are severe or may interrupt treatment within a few weeks, causing a high proportion of relapses.

Long-Term Treatment

The long-term use and risks of abuse of antianxiety agents are poorly evaluated. The U.S. Drug Enforcement Administration (DEA) and many state laws classify sedatives, including benzodiazepines, with controlled substances. Although suspected to occur sometimes, actual rates of tolerance to antianxiety effects and risks of habituation and dependence with the modern antianxiety agents are unknown, as are rates of abuse. The clinical dilemmas involved in long-term treatment of psychiatric populations can be especially difficult. Many patients for whom antianxiety agents are indicated have chronic or recurrent disorders; some also have unstable or impulsive personalities or have a history of abuse of alcohol or other central depressants. It is suspected that such patients present increased risks of engaging in prescribed or unauthorized escalation of doses, habituation or physical dependence, or acute overdosage. Risks such as these encourage conservatism in the long-term use of benzodiazepines and even more cautious long-term use of older sedatives. Reflecting such considerations and the lack of precise knowledge of risks involved with long-term use of antianxiety agents, the usual manufacturers' and U.S. Food and Drug Administration (FDA) guidelines are not to exceed four months of continuous use of a benzodiazepine. Although this may be a reasonable general guideline, it does not necessarily parallel actual patterns of use and may not fit all cases.

A 1979 national survey in the United States indicated that 80% of patients using a benzodiazepine did so for less than four months; nearly two-thirds of prescriptions were taken for less than two weeks, but nearly half were used intermittently on an "as needed" basis, often without further consultation with the prescribing physician, and about 15% of patients continued to use a benzodiazepine continuously for more than a year (Mellinger and Balter, 1981). The majority of long-term users were patients over age 50, and many of these had cardiac or other chronic physical disorders in addition to symptoms of anxiety; the great majority of them were given a benzodiazepine by a nonpsychiatric physician.

Among psychiatric patients with chronic or frequently recurring disorders marked by anxiety, most studies have found maximum benefits of a benzodiazepine within six weeks of treatment. Several studies and much clinical experience indicate that many severe anxiety disorders treated by psychiatrists have a high rate of relapse or chronicity and a high tendency to relapse when treatment is discontinued. Despite the likelihood that there are legitimate and safe indications for prolonged use of a benzodiazepine, this aspect of therapeutic use of these agents is very poorly evaluated through systematic, controlled clinical research.

A related area of ignorance is the optimal dosing pattern to advise in discontinuing a benzodiazepine after several months of use. This question is especially pertinent because symptoms of withdrawal from sedatives can mimic the relapse of anxiety disorders. Recent authoritative reviewers presented such disparate recommendations as reducing the dose of a benzodiazepine by as much as 10% per day, on the one hand, or by as little as the equivalent of 2 mg of diazepam per week, on the other. It seems reasonable to base such recommendations on the dose, duration of treatment, and type of agent given: higher doses and more prolonged use require a more cautious and protracted withdrawal. Long-acting agents such as diazepam, chlordiazepoxide, clorazepate, and prazepam require prolonged periods of withdrawal to clear the nervous system and other tissues of active agent, perhaps several weeks. On the other hand, their gradual clearance may also contribute to a reduced risk of severe reactions even with relatively rapid withdrawal. This issue is discussed further in the next section in connection with toxicity.

Influence of Age on Treatment

There is little reason to use barbiturates and other non-benzodiazepine sedatives in elderly patients for agitation or insomnia. The risks of paradoxical excitement and increased agitation, intoxication, fatal overdosage, and complex drug interactions from induction of hepatic enzymes outweigh the beneficial effects of barbiturates and the related nonbarbiturate sedative agents. Although benzodiazepines are relatively safer, they too are often associated with excessive sedation, intoxication and, occasionally, paradoxical excitation. Because of its rapid clearance, oxazepam may be particularly safe for use in elderly patients. Doses required by the elderly may be 10–20% of those typically administered to a young adult patient. One of the most common causes of *reversible confusional states* in the elderly is the overuse of sedatives, including even "small" doses of benzodiazepines. Such reactions are often misdiagnosed as examples of irreversible dementia, and there is a risk that accompanying agitation may lead to increased doses and even greater intoxication.

For children, barbiturates (and phenytoin) are used as anticonvulsants but should not be used as sedatives or behavior-modifying agents. When a hypnotic effect or the calming of severe, acute excitement is desirable, diphenhydramine (Benadryl) is commonly used in doses from 50 to 500 mg/day (2–20 mg/kg), and chloral hydrate is still used occasionally in doses from 500 to 2,500 mg (up to 50 mg/kg). Information concerning the use of benzodiazepines for the control of anxiety and behavioral disorders in children is scant; chlordiazepoxide (Librium) is the best evaluated agent of the class in this age group. This drug is not as useful as amphetamine in the control of hyperactivity, however. Chlordiazepoxide has been reported to have some beneficial effects, as have tricyclic and MAO-inhibitor antidepressants, on phobic states including school phobias, given in doses of 30–130 mg/day (1.0–5.0 mg/kg). There is probably an increased risk of paradoxical excitement and angry outbursts when benzodiazepines are given to brain-damaged children or those with a history of aggressive or impulsive behavior. Premature and newborn infants are strikingly intolerant of benzodiazepines, evidently reflecting their poorly developed ability to metabolize them by hepatic mechanisms.

Toxicology

For all sedatives, the most commonly encountered problem is daytime sedation with drowsiness, decreased mental acuity, some decrease in coordination, decreased occupational efficiency and productivity, and increased risk of accidents, particularly when sedatives are combined with alcohol. Autonomic and extrapyramidal side effects are rarely encountered with the sedatives. Liver damage and blood dyscrasias are also rare.

It would be a mistake to conclude that the benzodiazepines are totally innocuous. In rare cases overdoses equivalent to about a two weeks' supply, or even less if taken with alcohol, have led to death. The common use of chlordiazepoxide and diazepam in high doses to treat alcoholic withdrawal and the use of diazepam intravenously to control seizures or cardiac arrhythmias are occasionally complicated by apnea, ventricular arrhythmias, or cardiac arrest. Certain neurotic or psychotic patients, and even normal volunteers, occasionally become dysphoric, irritable, agitated, angry, or otherwise "disinhibited" while taking benzodiazepines. This effect resembles that of alcohol; it is most commonly ascribed to chlordiazepoxide, but is not unique to that agent. Such reactions may be more characteristic of benzodiazepines than of barbiturates or meprobamate.

The most serious problems of sedatives are related to their tendency to produce *tolerance* and *physiological dependence* (addiction) in addition to psychological habituation. Tolerance to the antianxiety and sedative effects of sedatives can contribute to innocent self-medication in increasing doses. Rapid intoxication and euphoria from large or parenteral doses of the rapidly acting barbiturates, most of the nonbarbiturate sedative-hypnotics, and especially diazepam among the benzodiazepines contribute to their abuse and to a brisk "black market" in these legally controlled agents.

It is currently a topic of debate whether the industrially developed societies of the world are overmedicated, and particularly whether the current medical use of drugs to treat mild neurotic reactions and even "normal" stresses and strains of living contributes to the abuse of psychotropic agents. While the debate continues, physicians can deal with the problems associated with sedative-tranquilizing agents by selecting those with less potential for abuse, addiction, and lethality and by using the drugs for clear indications, in adequate but not excessive doses, and for limited periods of time. Patients with a previous history of abuse of other sedatives or alcohol and with other antisocial or impulsive traits should be treated very cautiously with this class of agents. In general, the use of sedative-tranquilizers in patients with personality disorders and more chronic forms of anxiety disorders is unlikely to be helpful except in acute exacerbations of turmoil or anticipatory anxiety, and it is likely to engender abuse.

The probability that a patient will become physiologically dependent on a sedative increases with the daily dose of drug and the duration of its use. Meprobamate is potentially so highly addicting that its use is impractical except in moderate doses for brief periods. With short-acting barbiturates, some signs and symptoms of withdrawal (such as anxiety, agitation, anorexia, nausea and vomiting, tachycardia, postural hypotension, hyperreflexia, or tremor) can be expected after the intake of about four to five times the usual daily dose for more than a month; and severe withdrawal reactions, with hypotension, hypothermia, seizures, delirium tremens, and hallucinosis can be expected to occur two or three days after discontinuation of prolonged dosage more than five times the ordinary

Table 80   Principles of withdrawal in cases of addiction to barbiturates and other sedatives

1. A short-acting barbiturate (e.g., *pentobarbital,* Nembutal) has similar actions (cross-tolerance) to most of the sedative-tranquilizers in Table 79 (except the antihistamines, which rarely produce addiction) and can be used to withdraw from nonbarbiturates as well as all barbiturates, greatly simplifying the technique.

2. Withdrawal from barbiturate-type addiction (in contrast to opioid addiction) is a medically serious undertaking, best done *in hospital* and carried out *slowly* (especially with phenobarbital, glutethimide, and the benzodiazepines, although the withdrawal syndrome with most benzodiazepines is rarely severe).

3. *Estimate the amount of pentobarbital required* to protect against withdrawal symptoms after initial intoxication has cleared by giving a test dose of 200 mg. (A) If the patient is heavily sedated or falls asleep, there is probably no tolerance. (B) If mild intoxication is found (drowsiness, slurred speech, ataxia, incoordination, nystagmus), give 200 mg (preferably orally) in 6-hour intervals to induce repeated *mild* intoxication within an hour of each dose and to avoid prominent withdrawal symptoms, tremulousness, and hypotension 4–6 hours after each dose (if this occurs, increase the dose or decrease the interval to 4 hours). (C) If no intoxication occurs after the test dose, suspect significant tolerance and give 100 mg every 2 hours until intoxication occurs; then give the total in 6-hour intervals over the following 24 hours. In a 24-hour period, 800 to 2,400 mg is typically required; up to 400 mg/day of pentobarbital can be discontinued abruptly.

4. *Stabilization* continues for 2–3 days for most barbiturates and nonbarbiturate sedatives. The daily dose is given in four to six portions. Because of their tendency to produce severe withdrawal symptoms a week or more after withdrawal, a stabilization period of 7–10 days is recommended for phenobarbital and glutethimide, and following abuse of the benzodiazepines in very large doses.

5. *Withdraw* (over approximately 10–20 days) by removing not more than 100 mg of pentobarbital per day and *only* after stabilization is attained (mild intoxication and minimal withdrawal signs during a 24-hour period) and maintained for the recommended number of days. If withdrawal signs develop, stop withdrawal until the signs disappear and resume at 50 mg per day.

6. As an alternative to step 5, some experts recommend substituting *phenobarbital* (long-acting), 30 mg for each 100 mg of pentobarbital during the stabilization period and withdrawing it at the rate of 30 mg/day.

7. The short-acting barbiturates are not useful in the management of withdrawal from opiates. Even though there is cross-tolerance between alcohol and barbiturates, detoxification of alcoholics is usually accomplished with long-acting

Table 80 (continued)

benzodiazepines (chlordiazepoxide or diazepam). Addiction to meprobamate is often overcome by slow withdrawal of the offending agent by the same principles outlined above.

8. In mixed addictions involving a sedative plus an opioid, maintain the patient on methadone while carrying out the above protocol, the required doses being estimated by giving 10-mg doses to reverse increases of pulse and blood pressure and pupillary dilatation (rarely more than 40 mg/24 hours). In cases of mixed sedative and alcohol addiction, there is no general agreement on the ideal withdrawal procedure; the use of chlordiazepoxide alone is a reasonable choice, provided that enough is given initially to ensure mild intoxication (typically 100–400 mg/24 hours) and the withdrawal is carried out much more slowly than in simple alcohol addiction (typically over 4–5 days), with the steps and timing patterned after steps 4 and 5, withdrawing at 5–10% per day over 10–20 days. Some experts prefer to follow the protocol recommended in steps 3–6, with phenobarbital used during the withdrawal phase, especially when the history suggests that sedative addiction is the more important problem.

daily dose, and certainly above ten times this dose. The withdrawal syndrome is strikingly similar to that associated with alcohol. It is most important to realize that withdrawal from addiction to barbiturates and other sedatives is a serious and *life-threatening* medical problem, in contrast to withdrawal from narcotics, which is unpleasant but almost never fatal. Special measures to be taken in managing withdrawal from sedatives are outlined in Table 80.

Physical dependence on the benzodiazepines has been studied most extensively with the oldest agents of that group, chlordiazepoxide and diazepam, although the risk of tolerance, and possibly of dependence, may also be significant with the newer, shorter-acting benzodiazepines, especially those of high potency, such as alprazolam and lorazepam (see Table 78). While pharmacokinetic and drug metabolism mechanisms may contribute to tolerance to sedatives, the most critical mechanisms are believed to occur at the level of neuronal-cellular metabolism and function but are not known in detail. Addiction is not likely unless abuses reach at least ten, and more likely twenty, times the usual daily oral dose and continue for several months. This time can be shortened, however, if the drugs are taken intravenously, as has sometimes been done with diazepam in its recent abuse as a "street drug." The ordinarily delayed development of addiction to benzodiazepines in part reflects the prolonged half-life of these agents, much as the long-acting barbiturate phenobarbital infrequently leads to physical dependence and a withdrawal syndrome. Furthermore, the onset of the withdrawal syndrome with the benzodiazepines, glutethimide (Doriden), and phenobarbital is considerably later than with either the short-acting barbiturates and sedatives (two to three days) or alcohol (three to five days); it is usually seen at four to eight days, but as long as two weeks after withdrawal. Even when a withdrawal syndrome is encountered after abuse of the benzodiazepines, it is likely to be of only moderate intensity and is rarely associated with seizures.

The development of psychological and physiological dependence on sedative-hypnotic agents reflects a complex relationship between their pharmacology and sociological factors involved in their use. There is some evidence that the long-term use of benzodiazepines may be less frequent now than in the early 1970s, that doses may tend to decrease with duration of use, and that the use of antianxiety medication may decrease when patients are allowed to set their own dosage schedule according to their needs, in contrast to fixed dosage determined by the prescribing physician (Rickels, 1983). However, tolerance to the effects of this class of agents can encourage innocent increases in the amount of medication, and mild withdrawal reactions may be mistaken for relapse of a primary anxiety disorder. These considerations add further support to the conclusion that these agents are most safely used in acute anxiety and for brief periods, and that prolonged maintenance with antianxiety agents should be avoided when possible except when the unique responses to such treatment are adequately demonstrated and documented for an individual patient.

The benzodiazepines have a confortable margin of safety in comparison with other sedatives. Nevertheless, although it is commonly said that suicide is virtually impossible with a benzodiazepine, many deliberate overdoses involve more than one agent, typically whatever the victim has at hand, and can present complicated toxicologic crises that are difficult to manage. Alcohol is a common complicating factor. The problem is exacerbated when patients acquire a number of potentially lethal medications from more than one source or from one physician over time. Some of the problem could be eliminated by requiring that patients empty their medicine chests and bring *all* their medications to the physician, who should take the responsibility for disposing of the unnecessary or outdated ones before a new psychotropic chemical is prescribed. It is difficult to recommend a specific benzodiazepine supply that can be dispensed safely, since there are rare reports of deaths following the acute ingestion of 600–1,000 mg of chlordiazepoxide or diazepam, and reports of the survival of patients following doses of more than 2,000 mg. While antianxiety effects of diazepam have been associated with plasma benzodiazepine levels of 400–600 ng/ml, excessive sedation can occur in some patients at similar levels, and gross intoxication can be expected at levels above 900 ng/ml. As with other sedatives and hypnotics, as a general rule, the acute ingestion of ten days' supply of a benzodiazepine at once regularly produces severe intoxication and may be lethal, especially to a young child or an elderly person; the ingestion of twenty times the daily or hypnotic dose is likely to be fatal. Even though fatality is less likely and more unpredictable with acute overdoses of the benzodiazepines than with other sedative-tranquilizers, it is unwise to dispense more than perhaps two weeks' supply of a benzodiazepine or a week's supply of other sedatives. Moreover, continuing the use of any of these drugs for more than a few weeks calls for a critical appraisal of risks and benefits in individual cases. The routine dispensing of sedatives for "as needed" use at the discretion of the patient without close medical or psychiatric supervision also increases the risks of misuse and abuse.

The safety of sedative-tranquilizers in *pregnancy* is not established. There is some inconclusive evidence that the benzodiazepines may be teratogenic, inasmuch as cleft lip and palate have been suggestively associated with the use of a benzodiazepine in the first trimester of pregnancy; the risk involved is probably below that of birth defects overall (approximately 2%), and the defects are usually surgically correctable. The barbiturates can alter fetal hepatic metabolism and should be avoided. Claims have been made for the safety of meprobamate in pregnancy, but physiological dependence of the fetus on this agent or on barbiturate and non-barbiturate sedatives can be expected, with the attendant risk of a potentially fatal withdrawal reaction. Since the fetus and neonate are poorly defended against the CNS depressant effects of benzodiazepines, in part because of undeveloped hepatic metabolic mechanisms, the risk of neonatal intoxication or CNS depression is high.

In general, the clinical toxicity of the benzodiazepines is low. This factor contributes significantly to the enormous popularity of these agents and to the frequent suspicion that they are overused. Some nonspecific symptoms of patients treated with benzodiazepines, including weight gain, skin reactions, headaches, impairment of sexual function, and menstrual irregularity, have been described. Since these and other symptoms, such as light-headedness, difficulty in concentration, vertigo, and lethargy, overlap with the conditions for which a benzodiazepine might be used clinically, they are often difficult to assess. Temporary discontinuation or rapid dosage reduction may or may not help to resolve the question, since there is a risk that removal of the drug may lead to confusion of reappearance of the symptoms of primary anxiety disorder with mild withdrawal reactions that often include symptoms of anxiety and mild autonomic distress.

Drug interactions involving the older sedatives were common and sometimes significant. Those shared by the benzodiazepines are additive, or possible potentiating, interactions with other *CNS depressants,* including alcohol, other sedatives, other psychotropic agents, and opioid analgesics. The barbiturate and older, so-called non-barbiturate sedatives generally have potent inducing effects on hepatic microsomal and other drug-metabolizing systems, and can lead to reduced plasma levels and actions of many agents, including anticoagulants, hypoglycemic agents, and other psychotropic agents. For this reason, it is recommended that non-benzodiazepine sedatives or hypnotics not be combined with an antipsychotic or antidepressant agent, especially for long-term maintenance treatment. Benzodiazepines in ordinary doses are much less likely to increase the hepatic drug-metabolizing systems or to compete importantly with the metabolism of other agents, although moderate elevations of plasma levels of *phenytoin* and *digitalis* have been reported. On the other hand, there are several reports of interactions that alter the absorption, plasma levels, or effects of the benzodiazepines. Notable examples are the ability of several types of *antacids* to decrease the absorption of benzodiazepines; *anticholinergic agents* may have a similar effect (including antiparkinsonism, antidepressant, and over-the-counter sedative and decongestant agents). There are also reports that *cimetidine* (Tagamet) can increase plasma levels of some benzodiazepines, especially the longer-acting agents (such as diazepam, chlordiazepoxide, clorazepate, halazepam, prazepam, and flurazepam) with prominent microsomal metabolism. Interactions related to *alcohol* and alcoholism may also be important. The mixing of a benzodiazepine and alcohol can lead to severe intoxication, and alcohol may increase plasma levels of some benzodiazepines, including diazepam. Moreover, *disulfiram* (Antabuse), which is sometimes administered with chlordiazepoxide or other long-acting benzodiazepines in the treatment of alcoholism, may lead to increased plasma levels of the benzodiazepine by interfering with hepatic microsomal actions required for inactivation. It is also known that *food* can have complex effects on the gastrointestinal absorption of some benzodi-azepines; for example, decreased immediate absorption of diazepam has been reported, as well as increased total uptake over a period of several days.

Table 81 summarizes the interactions between benzodiazepines and other agents. As a general rule, the interactions involving hepatic metabo-lism of benzodiazepines appear to be more likely with the long-acting agents, the inactivation and clearance of which are likely to be decreased by agents that compete for hepatic microsomal systems. Benzodiazepines that are inactivated by conjugation reactions (such as oxazepam and lorazepam) have alternative routes not requiring hepatic microsomes and may be less likely to be involved in such interactions. Benzodiazepines are

Table 81   Interactions between benzodiazepines and other agents

Agent	Effect when combined with a benzodiazepine
Phenytoin and digitalis preparations	Plasma levels increased; best described as an effect of diazepam on pheny-toin and on digoxin; may occur with other long-acting benzodiazepines as well via hepatic metabolic interac-tions (including the anticonvulsant benzodiazepine clonazepam)
Antacids, agents with anticholinergic activity	Decreased absorption of benzodiaz-epines; best described with cloraze-pate, chlordiazepoxide, and diaze-pam
Alcohol; MAO inhibitors	Increased intoxication; plasma level of long-acting benzodiazepines may in-crease
Disulfiram (Antabuse) and cimetidine (Tagamet), but not other H$_2$ blockers (such as ranitidine)	Increased plasma levels of long-acting benzodiazepines, including chlordia-zepoxide but not short-acting con-geners (such as oxazepam and loraze-pam)
Food	Complex effects on absorption: initial decrease but gradual increases; best described with diazepam

unlikely to have important pharmacokinetic interactions with antipsychotic or antidepressant agents or lithium salts, but may increase the risk of excessive sedation or intoxication with any other CNS-active agent on an additive basis.

Alternative and Experimental Treatments

The clinical discussion in this chapter has suggested that, although the use of benzodiazepines and other sedatives is extraordinarily extensive in general medicine, their role in psychiatry remains limited and somewhat ambiguous. While there is no doubt that many cases involving severe symptoms of anxiety can benefit from treatment with a benzodiazepine, there are also a growing number of alternatives. In addition to the strong tradition in American psychiatry of relying on psychotherapeutic methods for many cases of disorders with prominent symptoms of anxiety, as well as of encouraging supportive, nonpharmacologic, interpersonal methods of assisting a patient through personal crises, there is a growing amount of research and clinical interest in refining the definitions of the syndromes classified as anxiety disorders, and in seeking more specific forms of treatment of each.

The current place of the benzodiazepines in the partial treatment of sustained, generalized, or anticipatory anxiety is secure. There is also evidence that some benzodiazepines may be effective in panic anxiety, and therefore beneficial in syndromes involving complexes of panic, anticipatory anxiety, phobias, and restricted activity (agoraphobia). *Alprazolam* (Xanax) has been especially extensively investigated in such syndromes recently, but it has not been proved that its effects, especially on panic reactions, are unique among the benzodiazepines. The anticonvulsant benzodiazepine *clonazepam* (Clonopin) may have a similar effect, but it is not known whether other anticonvulsants may also have useful effects in anxiety or panic disorders.

The major alternatives to a benzodiazepine for panic disorder currently are the tricyclic-type antidepressants (especially *imipramine* and possibly also *clomipramine*) or an *MAO inhibitor*. It is not established that any of these choices is consistently more effective than the others; for this reason, some clinicians and patients prefer to initiate treatment with a benzodiazepine, perhaps alprazolam, then to try a tricyclic antidepressant, and finally to resort to an MAO inhibitor if the preceding trials lead to unsatisfactory results. This recommendation is based on the relative simplicity and safety of the three choices, and may be modified as further research evidence is gained from direct comparisons of the efficacy of these or alternative treatments of panic and agoraphobic disorders. The additional hypothesis that alprazolam and other *triazolobenzodiazepines* may have unique properties not only in anxiety disorders, panic disorder, and phobias but also in depression requires further study, especially for cases of severe major depression, in which the efficacy of sedative-antianxiety agents is least well demonstrated.

Partly as a result of laboratory research implicating the locus ceruleus and other CNS centers for the control of the autonomic nervous system in panic and anxiety reactions, there is a strong interest in the evaluation of agents with central antiadrenergic actions in the treatment of anxiety disorders. Perhaps the best-known example is the beta-adrenergic antagonist *propranolol,* which may have useful and safe antianxiety effects in doses similar to, or even smaller than, those used in cardiology. This agent, unlike many of the newer beta-blockers designed specifically for peripheral cardiovascular actions (that is, with selective anti-β_1 actions and relatively low lipophilicity and penetration into the CNS), is effective at both of the major known subtypes of beta receptors and penetrates the blood-brain barrier relatively well at ordinary clinical doses. These pharmacologic characteristics, especially access to the CNS, may be desirable in an antianxiety agent, although the role of beta-adrenergic, as opposed to alpha-adrenergic, receptors in anxiety remains unclear. Propranolol, while considered investigational for the treatment of anxiety disorders, is officially approved by the U.S. Food and Drug Administration for general clinical use and has been used in anxiety disorders in a large number of patients. Its main benefits appear to involve reduction of somatic, autonomic features of anxiety reactions, such as tachycardia and palpitations, sweating, and tremor, although its effects on the more subjective, psychic aspects of anxiety disorders (fear, anticipation, dread, tension, dysphoria) are less clear and probably less prominent. Propranolol has been reported in clinical anecdotes to have particular benefits in predictable, acute, situational anxiety reactions, such as those associated with public speaking ("stage fright") and possibly other specific or situational phobias. Such benefits have led to some efforts to treat panic disorder, with its prominent autonomic symptoms, as well as agoraphobia which is often associated with panic reactions, with propranolol when a benzodiazepine or antidepressant has proved ineffective, but results have been inconsistent.

Further interest in antiadrenergic compounds has included limited experience with *clonidine* (Catapres), an antihypertensive agent with a complex pharmacology and a remarkable range of actions. It is believed to act mainly as an agonist of presumably presynaptic α_2 autoreceptors that throttle the production and release of norepinephrine, and to do so importantly at the locus ceruleus of the brainstem, a major adrenergic center of regulation of the sympathetic nervous system (see Chapter 4). The net effect of this agent is evidently to diminish the availability of norepinephrine at all types of receptors, both alpha and beta, in the central nervous system. This drug was referred to in Chapter 2 with respect to its possible benefits in Gilles de la Tourette's syndrome and in akathisia induced by neuroleptic agents. It has also been reported to reduce the agitation and autonomic responses during withdrawal from opioids, ethanol, and nicotine. The potential utility of clonidine in anxiety disorders is not yet well evaluated, but there is some preliminary clinical experience to indicate that it may have useful antianxiety actions at doses (0.1–0.2 mg/day) with only mild hypotensive effects, but possibly with rapid development of tolerance. Whether these actions will be limited to reducing the physical, sympathetic responses in panic or other anxiety disorders, or may also include the subjective, psychic aspects of anxiety as well, remains to be better investigated. Other agents, especially selective α_1 antagonists with CNS activity, might also be worthy of investigation in the anxiety disorders.

The well-established phenomenon of inducing panic or severe anxiety reactions in susceptible patient-subjects by intravenous *infusions of lactate* may also present an opportunity to test novel treatments of anxiety disorders. The physiology of the response to lactate is not established; it may involve altered availability of calcium ion or other effects on membrane functions related to changes in plasma pH. Agents with selective effects on ion transport, such as the calcium channel blockers, might be of interest for their possible effects in anxiety but have not yet been evaluated. Although the deliberate induction of severe anxiety by a chemical challenge such as lactate infusion presents an ethical dilemma, this procedure has been remarkably well tolerated in research patients, who are often disabled by severe anxiety and panic, and the short-lasting responses can be terminated by stopping the infusion or administering intravenous diazepam. Another emerging area of investigation into experimentally induced anxiety is the study of new agents that seem to act as *antagonists of the benzodiazepines,* possibly through interactions at specific receptor sites in the brain. These compounds include benzodiazepine analogues as well as β-carboline compounds. Some of these agents are capable of inducing reactions that resemble severe anxiety in animals, including primates, and possibly also in man. Such agents may offer additional experimental models with which to test potential new antianxiety agents under controlled conditions, as is being done with the lactate infusion technique.

A new type of agent with antianxiety effects but limited sedation is *buspirone* (Buspar), about to be released for general use in the United States (see Figure 20 and Table 78). The basis for its activity is unclear; it does not appear to interact with GABA receptors or benzodiazepine binding sites in brain tissue or to show cross-tolerance with other sedatives or alcohol. Clinical trials have provided support for its effectiveness in generalized anxiety, but its possible effects in panic, phobic, or obsessive-compulsive disorders are unclear. Unlike other sedative or antianxiety agents, there is some evidence that buspirone may exert antidopaminergic actions in the forebrain, although the limited clinical experience with it to date does not suggest that it can induce extrapyramidal or other effects typical of neuroleptic antidopaminergic agents.

Interpretation of the possible significance of the putative antidopaminergic actions of buspirone is further complicated by recent clinical experience suggesting that the dopamine agonist *bromocriptine* (Parlodel), in centrally effective doses above 10 mg/day, may exert beneficial effects in some conditions marked by anxiety, and particularly in *obsessive-compulsive disorder*. This beneficial effect may undergo tolerance in many cases, however, and in general this condition remains particularly hard to treat by any available method — pharmacologic or behavioral. A better understanding of the actions of buspirone and bromocriptine in anxiety disorders and "neuroses" may lead to the development of additional new treatments with effects unlike those of older sedatives or of the benzodiazepines.

A final point concerning the treatment of anxiety disorders and the growing number of allied syndromes (panic disorder, agoraphobia, specific phobias, anxious depression, obsessive-compulsive disorder) is that simple pharmacologic interventions are rarely curative, even though they help many patients and minimize some symptoms or features of these often complex and chronic or frequently recurrent disorders. At the present time, it is reasonable to try treating such disorders with adequate doses of the various agents discussed in this chapter, serially for at least several weeks. In addition, comprehensive treatment programs require consideration of additional therapeutic modalities, including psychotherapies and behavioral methods. For example, although an antidepressant can often minimize or even block the expression of panic, anticipation of further panic attacks, with sustained or situational anxiety, typically persists, and phobic or avoidant behaviors aimed at minimizing risks and dangers attendant on the feared loss of control during a panic attack may not be modified at all. A benzodiazepine may modify the anticipatory anxiety partially, but full treatment of the panic-agoraphobic-anxiety syndrome usually requires behavioral and psychological treatments as well, especially in order to "unlearn" the associations of panic with certain situations and to undo the acquired self-defensive, avoidant-phobic patterns of behavior, as well as to understand or rationalize the behavior patterns and emotional responses involved in this common, complex, and often severe and incapacitating illness.

Summary and Conclusions

Anxiety and dysphoria are ubiquitous human experiences. They are most effectively and appropriately treated with chemotherapy when they represent acute and severe symptoms of "neurotic" psychiatric illness, or reactive or anticipatory features of medical or surgical illness. Antianxiety medications should ideally be used for brief periods of time because tolerance to their antianxiety and sedative effects may develop and contribute to the risk of psychological habituation and even physical dependence. However, psychiatrists treat a growing number of patients with severe, chronic, or frequently recurring anxiety disorders that may require long-term treatment with a benzodiazepine or an antidepressant. Routine and sustained use of sedatives for psychiatric patients with personality disorders is often of questionable value and presents increased risk of abuse.

The history of psychopharmacology has been marked by the partially successful search for more effective and less toxic antianxiety agents; significant developments have been the replacement of alcohol and the bromides by the barbiturates in the early twentieth century, and the later addition of nonbarbiturate sedatives, including the propanediols. All of these sedative agents are severely toxic and potentially lethal when taken acutely in doses above ten times the usual daily dose, and are physically addicting when used for several months at doses only a few times above the daily dose. Withdrawal can be managed by use of the addicting agent itself or substitution of a barbiturate and its *slow* withdrawal. Reactions to rapid withdrawal of an antianxiety agent can be confused with relapse of the primary disorder.

Since the 1960s, the benzodiazepines have become the most useful antianxiety agents with the widest margin of safety and a limited potential for addiction. They also have useful hypnotic, anticonvulsant, and muscle-relaxant effects. The "metapharmacologic" aspects of anxiolytic agents, including psychosocial characteristics of patients and physicians using them, contribute to their efficacy, which depends at least partly on suggestion and placebo effects.

Antidepressants of the tricyclic or MAO inhibitor type are useful in panic disorders. New or experimental treatments include buspirone, antiadrenergic agents with CNS activity, and anticonvulsants. Comprehensive treatment of severe anxiety disorders includes use of psychotherapy and behavioral techniques as well as effective medication.

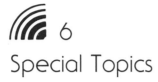 6

Special Topics

This final chapter deals with several specialized topics that pertain to the use of any chemotherapy in psychiatric practice. These topics include the special considerations required in the treatment of geriatric and pediatric patients; the unique circumstances of outpatient treatment programs; legal, regulatory, and ethical aspects of medical treatment of psychiatric conditions; the need for objectivity and common sense in the safe and effective use of psychotropic agents; and the future needs for the field of chemotherapy in psychiatry.

Pediatric and geriatric psychopharmacology are two of the least well developed aspects of the field. The uncertain categorization of behavioral disorders in children and resistance to experimentation with these patients have limited the development of pediatric psychopharmacology. It is only beginning to be understood that, in contrast to older notions that children require small doses of many drugs, children are often more efficient in metabolizing and eliminating psychotropic agents than are adults. The elderly encounter problems with inadequate differential evaluation of their psychiatric problems, an often pessimistic view about their treatment, and markedly increased risk of toxic effects of all chemotherapeutic agents.

The effectiveness and safety of chemotherapy can be enhanced greatly by attention to the psychological and social aspects of the individuals involved and the setting in which the treatment is carried out. Special sensitivity is required when the locus of control shifts from the clinical staff in an inpatient setting to the patient and family in an outpatient program, particularly in maximizing compliance with the prescribed treatment. Psychiatric treatment occurs in settings that are increasingly heavily influenced by legal and ethical constraints and guidelines, with a significant impact on the wise application of chemical as well as psychological treatments. The safety and effectiveness of chemotherapy in psychiatry can be enhanced greatly by simplification and objective evaluation of the need for chemotherapy and responses to it. Application of judgment and common sense, as well as sensitivity to the needs and circumstances of individual patients, can increase adherence to, and success of, treatment.

Future needs for improved treatments of psychiatric disorders include continued study of the natural history and differential categorization of disorders, continued searches for pathophysiologic and etiologic factors, and the development of additional agents that are more effective and safer than available drugs — most of which were developed empirically in the 1950s. There is a need to break away from the highly conservative constraints that have impeded progress in the field, and to move earlier to imaginative, brief clinical trials.

Geriatric and Pediatric Psychopharmacology

The use of psychiatric chemotherapy in patients at the extremes of the age spectrum raises several special considerations. Although geriatric psychopharmacology remains a relatively underdeveloped area of investigation, the elderly represent an increasingly large proportion of psychiatric as well as general medical patients, partly as a reflection of their increased representation in the population. Between 1900 and 1970 the rate of increase of persons over age 65 was about seven times greater than that of the total population, and the number of elderly citizens in the United States now exceeds 20 million. Among elderly nursing home residents, 90% or more are estimated to have clinically significant neuropsychiatric disabilities, and about 75% of these receive psychotropic medications. Many specific aspects of the use of antipsychotic, antimanic, antidepressant, and antianxiety agents in the elderly have already been discussed.

In addition, attempts have been made to develop chemical treatments for the loss of cerebral function that is characteristic of advanced age as well as symptomatic of dementias of the Alzheimer or multi-infarct types. Thus, a special application of psychopharmacology in aged patients is the use of mild *stimulants* and putative *cerebral vasodilators* in an effort to improve senile mentation. Stimulants such as amphetamine or methylphenidate (Ritalin) often induce agitation and unwanted side effects in elderly patients, and controlled studies offer little support for their efficacy in cognitive aspects of dementia, although they may reduce with-

Table 82 Proposed treatments for dementia

Agents	Comments
Cerebral vasodilators	
Hydrogenated ergot alkaloids (Hydergine, Deapril-ST)[a]	Commonly used in Europe; has anti-α-adrenergic effects and some direct poorly defined CNS effects; 7/13 controlled studies indicate better than placebo for up to 15 months, especially if dose 4.5 mg/day or more; may not increase CBF; has more effect on mood and activity than cognition; sublingual dosing difficult
Smooth muscle relaxants: papaverine[a] (Pavabid),[a] hexobendine	Direct actions on arteriolar smooth muscle, in part via cyclic-AMP; increases CBF but effects on cognition less clear; a few controlled studies suggest efficacy up to two years
Beta agonists: cyclandelate[a] (Cyclospasmol),[a] isoxuprine[a] (Vasodilan)[a]	May have beta-agonistic action and perhaps other smooth muscle effects; probably increase CBF; a few controlled trials fail to provide strong support of efficacy in cognition
Xanthines: caffeine, theophylline,[a] Cosaldon (contains hexyl-methyl-xanthine and nicotinic acid)	Poorly evaluated with mixed results; may actually decrease CBF, especially with increased peripheral flow; may have mild stimulant-like effects
Acetic anhydrase inhibitors: acetazolamide[a] (Diamox)[a]	Poorly evaluated; can increase CBF
Beta antagonists: propranolol (Inderal)[a]	Poorly evaluated
Anticoagulants	
Coumarins and others[a]	Poorly evaluated; potentially dangerous; theoretically indicated for multi-infarct dementia only
Psychostimulants	
Amphetamines,[a] methylphenidate (Ritalin),[a] fencamfamine	Can increase agitation; some effects on mood and activity; little support for cognitive benefits in few controlled trials

Table 82 (continued)

Agents	Comments
Pemoline (Cylert)[a]	Some support for benefits over placebo; effects probably mainly on mood and activity
Pentylenetetrazol (Metrazol)	7/17 controlled trials suggest some benefit at subconvulsant doses
Cerebral metabolic stimulants	
Meclofenoxate (Lucidril), naftidrofuryl (Praxilene), pyritinol (Encephabol), hopate	Several controlled trials suggest some benefits, but may have stimulant-like actions; pharmacology not well understood
Antidepressants	Imipramine[a] and congeners (especially nortriptyline[a] and desipramine)[a] may have mood-elevating and nonspecific effects in some cases; MAO inhibitors are excessively risky and hypotensive
Procaineamide preparations	
Gerovital H-3	Contains other unknown ingredients; may have weak MAO inhibitor effect; probably weakly stimulant-like; cognitive effects poorly supported
Noötropic agents	
Piracetam (Noötropil) and congeners (aniracetam, oxiracetam, pramiracetam, etc.)	GABA analogue, but may have cholinergic actions; has unique, poorly understood CNS actions and little else; slightly improved cognition in mild dementia in 2/3 controlled trials; term *noötropic* ("toward the mind," cognition-enhancing) is unique to piracetam or other agents like it
Neuropeptides	
ACTH, $ACTH_{4-10}$ (ORG-2766); MSH; vasopressin and analogues (DG-LVP); enkephalins (*met* and *leu)*	Main support for enhanced learning is from animal behavioral studies; may also produce nonspecific arousal; clinical studies of ACTH fragments are few and inconclusive or negative, especially re cognition in man, but

Table 82 (continued)

Agents	Comments
	vasopressin may be active; most are peptide sequences contained in β-lipotropin and other large peptide precursors of ACTH; most require injections or nasal inhalation
Cholinomimetics	
Choline, lecithin	Doses up to 20 g/day have yielded inconclusive or negative results, especially regarding cognition, despite good evidence of a specific ACh deficit in Alzheimer-type dementia; ability to increase ACh synthesis and use in CNS not proved
Deanol (Deaner)[a]	Choline analogue, increases choline levels, effects on CNS ACh systems not proved; may have mild stimulant-like effects; clinical trials in dementia inconclusive
Physostigmine,[a] tetrahydroaminoacridine, galanthamine	Only reversible anticholinesterases with CNS actions; results inconclusive with injected physostigmine; oral physostigmine and other agents of this type are not yet adequately evaluated

Abbreviations: ACh (acetylcholine); ACTH (adrenocorticotropic hormone); $ACTH_{4-10}$ (heptapeptide fragment containing amino acids 4–10 in the ACTH peptide sequence); CBF (cerebral blood flow); CNS (central nervous system); enkephalins (*leu:* leucine-containing; *met:* methionine-containing); MSH (melanocyte-stimulating hormone).

Note: The categories are somewhat arbitrary, since the pharmacology of some agents is unclear or ambiguous; many of the agents with at least strongly suggestive evidence of clinical activity in aged or demented patients have stimulant-like effects on arousal, general activity, and mood, although their effects on cognition are not as clear. Hydergine and piracetam seem especially promising; studies of peptides are still highly preliminary. Hyperbaric oxygen is ineffective and impractical; use of nitrites actually reduces CBF.

Use of such agents presumes that potentially treatable forms of dementia have been ruled out or treated more specifically (including hypothyroidism, congestive heart failure or other organ failures; poor nutrition; or intoxication with an agent such as a cardiac, hypotensive, sedative, andidepressant, antiparkinsonism, neuroleptic, or other drug; and other reversible neuromedical conditions).

For reviews of this topic, see Cole and Branconnier, *McLean Hosp. J.* 2:210, 1977; Goodnick and Gershon, *J. Clin. Psychiatry* 45:196, 1984.

a. Agents available for clinical use in the United States by brand name or as generic agents.

drawal and lassitude. Pemoline (Cylert) might increase intellectual function in addition to having stimulant effects, but its efficacy is not well established. However, vasodilators such as papaverine (Pavabid), cyclandelate (Cyclospasmol), isoxuprene (Vasodilan), and hexobendine (investigational); ergot alkaloids (especially Hydergine); and beta-adrenergic blocking agents such as propranolol (Inderal) have all been claimed to produce improvement in behavior, mood, and cerebral cognitive functions. A novel type of agent (*noötropic*) with selective CNS effects of uncertain basis is *piracetam,* which may also have benefits in dementia. Although all of these antidementia and noötropic agents have some promise, their effectiveness is not well established by rigorously controlled studies. Some of the putative cerebral vasodilators, as well as *procainamide* preparations (such as the European drug Gerovital), may also have euphoriant properties, and all drugs of this type no doubt have placebo effects in addition to any specific pharmacologic activity they may possess. A summary of these and other investigational treatments of dementia is provided in Table 82. Of the available agents, Hydergine and piracetam and their congeners appear to be especially promising, especially in mild dementia.

The physiological characteristics of elderly patients contribute to an increased risk of severe *toxic effects* of all medications. Patients in their seventies and eighties have been reported to experience side effects from many drugs two to three times more frequently than patients in their forties, and up to seven times more than patients in their twenties; adverse reactions occur in at least 25% of patients over age 80 treated with medications of all kinds. The most common untoward effects are lethargy, confusion, and disorientation, or restlessness, agitation, and aggression; hypotension; urinary retention and ileus; and diminution of respiration. These reactions are particularly likely with drugs that act on the central nervous system, such as antipsychotic and antidepressant agents and anxiolytic sedative-tranquilizers. In elderly subjects the absorption, distribution, metabolism, and excretion of many drugs are decreased. An increased ratio of fat to lean body mass increases the retention of many centrally active drugs, including antipsychotic and antidepressant agents. There may also be an increased sensitivity to exogenous adrenergic agents. Generally, with advancing age there is a strikingly decreasing dosage requirement (or, more precisely, *decreased tolerance*), and a narrowing of the therapeutic index.

At the other end of the age range, pediatric psychopharmacology, like geriatric psychopharmacology, is an underdeveloped area, marked by less rigor and fewer controlled trials of medications than exist for adults. There are a number of reasons for this situation. The differential diagnosis and even the classification of childhood mental illnesses are much less firmly established than for adults. The models of illness developed in adult psychiatry are not readily adapted to childhood, since children tend to respond with alterations of behavior or development such as irritability, temper tantrums, hyperactivity, aggressiveness, withdrawal, regression, negativism, misbehavior or "acting up," poor school performance, intellectual deterioration, or slow development. Such reactions are much more typical than the classical forms of depression, thought disorder, or mania seen in adults. For example, the term "schizophrenia" when applied to children has been used especially loosely, and has different meanings in various psychiatric centers. Similar signs and symptoms can be associated with a wide range of problems: for example, minimal brain dysfunction, gross brain pathology, retardation, aphasia, autism, sensory deficits, functional psychosis, and reactions to neglect or environmental turmoil may all have many similar clinical features. Another factor apparently contributing to the underdevelopment of pediatric psychopharmacology is that many psychiatrists interested in children have been strongly committed to psychosocial and developmental concepts in their therapeutic strategies. There is also a general tendency for adults to be protective of children, to be conservative about permitting the investigation of new therapies for them, and to be suspicious of medications that alter behavior or that may diminish intellectual, physical, or social skills.

Since pediatric doses are often recommended in units of body weight, a table of typical body weights in pounds and kilograms, by age, for girls and boys is provided in Table 83. It was noted in Chapters 2–5 that recent research and clinical experience indicate that effective doses of psychotropic agents used for severely mentally ill, school-age children (especially antipsychotic, antimanic, and antidepressant agents) resemble or may even exceed those for adults on a mg/kg basis and overlap the adult range on a mg/day basis. Earlier chapters have also provided comments on the use of specific classes of psychotropic agents in children and the elderly.

Medicolegal Issues

There are many points of contact between research and clinical practice in psychopharmacology, on the one hand, and the legal or regulatory systems as well as the ethical standards of the practice of psychiatric medi-

Table 83 Body weight for girls and boys by age

Age (years)	Girls		Boys	
	Pounds	*Kilograms*	*Pounds*	*Kilograms*
0.5	14–19	6.4–8.6	15–19	6.8–8.6
1.0	18–25	8.2–11.3	20–25	9.1–11.3
1.5	21–28	9.5–12.7	22–29	10.0–13.2
2.0	24–32	10.9–14.5	25–32	11.3–14.5
2.5	26–34	11.8–15.4	27–35	12.2–15.9
3.0	28–36	12.7–16.3	29–37	13.2–16.8
4.0	31–41	14.1–18.6	32–43	14.5–19.5
5.0	35–48	15.9–21.8	36–48	16.3–21.8
6.0	39–53	17.7–24.0	40–54	18.1–24.5
7.0	43–60	19.5–27.2	44–62	20.0–28.1
8.0	47–68	21.3–30.8	48–70	21.8–31.8
9.0	52–78	23.6–35.4	53–80	24.0–36.3
10	57–88	25.8–39.9	60–88	27.2–39.9
11	63–99	28.6–44.9	65–100	29.5–45.4
12	70–110	31.8–49.9	71–111	32.2–50.3
13	79–125	35.8–56.7	78–126	35.4–57.2
14	90–133	40.8–60.3	90–137	40.8–62.1
15	97–138	44.0–62.6	99–148	44.9–67.1
16	101–141	45.8–64.0	111–157	50.3–71.2
17	103–143	46.7–64.9	118–165	53.5–74.8
18	104–145	47.2–65.8	120–169	54.4–76.7

Source: Data are adapted from W. E. Nelson, ed., *Textbook of Pediatrics* (Saunders, Philadelphia, 1959), pp. 45–55; based on data pooled from several studies in Massachusetts and Iowa. The ranges represent the 10th and 90th percentiles. 1 pound = 0.4536 kg; 1 kg = 2.205 pounds.

cine, on the other. A few selected points are raised here that have special pertinence to the use of medical treatments for psychiatric patients. The first issue involves the procedures for development of new medicines, particularly in compliance with the standards of the U.S. Food and Drug Administration (FDA). These procedures were outlined in Chapter 1; however, some important additional points require clarification, especially since they have been accompanied by some confusion in recent years. The decision to bring a new medicine into general clinical use is fundamentally a business decision made by its manufacturer, with the approval of the FDA, following federal requirements to show adequate safety as well as efficacy. In fact, the matter of safety is at best tentative and incompletely resolved when a new agent is released for general use, even following the several phases of clinical investigation described in Chapter 1. Many toxic problems have been discovered only in the "postmarketing" phase of investigation and experience with the new agent in actual clinical practice (phase IV). Sometimes such new knowledge markedly alters or limits the clinical use of a drug, or may even lead to a decision by the FDA or its manufacturer to withdraw it from further distribution, especially if the newly discovered problems appear to be excessive from the point of view of the risk of morbidity to patients, or of financial losses or liabilities to the manufacturer.

A sometimes more complex matter is that of defining "efficacy" in the postmarketing phase of evaluating a new or even a well-established agent. Currently, efficacy is typically established for a limited range of *indications,* concerning which a business decision must be made as to whether to invest in further studies in order to support new or expanded indications. There has been a tendency to consider any use (or dose) of a drug not explicitly or officially "approved" (as documented in the language of the product insert and as compiled in reference works such as the *Physicians' Desk Reference*) as "investigational." This latter term has taken on legalistic and somewhat threatening implications, suggesting, in fact, disapprobation or a high risk of censure, lawsuit, or other action against the physician, usually from ill-defined sources. Recent statements by the FDA as well as current standards of medical practice in the United States help to clarify this issue. When an agent is made available for general clinical use, the manner of use (indications and doses) falls to the *responsibility of the practicing physician,* who is expected to follow rational and ethical practices based on judgments arising from the available medical and research literature, personal experience and that of competent colleagues, and the apparent requirements and progress of individual cases. The "official" recognition of a new use of an approved agent may not be sought by the manufacturer. The process of obtaining such recognition is time-consuming and expensive, and marketing decisions may play a dominant role in such decisions. Pharmaceutical manufacturers balance the need or potential profitability of a new indication against the effort and expense of seeking FDA approval, as well as against possible extension of their liability as their recommendations are broadened. The point is not that a physician should feel free to do whatever he or she may please in the use of a licensed drug, but that the physician should be prepared to accept the responsibility for making an informed professional judgment concerning a novel use of a drug. Some examples of "unofficial" indications for psychotropic agents that are commonly employed and recommended elsewhere in this book include the use of low doses of propranolol for akathisia; a broadening of the range of several agents and doses appropriate for pediatric use; the use of tricyclic and MAO-inhibitor antidepressants for the treatment of several conditions other than acute major depression; the use of lithium for long-term treatment of disorders other than classic bipolar illness; the use of carbamazepine as a mood-stabilizing agent; and a broadening of possible indications, doses, and durations of use of benzodiazepines.

The matter of clinical use of *truly investigational agents* is quite separate and is, appropriately, restricted by regulatory and ethical procedures. Currently, such agents in phases II and III of development (see Chapter 1)—and thus needing data to demonstrate their efficacy for specific, limited indications, as well as to support their safety—are almost always restricted to specific research protocols prepared by an individual investigator or pharmaceutical sponsor. Such protocols require the informed consent of each participating patient-subject, with written documentation, as well as review and prior approval by the sponsoring institution (usually a hospital or medical center) and its independent Investigations Review Board (IRB), which makes periodic reviews of the progress of each study and of unexpected outcomes. In addition to review by an IRB for ethical considerations of the study, it is usual for research protocols to be reviewed by experts in medical research to evaluate their scientific quality, whether through the grant support process or through advisers available to a pharmaceutical sponsor. In this situation, deviations from an approved protocol may be considered unethical or expose the physician to liability.

In recent years there have been repeated suggestions that, like investigational agents or some (usually surgical) procedures of high risk, some psychotropic agents may require special "protections" for patients, physicians, medical institutions, or pharmaceutical manufacturers. One such suggestion is that the routine use of a written document to demonstrate *informed consent* be employed in the long-term use of antipsychotic drugs, as is now a common practice in the use of ECT. This is a curious proposal that probably says more about perceptions of psychiatric patients or the psychiatric profession than about the risks involved in such routine practices, which are discussed in detail in Chapter 2. Similar suggestions have not been entertained seriously for many medical treatments or procedures in general medicine that carry a finite risk of serious morbidity or even fatality. The case of ECT is a separate matter because, as currently practiced, it is essentially a surgical procedure involving general anesthesia and temporary life support. The suggestion concerning routine written documentation of the consent and patient-education process with respect to certain psychotropic agents, and particularly the long-term use of antipsychotic agents, may arise from concerns about the potential vulnerability of chronically psychotic patients to accepting bad advice or making an unwise decision, or from concern that some systems —largely within public institutions and programs—are not likely to provide competent medical care for the chronically, severely mentally ill. To the extent that this suggestion arises from an urge to "protect" the mentally ill from potentially ill-advised or abusive use of psychotropic agents, it is not only likely to be ineffectual (based on several recent research studies and clinical experience) but may represent a precedent-setting extension of both legal and ethical standards involved in the consent process. Alternatives to legalistic steps such as requiring routine written documentation of the consent procedure with a signed document are suggested in Chapter 2. The essential point, again, is that informed consent for any medical treatment remains a standard of sound and ethical practice: it is the responsibility of the physician to inform and advise the patient, but it is up to the patient to accept or reject that advice. In addition, written notes in the case records to document specific discussions and reviews of matters involving unusual risks are advisable, if only to protect the physician from accusations of malpractice in the future, especially following an unwanted outcome.

If a patient appears to be truly *incompetent* to provide consent to treatment or to manage his affairs, then it is appropriate and usual practice to seek adjudication of this essentially legal question and to seek a court-appointed guardian or the court's assistance in deciding whether treatment will be accepted—even forced—deferred, or rejected.

An even more complex and still-evolving area of medicolegal influence on medical treatments in psychiatry, which involves laws and regulations concerning commitment of psychiatric patients to hospitals or treatment programs, determination of competence, provision of guardianship, and coercion to accept treatment, is beyond the scope of this book. Much of the controversy and debate in this field, as in the matter of consent, appear to arise partly from a view of psychiatric patients as being more vulnerable or less able to make informed judgments than other medical patients, or a view that some psychiatric institutions and programs may be inferior to those usually available in general medicine. Because the guidelines for handling these issues vary widely among local jurisdictions, the physician must be guided by the local legal and medical standards of practice.

Given the recent increase in intensity of involvement of the federal and local courts in matters pertaining to the practice of psychiatric chemo-therapy, and the growing number of lawsuits arising from accusations of malpractice through coercive uses or toxicity of psychotropic agents, the physician is well advised to follow practices that are beyond reproach. These include a commitment to continued education and updating on new knowledge through the medical literature and postgraduate pro-grams, thoughtful selection of treatments and their repeated, objective review, and adequate documentation of findings and decisions in the patient's medical records.

There is an unusually high risk of abuse of psychotropic substances, both through medical and illicit channels of distribution. There are many local and state regulations that bear on the use and availability of such agents, but the most stringent regulations in this country arise from the Comprehensive Drug Abuse Prevention and Control Act of 1970, which categorizes agents of potential abuse into five "schedules" in order of descending putative risk of abuse or addiction according to criteria that have evidently been determined by political and administrative as well as pharmacologic principles and characteristics of the agents so categorized. In order to obtain or prescribe a drug controlled in this manner, a physi-cian must be registered with the federal Drug Enforcement Administra-tion (DEA), a branch of the U.S. Department of Justice, and must comply with various requirements for record keeping, inventories, and the like. The "schedules" for controlled substances emerging from this federal program include the following. *Schedule I* includes agents that have no currently accepted, noninvestigational medical use in the United States (examples include some opioids and most hallucinogens) and cannot be prescribed. *Schedule II* includes agents considered to have a high poten-tial for abuse, such as the amphetamines and methylphenidate, short-act-ing barbiturates, and the sedative methaqualone (Quäälude), as well as certain opioids. *Schedule III* includes agents considered to have a lesser risk of abuse, including certain opioids but also methyprylon (Noludar) and glutethimide (Doriden and others) and some barbiturates. *Schedule IV* includes agents with a low potential for abuse, such as long-acting barbiturates, benzodiazepines, paraldehyde, and ethinamate (Valmid), but also ethchlorvynol (Placidyl) and meprobamate (Miltown and others). *Schedule V* includes agents such as certain antitussive and antispasmodic opioids with a very low potential for abuse that may even appear in nonprescription preparations.

Outpatient Psychiatric Chemotherapy

Several general features of chemotherapy in an outpatient psychiatric setting are somewhat different from those in a more controlled hospital inpatient unit, and require further consideration. Outpatient psychiatric treatment, including chemotherapy, has become increasingly important since the 1950s in preventing hospitalization and in providing long-term care following hospitalization of seriously ill psychiatric patients, particularly since chemotherapy has had its greatest impact on the more severe illnesses.

A crucial aspect of outpatient practice involving medications is the patient's *cooperation* at the initiation of treatment and during the sometimes prolonged medical regimen that may be required. Outpatient and inpatient psychiatric services differ in the degree to which the patient collaborates in the planning and execution of his treatment program. In the outpatient setting it is the *patient,* not the staff, who ultimately controls the decision to accept medication, ordinarily administers the medication, and is usually the first to detect beneficial or unwanted effects of a drug. Since the patient's cooperation is required, the routine or indifferent prescription of a medical treatment, particularly by a physician who may not know the patient well and may not follow his progress by close personal contact, will have little chance of success even if the right drug is prescribed at the optimal dose — particularly if the patient is depressed, confused, or suspicious. Thus, considerable sensitivity and diplomacy are required to elicit the patient's informed cooperation. An authoritarian approach to medication may occasionally be warranted in an outpatient setting, for example when the physician is attempting to interrupt a psychotic, manic, or acute depressive illness that might otherwise require hospitalization or end in suicide. Generally, however, a flexible, open-minded "advisory" attitude will more often lead to the acceptance of a medical regimen. A goal of treatment should be to encourage the development of positive feelings of the patient to the clinician most directly involved with the patient's care, and not to rely on exaggerated expectations of the efficacy of the chemotherapy. In this way a cooperative working relationship can develop, and there is a greater likelihood that medication will be accepted, that minor side effects will be tolerated, and that necessary modifications in the treatment can be made efficiently. The alternative is a dissatisfied and inadequately treated patient who may decline further care and encourage dissatisfaction and resentment in other patients.

It is important to provide the outpatient and his family with detailed *information* and *education* about the use of medications so that they can arrive at informed consent to the treatment. Such information may be even more crucial in an outpatient setting than in an acute inpatient service, particularly when potentially toxic and expensive drugs must be used for prolonged periods, sometimes indefinitely. It is not only more humane and legally wise to practice chemotherapy in this manner, but it will also improve the safety of treatment by encouraging earlier recognition of drug side effects, and will contribute to a relationship between patient and doctor that is more likely to endure. Some clinicians provide and discuss written lists of specific warnings about the symptoms of drug toxicity, the description and dosage of medication, and conditions that might represent increased medical risks to patients. Some points to be included in such an approach are suggested in Table 84. It is possible to discuss these matters without being unnecessarily alarming; indeed, since some side effects are common, it is unrealistic and misleading to avoid discussing them. At times when a patient is too confused, suspicious, or depressed to manage his own medication safely, a family member may be instructed about the effects of a drug and given responsibility for storing and dispensing it.

With the prolonged use of medication in the clinical management of patients, there is a risk of gradual diminution of thoughtful objectivity in the conduct of the treatment, which may degrade into a routine of occasional superficial "check-ups" and reissuing of prescriptions. This pattern derives from unrealistic and simplistic expectations of chemotherapy, is demoralizing to patients as well as to psychiatrists and their colleagues, and contributes to high dropout rates and often to the failure of treatment programs. Moreover, such a pattern of indifferent and routine care probably contributes to increased rates of toxic side effects of antipsychotic, antimanic, and antidepressant drugs and to the abuse of antianxiety agents. In a busy clinic or office practice, it is particularly tempting to allow the "ritualization" of chemotherapy to displace sensitive and honest attention to painful and difficult psychological and social issues, needs, and wishes of patients. Ritualization of chemotherapy can also encourage patients to overvalue the importance of medications to their continued well-being, and to resist necessary changes of medication. To some extent,

Table 84 Information to elicit regularly from patients about drug side effects

Antipsychotic agents
• Sedation, "depression"
• Dry mouth, blurred vision, constipation, urinary hesitation
• Restlessness, muscle spasms, awkwardness, sluggishness, shaking
• Itching; color of urine, stool, and skin; sun sensitivity
• Sore throat, malaise, fever
• Pregnancy
• Sexual dysfunction
• Weight gain

Lithium
• Ascertain whether patient is following prescription and blood testing protocols closely
• Nausea, vomiting, diarrhea, metallic taste
• Trembling, awkwardness, unsteadiness, confusion (especially in the elderly)
• Thirst, urinary frequency
• Enlargement of thyroid
• Skin rashes and acne; hair loss
• Pregnancy
• Weight gain

Antidepressants
• Sedation, confusion (especially in the elderly)
• Dizziness, fainting
• Dry mouth, vile taste, blurred vision, urinary hesitation, constipation
• Other medications used
• Skin rashes; sunburn; color of urine, stool, and skin
• Sexual dysfunction
• Pregnancy
• Weight gain

Antianxiety agents
• Ascertain whether patient is following prescription closely
• Excessive sedation, unsteadiness (especially in the elderly)
• Other medications used
• Skin rashes
• Pregnancy
• Weight gain

such an impasse can be avoided by the encouragement of positive feelings toward the psychiatrist or clinic staff as people rather than emphasizing the "magical" pills they provide. Another useful principle is to be prepared to offer something (more time or other psychological support) in place of what the patient feels deprived of, and to discontinue a cherished agent gradually, or substitute a more innocuous agent for a more toxic one temporarily.

Medical Responsibility and Shared Clinical Responsibility

The management of psychiatric chemotherapy — a medical treatment — is further complicated by the *sharing of responsibility* for patients and clients among professional and paraprofessional colleagues, many of whom are not medically trained. Treatment by psychiatric teams representing vastly different backgrounds and experience is presently encountered frequently in private as well as public psychiatric services, especially in ambulatory care settings. Arrangements for the sharing of clinical responsibilities in outpatient services, as in all forms of psychiatric care, are heavily influenced by forces that are not directly medical or scientific, including the administrative and financial environment. For example, clinical teams representing several disciplines are common in public institutions, hospital clinics, community mental health centers, and some private group practices. Often these arrangements have arisen in part because of the manpower needs and limited funds available for rapidly expanded community mental health services. Economic forces that encourage reliance on clinicians without medical training include support by public funds or grants, rather than by private or insured fees. Meeting the requirements of responsible and medically safe care in such a complex environment is not a simple matter.

Treatment with prescription drugs is the medical and legal responsibility of a psychiatrist or other physician on the treatment team, and in this way chemotherapy differs from the psychological, social, and rehabilitative aspects of work with psychiatric outpatients and clients. Furthermore, a physician is important in the initial evaluation of psychiatric patients, particularly those with psychotic or neuropsychiatric symptoms of other disorders that require consideration of medical conditions in their differential diagnosis and treatment. In addition, a physician is required to prescribe medications, to regulate dosages, to evaluate medically the subsequent responses of the patient, and to manage the treatment when other medical illnesses coexist with psychiatric conditions. Such activities related to chemotherapy have contributed greatly to the strong medical orientation of general psychiatrists trained since the 1950s.

The administrative mechanisms by which these requirements are met vary considerably with patients' requirements and the personnel and facilities available. When availability of the services of psychiatrists or other physicians is severely limited, the effectiveness of a physician can be increased by his serving in a supervisory capacity, in addition to providing an initial examination and at least brief subsequent direct contacts with patients. In order to carry out such interdisciplinary outpatient programs, it is increasingly necessary for colleagues without medical training to gain some appreciation for the actions, pharmacology, and toxic effects of drugs used to treat psychiatric patients, as discussed in this book. Thus, a crucial role for the psychiatrist on an outpatient psychiatric treatment team is staff education and, directly or indirectly, patient education as well. In order to achieve adequate medical care in a complex multidisciplinary setting, the effectiveness and safety of chemotherapy and continuing requirements for it are sometimes monitored by the use of explicit and detailed treatment protocols and checklists with which a nonphysician staff member trained in their use can evaluate a patient on a clinic visit. These checklists typically include behavioral and psychological ratings tailored to the syndrome being treated, along with a record of the medication given, doses, drug blood levels (when available), timing, and the responses of the patient to a specific list of questions (incorporating at least the items listed in Table 84), as well as the clinician's observations appropriate to the medication in question. During each clinic visit, in every case, the protocol is evaluated by a psychiatrist or other physician, and appropriate steps are taken before the patient leaves the clinic the same day. A medical evaluation can often be conducted with enhanced benefit to all concerned by inviting the involved staff members to participate in the examination.

Cooperation with Treatment

A topic related especially to the long-term treatment of patients in an outpatient or office setting is that of *compliance* with the prescribed treatment. Since this term carries an implication of an authoritarian rather than a professional-advisory relationship of a physician with a patient, the term *adherence* is an appropriate alternative in that it is more neutral and

Table 85   Conditions that may reduce adherence with treatment

- Excessively complex regimen (multiple agents, multiple small doses)
- Early onset and persistence of side effects
- Slow onset of beneficial effects
- Low apparent relapse risk experienced if treatment is interrupted
- Psychosis, confusion, dementia, pseudodementia, low intelligence, impaired hearing or vision, illiteracy
- Simple ignorance; need for patient education
- Financial hardship; conflicting obligations of time or money
- Resentment; lack of confidence or trust
- Specific psychopathology: paranoid delusions, hopelessness, masochism, anxiety and fear, ambivalence, control, splitting, passive aggression, passive dependence, denial, sociopathy, substance abuse
- Involvement of multiple clinicians
- Clinician who is authoritarian, aloof, rigid, passive, angry, denying, or ignorant
- Inevitable human error

more in line with the view that the patient is essentially in control of the treatment. There have been many studies of patterns of nonadherence to medical treatments of all kinds, including the use of psychotropic agents. Generally, the risk of nonadherence is increased with increasing duration of treatment, and some surveys suggest that the impression that perhaps half of patients take half of the recommended long-term medication half of the time is not excessively cynical. Such patterns of nonadherence are well known in the use of antihypertensive agents, cardiac drugs, antibiotics, and other medications as well as antipsychotic agents and antidepressants or lithium salts. Adherence with the long-term use of lithium salts may be somewhat better because of the repeated assays of blood levels and unusual concern about the potential toxicity involved. Assays of plasma levels of other psychotropic agents can also be used to monitor adherence, but there are many psychological and general commonsense issues that should be addressed routinely in attempting to maximize adherence to a recommended treatment program. Some of these issues are summarized in Table 85.

Psychological Factors in Chemotherapy

Traditionally psychiatry has been preoccupied with the *process* of psychiatric treatment, and usually that has meant psychotherapy. This concern has arisen in part from psychoanalytic suggestions that the behavior, utterances, and feelings of patients in any setting to some extent reflect typical or characteristic reactions, or even earlier experiences. However, the personal, psychological, and sociological aspects of medical treatments are at least as important as they are to psychotherapy. *Characterological traits* of patients and the nature of their acute *psychological problems* color their way of dealing with medications, and their reactions to chemotherapy and other aspects of their care. For example, obsessional patients may worry and fuss about details of their treatment and their reactions to it, and may provoke sticky controversies and debates over their treatment. Hysterical or impulsive patients may react to side effects in an exaggerated manner, or abuse medications impulsively. Narcissistic or hypomanic patients are often bothered by any loss of mental or physical capacity perceived as resulting from drug treatment, or may refuse to accept the "crutch" of medication at all. Depressed patients may be reluctant to accept medication because of their feelings of hopelessness, worthlessness, or anger, and side effects may contribute to their hypochondriacal preoccupations. Schizophrenic patients may cooperate poorly because of suspiciousness, delusions, autistic preoccupation, and perplexity or may become unrealistically dependent on the treatment program and rigidly resistant to changes in it. Sociopathic patients may abuse sedatives, try to involve a number of clinicians in their abuses, or embroil the clinicians in struggles for control and dominance over the patient or with each other.

Simplification of Chemotherapy

Chemotherapy can be conducted with greater accuracy, safety, and success by *simplification* of the regimen. Multiple medications should be avoided, not only because of the increased risk of complex and sometimes obscure toxicity and drug interactions but also because multiple prescriptions are too difficult to follow faithfully over a long time. Moreover, since antipsychotic agents and antidepressants (in contrast to lithium salts and some sedatives) have a relatively long half-life in the body as well as a safe therapeutic index, it is often possible to take an entire day's dose at bedtime, thus simplifying the regimen and at the same time minimizing excessive daytime sedation and autonomic side effects. In addition, for simplicity and saving in cost, the largest available unit of medication (milligrams per pill) should be prescribed, and small quantities should be dispensed until it is certain that the drug will be used for prolonged periods. At the start of outpatient chemotherapy, it is a good idea to insist that the patient or a family member bring to the clinician *all* bottles of medications of all types that are at home in order to avoid continued use of unnecessary medications, reduce suicidal risks, and avoid potential drug interactions. In addition, a list should be made of all the other physicians involved in the patient's care, and this list and an outline of other coexisting medical treatments should be updated frequently.

Simplification of another type is also important to both inpatient and outpatient psychiatrists. Since many agents in each of the classes discussed in the preceding chapters are more similar than different, and since it is difficult to become clinically and pharmacologically expert on every agent available, it is reasonable for a psychiatrist to select a limited number of agents for inclusion in his *personal pharmacopoeia*. Certain general principles can be followed in making such selections. Only those agents that have been exposed to extensive clinical testing should be selected, unless there are compelling indications that a new agent has something special to offer. Although it is tempting to try every new agent that comes along, if only out of dissatisfaction with older drugs or to make use of novelty for its own sake, optimistic expectations of new agents in psychopharmacology have often been unrealistic. An important point to reiterate about the past several decades of drug development in this field is that there have been remarkably few fundamentally new developments since the 1950s. It is also advisable to use agents that are readily available in several forms for oral and parenteral use, and to select drugs that are available as generic chemicals, or whose price is known to be competitive locally.

The list of drugs used should include at least one representative of the major chemical classes in each division. Thus, among the antipsychotic agents, one aliphatic (for example, chlorpromazine) and one piperidine (for example, thioridazine) low-potency phenothiazine might be selected, as well as one or two high-potency phenothiazines (such as fluphenazine and perphenazine), including a depot form, and a butyrophenone (haloperidol). It is important to be aware of the availability of loxitane and molindone if allergic toxic reactions require the use of a chemically unique agent. Lithium can be used as the generic carbonate salt or a slow-release carbonate, and occasionally the liquid citrate may be useful. Among the antidepressants, only two or three with the best overall results in clinical trials are necessary; these might include one or two tertiary amines (including imipramine) as well as desmethylated agents (including nortriptyline and desipramine). Although the MAO inhibitors are not used frequently, one should be familiar with tranylcypromine and phenelzine. Among the large sedative-antianxiety group of agents, familiarity with only a short-acting barbiturate and phenobarbital, as well as diphenhydramine among the antihistamines, is usually adequate. Heavy reliance should be placed on not more than five benzodiazepines, including alprazolam, lorazepam, oxazepam, and either diazepam or chlordiazepoxide, as well as temazepam or triazolam as a hypnotic. To manage neurological side effects of the antipsychotic agents, diphenhydramine can be used for dystonia; propranolol for akathisia; and trihexiphenidyl, benztropine, or their equivalent for dystonia, parkinsonism, and akathisia; one should also be familiar with amantadine and bromocriptine (Parlodel) for treating side effects of neuroleptics and with propranolol for tremor.

An additional consideration in the selection of specific agents is that, as time passes, more and more pioneer psychotropic agents are being made available as generic products. These are often lower in price. Several generic products of the antidepressants imipramine and amitriptyline, as well as the antipsychotic phenothiazines chlorpromazine and thioridazine, are currently available. The "bioequivalence" of various preparations of such agents is difficult to demonstrate precisely, and it should not be assumed that all preparations produce identical tissue levels of active agent or its pharmacologically active metabolites. Since pharmaceutical preparations are almost never identical, it is reasonable to assume that some differences in rates of absorption or metabolism might occur between different brands of the same agent, even at the same dose. Clinically important consequences of changing brands or preparations of an agent are not easily proved, but this factor should be considered when a patient fails to respond as expected or develops apparent toxicity following a change between a specific brand and a generic preparation of the same agent.

Objectivity and Circumspection in Chemotherapy

The success of psychiatric chemotherapy has led to a class of problems that have been mentioned in previous chapters but warrant further discussion. In this book the very term "chemotherapy" has been chosen rather than more fashionable alternatives such as "psychopharmacology" to emphasize the point that these treatments involve the introduction of foreign chemical substances into the body with the hope of modifying the brain, behavior, and feelings in beneficial ways. Despite their sometimes impressive successes, these treatments are limited in efficacy, are potentially toxic, and are not to be undertaken lightly or pursued relentlessly. The general effectiveness and relative simplicity of chemotherapy are highly attractive — so attractive that it is sometimes difficult to know when to stop using it. As in any other form of medical or psychiatric treatment, it is important to work constantly toward an honest and objective assessment of the continuing need for a given treatment, and of its efficacy, safety, and economy. Although such advice may sound almost trivially obvious, its acceptance in practice is often incomplete and sometimes painfully difficult.

Many psychiatric conditions are not suitable for medical treatment, or else respond poorly to such treatment. For example, it is not reasonable to use antipsychotic agents in cases of mild stresses and strains of life, adolescent turmoil, or most personality disorders. Antianxiety agents are only occasionally indicated for prolonged use in such conditions, although they are reasonably used for brief periods in episodes of acute anxiety. Lithium is another agent currently at high risk for medical misuse, as more and more cases are inappropriately considered to represent manic-depressive illness. Chronic schizophrenia is often helped greatly by antipsychotic agents, but many patients are not convincingly benefited except during periods of acute psychotic turmoil and disorganization, and even those who do seem to benefit require regular reevaluations to determine their continuing need for the medication. Antipsychotic agents are sometimes given in grossly excessive doses on a short-term as well as a long-term basis. Antidepressants and stimulants are to be avoided in cases of chronic fatigue or most cases of chronic, characterological dysphoria. Reasonable long-term uses of antidepressants are limited at present: they include indubitable, severe, recurrent, unipolar, major depressive illness (at least for several months at a time); cases of panic disorder or obsessive-compulsive disorder; and possibly eating disorders found to respond to such treatment and to relapse without it.

Another important aspect of excessive zeal in the use of medication is the use of excessive numbers of medications as well as of unnecessarily high doses. One cause of this problem is the naïve use of drugs for theoretical or wishful reasons rather than objectively demonstrated indications with clearly demonstrable, beneficial responses and adequate lack of toxicity. Examples include treating a "depressed" schizophrenic with an antidepressant, provoking clinical worsening, and then compounding the problem with more antipsychotic drug; giving an antipsychotic agent or more antidepressant to a depressed patient who becomes agitated and mildly delirious with high doses of an antidepressant; using an antiparkinsonism medication "prophylactically," routinely, and indefinitely with an antipsychotic agent, whether it is needed or not; increasing the dose of an antipsychotic agent for a schizophrenic patient who is doing poorly, and not changing the treatment even though no further progress is obtained for months; using high doses of a neuroleptic in a manic patient who seems intolerant of its side effects; prescribing lithium for indefinite use after an episode of mild depression, with a history of a similar illness many years previously; adding a barbiturate or flurazepam at bedtime for a schizophrenic patient who receives several doses of chlorpromazine a day; using antipsychotic agents routinely to sedate angry, troublesome, brain-damaged, or retarded hospitalized or institutionalized patients for prolonged periods; using small doses of antipsychotic agents in place of lithium in the prophylactic treatment of affective disorders.

One of the most difficult concepts for many psychiatrists and other psychiatric professionals to grasp is the requirement of thinking about the vicissitudes of a patient's clinical progress *differentially,* and to avoid the temptation to substitute "understanding" for examination, and an interpretation or glib rationalization for medical appraisal and treatment. Nowhere is this problem more common or more dangerous than in the use of medications. Many cases of intoxication with antipsychotic agents, lithium, antidepressants, or sedatives could be avoided or minimized if early changes in the patient's mental status as evaluated in even a superficial medical examination were recognized as organic, although superimposed upon a functional mental illness. A common error in this situation is to recognize clinical worsening, but to assume that worsening must be an exacerbation of the primary diagnosis. The mistreatment that follows often includes inappropriate increases of the dose of one drug or the addition of other toxic agents to complicate matters further. The best protection against this kind of trap is to maintain a high index of suspicion about toxic responses to medication, and then to *stop the treatment* if there is any doubt about the diagnosis. There is little chance that being proved wrong in this decision will be as dangerous as persisting in, or increasing, a toxic treatment.

A final, somewhat ironic aspect of the need for objectivity and circumspection in the differential evaluation and treatment of patients with serious psychiatric disorders is that *modern treatments often modify the clinical presentation* in confusing and potentially misleading ways. As the use of psychotropic agents by general physicians has been increasing even for patients with major psychiatric illnesses, it is now unusual to encounter a patient in a psychiatric referral center who has not already been partially treated with chemotherapy. Psychiatric trainees now see correspondingly fewer untreated, severely ill patients. Cases that might be more clear-cut and classic given a period of observation without medication can be obscured by early treatment. For example, when mania is modified by a lithium salt, antipsychotic agent, or sedative, the excitement and overtalkativeness may be limited, while psychotic, irrational thinking may continue; another risk is that dysphoria may predominate, and the addition of an antidepressant may increase psychotic agitation. Lack of knowledge of such a patient's past and family history might lead to the misdiagnosis of an exacerbation of schizophrenia or of schizophreniform psychosis, or of psychotic, agitated depression. Neuroleptic agents seem especially likely to have such an effect in psychotic affective disorders, since they tend to diminish excitement and agitation earlier than they reduce disorganized or psychotic patterns of thinking. Much confusion can arise in the differentiation of neurobehavioral side effects of antipsychotic and other medications from primary clinical manifestations in schizophrenic and other psychotic patients; drug-induced akathisia can be misdiagnosed as worsening of "psychotic agitation" and might lead to the use of even more medication; bradykinesia, posturing, and inexpressiveness can be accepted erroneously as usual and expected behavior in many chronically schizophrenic patients and thus contribute to *increased* disability. Depression may also be modified, especially by reduction of agitation and acute turmoil, or by adding sedation or confusion to suggest an organic mental syndrome. One may also be misled as to the severity of illness and its full symptomatology after partial or premature treatment, thus depriving the patient of an adequate assessment and the clinician of clear guidelines to later progress. In such situations, generally early in the evaluation of any severely ill psychiatric patient, and routinely in an inpatient setting with an unfamiliar patient, it is sound practice to *delay treatment* until an adequate medical and psychiatric assessment has been undertaken. Pressures to avoid interrupting or deferring treatment are common in such circumstances, but should be resisted.

Needs for the Future

There are many remaining problems and limitations of available treatments for psychiatric disorders. As the patent protection of many older psychotropic agents is running out, some pharmaceutical laboratories and academic psychopharmacologists are starting to question the potential for substantive progress without more coherent biological theories of the pathophysiology or etiology of major mental illnesses, the study of which has led to decades of effort with few solid gains and many false leads. It has been extremely difficult to break out of the cycle of pursuing characteristics of older agents to find additional similar drugs. Indeed, it is not known what characteristics of most available agents are both necessary and sufficient for their beneficial actions in psychiatric disorders, despite the impressive progress in neuropharmacologic research in recent years. Although better and more efficient screening methods for psychopharmaceutical development are desirable and may be forthcoming, it may also be useful to encourage more open-ended exploration of novel agents in small clinical trials as a means of stimulating new discoveries and novel concepts.

Specific needs for the future include the following: highly effective and nontoxic antidepressants; effective antipsychotic agents that are not neurologically or systemically toxic and that can be given with impunity and with sustained benefit for an indefinite time; antianxiety agents with little or no risk of tolerance, dependence, or abuse; mood-stabilizing agents that are effective in the many patients with recurrent major mood disorders who do not respond well to existing treatments; and agents that are safe and effective in the long-term treatment of neuroses and eating disorders.

Further progress should be greatly assisted by the current worldwide ferment in psychiatric nosology and epidemiology. The status of differential diagnosis in psychiatry remains primitive and largely arbitrary, but the attempt to combine information of all kinds (descriptive, historical, genetic, longitudinal, treatment-response) in the formulation of diagnostic categories is a promising trend. This trend should also help to increase the precision and rationality of seeking and prescribing specific treatments for specific conditions.

Bibliography

Index

Bibliography

General Reviews and Monographs

American Medical Association Department of Drugs. *AMA Drug Evaluations*, 4th ed. John Wiley and Sons, New York, 1980, and in press.

American Pharmaceutical Association. *Evaluation of Drug Interactions*, 2nd ed. American Pharmaceutical Association, Washington, D.C., 1976.

American Psychiatric Association. *Diagnostic and Statistical Manual*, 3rd ed. (DSM-III). Washington, D.C., American Psychiatric Association, 1980.

Appleton, W. S., and Davis, J. M. *Practical Clinical Psychopharmacology*, 2nd ed. Williams and Wilkins, Baltimore, 1980.

Ayd, F. J. *Rational Psychopharmacotherapy and the Right to Treatment*. Ayd Medical Communications, Baltimore, 1974.

Ayd, F. J., and Blackwell, B., eds. *Discoveries in Biological Psychiatry*. Lippincott, Philadelphia, 1970.

Baldessarini, R. J. *Chemotherapy in Psychiatry*. Harvard University Press, Cambridge, Mass., 1977.

——— *Biomedical Aspects of Depression and Its Treatment*. American Psychiatric Press, Washington, D.C., 1983.

——— Clinical pharmacology and side-effects of antipsychotic and mood-stabilizing drugs used in the treatment of psychiatric patients with chronic or recurrent illnesses. In *The Chronic Psychiatric Patient in the Community: Principles of Treatment*, ed. I. Barovsky and R. D. Budson, Jamaica, N.Y., Spectrum Publications, 1983, pp. 321–381.

——— Drugs and the treatment of psychiatric disorders. In *The Pharmacological Basis of Therapeutics*, 7th ed., ed. A. G. Gilman and L. S. Goodman, Macmillan, New York, 1985.

Ban, T. A. Clinical pharmacology and psychiatry. *Dis. Nerv. Syst.* 36:612–616, 1975.

Barchas, J. D., Berger, P. A., Ciaranello, R., and Elliott, G. R., eds. *Psychopharmacology: From Theory to Practice*. Oxford University Press, New York, 1977.

Bassuk, E. L., Schoonover, S. C., and Gelenberg, A. J. *The Practitioner's Guide to Psychoactive Drugs*, 2nd ed. Plenum Medical Book Co., New York, 1983.

Bente, D., and Bradley, P., eds. *Neuropharmacology*. Elsevier, Amsterdam, 1965.

Clark, W. G., and Del Guidice, J., eds. *Principles of Psychopharmacology*, 2nd ed. Academic Press, New York, 1978.

Cook, L., and Weidley, E. Behavioral effects of some psychopharmacological agents. *Ann. N.Y. Acad. Sci.* 66:740–752, 1957.

Cooper, J. R., Bloom, F. E., and Roth, R. H. *The Biochemical Basis of Neuropharmacology*, 3rd ed. Oxford University Press, New York, 1979.

Cooper, T. B., Simpson, G. M., and Lee, H. J. Thymoleptic and neuroleptic drug plasma levels in psychiatry: Current status. *Int. Rev. Neurobiol.* 19:269–309, 1976.

Costa, E., ed. *The Benzodiazepines: From Molecular Biology to Clinical Practice.* Raven Press, New York, 1983.

Detre, T. P., and Jarecki, H. G. *Modern Psychiatric Treatment.* Lippincott, Philadelphia, 1971.

DiMascio, A., and Shader, R. I. *Clinical Handbook of Psychopharmacology.* Science House, New York, 1970.

Efron, D. H., ed. *Psychopharmacology: A Review of Progress, 1957–1967.* U.S. Public Health Service Publication no. 1836. Government Printing Office, Washington, D.C., 1968.

Eisenberg, L., and Conners, C. K. Psychopharmacology in childhood. In *Behavioral Science in Pediatric Medicine*, ed. N. B. Talbot, J. Kagan, and L. Eisenberg. Saunders, Philadelphia, 1971.

Gittelman, R. K., Klein, D. F., and Pollack, M. Effects of psychotropic drugs on long-term adjustment: A review. *Psychopharmacologia* 5:317–338, 1964.

Goldberg, H. L., and DiMascio, A. Psychotropic drugs in pregnancy. In *Psychopharmacology: A Generation of Progress*, ed. M. A. Lipton, A. DiMascio, and K. F. Killam. Raven Press, New York, 1978, pp. 1047–1055.

Gordon, M., ed. *Psychopharmacological Agents.* Academic Press, New York, 1964 and 1974.

Hansten, P. D. *Drug Interactions*, 4th ed. Lea and Febiger, Philadelphia, 1979.

Herrington, R. N., and Lader, M. H. Antidepressant drugs (chap. 1) and Lithium (chap. 2). In *Handbook of Biological Psychiatry, Part V: Drug Treatment in Psychiatry—Psychotropic Drugs*, ed. Van Praag. M. Dekker, New York, 1981, pp. 1–72.

Hollister, L. E. *Clinical Pharmacology of Psychotherapeutic Drugs.* Churchill Livingstone, New York, 1978.

Irwin, S. How to prescribe psychoactive drugs: The uses and relative hazard potential of psychoactive drugs. *Bull. Menninger Clin.* 38:1–48, 1974.

Iversen, L. L., Iversen, S. D., and Snyder, S. H. *Handbook of Psychopharmacology* (17 vols.). Plenum Press, New York, 1975–1983.

Karasu, B., ed. *The Psychiatric Therapies.* The American Psychiatric Press, Washington, D.C., 1984.

Klein, D. F. Importance of psychiatric diagnosis in prediction of clinical drug effects. *Arch. Gen. Psychiatry* 16:18–26, 1967.

———*Psychiatric Case Studies: Treatment, Drugs and Outcome.* Williams and Wilkins, Baltimore, 1972.

Klein, D. F., and Davis, J. M. *Diagnosis and Drug Treatment of Psychiatric Disorders.* Williams and Wilkins, Baltimore, 1969.

Klein, D. F., Gittelman, R., Quitkin, F., and Rifkin, A. *Diagnosis and Drug Treatment of Psychiatric Disorders: Adults and Children*, 2nd ed. Williams and Wilkins, Baltimore, 1980.

Levitt, R. A., ed. *Psychopharmacology, A Biological Approach.* John Wiley, New York, 1975.

Lipton, M. A., DiMascio, A., and Killam, K. F., eds. *Psychopharmacology: A Generation of Progress.* Raven Press, New York, 1978.

Popper, C. W. Child and adolescent psychopharmacology. In *Psychiatry*, ed. J. O. Cavenar. J. B. Lippincott, Philadelphia, 1985.

Rech, R. H., and Moore, K. E., eds. *An Introduction to Psychopharmacology.* Raven Press, New York, 1971.

Shader, R. I., ed. *Manual of Psychiatric Therapeutics: Practical Psychopharmacology and Psychiatry.* Little Brown, Boston, 1975.

Solomon, P. *Psychiatric Drugs.* Grune and Stratton, New York, 1966.

Usdin, E., and Efron, D. E., eds. *Psychotropic Drugs and Related Compounds.* U.S. Public Health Service Publication no. 1589. Government Printing Office, Washington, D.C., 1967.

——— *Psychotropic Drugs and Related Compounds*, 2nd ed. Public Health Service Publication no. 72–9074. Government Printing Office, Washington, D.C., 1972.

Valzelli, L. *Psychopharmacology: An Introduction to Experimental and Clinical Principles.* Spectrum, Flushing, N.Y., 1973.

Van Praag, H. M. *Psychotropic Drugs: A Guide for the Practitioner.* Brunner/Mazel, New York, 1978.

——— Drug treatment in psychiatry: Psychotropic drugs, part IV. In *Handbook of Biological Psychiatry.* Marcel Dekker, New York, 1981.

Werry, J. S., ed. *Pediatric Psychopharmacology: The Use of Behavior Modifying Drugs in Children.* Brunner/Mazel, New York, 1978.

Wheatley, D., ed. *Psychopharmacology of Old Age.* Oxford University Press, New York, 1982.

World Health Organization. *Manual of the International Statistical Classification of Diseases, Injuries, and Causes of Death*, ninth revision, vol. 1 (ICD-9). Geneva, World Health Organization (WHO), 1977.

General Aspects of Psychopharmacology

Altman, H., Mehta, D., Evensen, R., and Sletten, I. W. Behavioral effects of drug therapy on psychogeriatric in-patients. *J. Am. Geriatr. Soc.* 21:241–252, 1973.

American Psychiatric Association (APA). *Diagnostic and Statistical Manual of Mental Disorders*, 3rd ed. (DSM-III). APA Press, Washington, D.C., 1980.

Ananth, J. Side effects in the neonate from psychotropic agents excreted through breastfeeding. *Am. J. Psychiatry* 135:801–805, 1978.

Appleton, W. S. Legal problems in psychiatric drug prescription. *Am. J. Psychiatry* 124:877–882, 1968.

Baldessarini, R. J. Frequency of diagnosis of schizophrenia vs. affective disorders from 1944–1968. *Am. J. Psychiatry* 127:759–763, 1970.

——— Biogenic amine hypotheses in affective disorders. In *The Nature and*

Treatment of Depression, ed. F. F. Flach and S. C. Draghi. John Wiley, New York, 1975, pp. 347–385.

Bender, A. D. Pharmacodynamic principles of drug therapy in the aged. *J. Am. Geriatr. Soc.* 22:296–303, 1974.

Biederman, J., and Jellinek, M. S. Psychopharmacology in children. *N. Engl. J. Med.* 310:968–972, 1984.

Bok, S. The ethics of giving placebos. *Sci. American* 231:17–23, 1974.

Blackwell, B. Patient compliance with drug therapy. *N. Engl. J. Med.* 289:249–252, 1973.

Caldwell, A. E. History of psychopharmacology. In *Principles of Psychopharmacology*, 2nd ed., ed. W. G. Clark and J. Del Guidice. Raven Press, New York, 1978, pp. 9–40.

Cantwell, D. P. Pediatric psychopharmacology, parts I and II. In *Directions in Psychiatry*, vol. 3 (31, 32), ed. F. F. Flach. The Hatherleigh Co., New York, 1983, pp. 1–7.

Comfort, A. Effects of psychotropic drugs on ejaculation. *Am. J. Psychiatry* 136:124–125, 1979.

Cronnie, B. W. The feet of clay of the double-blind trial. *Lancet* 2:994–997, 1963.

Davis, J. M. Psychopharmacology in the aged: Use of psychotropic drugs in geriatric patients. *J. Geriatr. Psychiatry* 7:145–159, 1974.

DeFelice, S. An analysis of the relationship between human experimentation and drug discovery in the United States. *Drug Metab. Rev.* 3:167–184, 1974.

Efron, D. H., Holmstedt, B., and Kline, N. S., eds. *Ethnopharmacologic Search for Psychoactive Drugs*. Public Health Service Publication no. 67–1645. Government Printing Office, Washington, D.C., 1967.

Eisdorfer, C., and Fann, W. E., eds. *Psychopharmacology and Aging*. Plenum, New York, 1973.

Hardesty, A. S., and Burdock, E. I. Quantitative clinical evaluation in psychopharmacology. In *Psychopharmacology: A Generation of Progress*, ed. M. A. Lipton, A. DiMascio, and K. F. Killam. Raven Press, New York, 1978, pp. 871–878.

Irwin, S. Psychoactive drug evaluation. In *Search for New Drugs*, ed. A. A. Rubin. Marcel Dekker, New York, 1972, pp. 201–232.

Itil, T. M. Effects of psychotropic drugs on qualitatively and quantitatively analyzed human EEG. In *Principles of Psychopharmacology*, 2nd ed., ed. W. G. Clark and J. Del Guidice. Academic Press, New York, 1978, pp. 261–277.

Jarvik, L. F., Greenblatt, D. J., and Harman, D., eds. *Clinical Pharmacology and the Aged Patient (Aging, vol. 16)*. Raven Press, New York, 1981.

Lasagna, L., Mosteller, F., Felsinger, J., and Bucher, H. A study of the placebo response. *Am. J. Med.* 16:770–779, 1954.

Levenson, A. J., ed. *Neuropsychiatric Side Effects of Drugs in the Elderly (Aging, vol. 9)*. Raven Press, New York, 1979.

Levine, J., Schiele, B. C., and Bouthilet, L., eds. *Principles and Problems in Establishing the Efficacy of Psychotropic Agents*. Public Health Service Publication no. 2138. Government Printing Office, Washington, D.C., 1971.

Lewin, L. *Phantastica, Narcotic and Stimulating Drugs: Their Use and Abuse.* [Berlin, 1924]; English translation, E. P. Dutton, New York, 1931.

Lipman, R. S. Pharmacotherapy of children (bibliography). *Psychopharmacol. Bull.* 7:14–30, 1971.

Longo, V. G. Effects of psychotropic drugs on the EEG of animals. In *Principles of Psychopharmacology*, 2nd ed., ed. W. G. Clark and J. Del Guidice. Academic Press, New York, 1978, pp. 247–260.

McKinney, W. T., and Moran, F. C. Animal models. In *Handbook of Affective Disorders*, ed. E. Paykel, The Guilford Press, New York, 1982, pp. 202–211.

Meltzer, H. Y., Goode, D. J., and Fang, V. S. The effect of psychotropic drugs on endocrine function. In *Psychopharmacology: A Generation of Progress*, ed. M. A. Lipton, A. DiMascio, and K. F. Killam, eds. Raven Press, New York, 1978, pp. 509–529.

Merlis, S., Sheppard, C., Collins, L., and Fiorentino, D. Polypharmacy in psychiatry: Patterns of differential treatment. *Am. J. Psychiatry* 126:1647–1651, 1970.

Morselli, P. L. Psychotropic drugs. In *Drug Disposition during Development*, ed. P. L. Morselli. Spectrum Publications, New York, 1977, 431–474.

Muller, C. The overmedicated society: Forces in the marketplace for medical care. *Science* 176:488–492, 1972.

O'Connell, R. A. Psychological and social aspects of psychopharmacologic treatment. In *Directions in Psychiatry*, vol. 1 (3), ed. F. F. Flach. The Hatherleigh Co., New York, 1981, pp. 1–7.

Park, L. C., and Imboden, J. B. Chemical and heuristic value of clinical drug research. *J. Nerv. Ment. Dis.* 151:322–340, 1970.

Plutchik, R., Platman, S., and Fieve, R. Three alternatives to the double-blind. *Arch. Gen. Psychiatry* 20:428–432, 1950.

Prien, R. F. Chemotherapy in chronic organic brain syndrome: A review of the literature. *Psychopharmacol. Bull.* 9:5–20, 1973.

Prien, R. F., and Cole, J. O. The use of psychopharmacological drugs in the aged. In *Principles of Psychopharmacology*, 2nd ed., ed. W. G. Clark and J. Del Guidice. Academic Press, New York, 1978, pp. 593–605.

Quay, H. C., and Werry, J. S., eds. *Psychopathological Disorders of Childhood.* John Wiley, New York, 1972.

Raskin, A., Robinson, D. S., and Levine, J. *Age and the Pharmacology of Psychoactive Drugs.* Elsevier–North Holland, New York, 1981, 212 pp.

Reisberg, B., Ferris, S. H., and Gershon, S. An overview of pharmacologic treatment of cognitive decline in the elderly. *Am. J. Psychiatry* 138:593–600, 1981.

Rickels, K. *Non-specific Factors in Drug Therapy.* Charles C Thomas, Springfield, Ill., 1968.

Rosenthal, R. Experimenter outcome-orientation and the results of the psychological experiment. *Psychol. Bull.* 61:405–412, 1964.

Ross, S., Krugman, A., Lyerly, S., and Clyde, D. Drugs and placebos: A model design. *Psychol. Rep.* 10:383–392, 1962.

Sachar, E. J. Neuroendocrine responses to psychotropic drugs. In *Psychopharmacology: A Generation of Progress*, ed. M. A. Lipton, A. DiMascio, and K. F. Killam. Raven Press, New York, 1978, pp. 499–507.

Salzman, C. A primer of geriatric psychopharmacology. *Am. J. Psychiatry* 139:67–74, 1982.

Schildkraut, J. J. *Neuropsychopharmacology and the Affective Disorders.* Little, Brown, Boston, 1970.

Schultes, R. E. Ethnopharmacological significance of psychotropic drugs of vegetal origin. In *Principles of Psychopharmacology*, 2nd ed., ed. W. G. Clark and J. Del Guidice. Academic Press, New York, 1978, pp. 41–70.

Seeman, P. The membrane actions of anesthetics and tranquilizers. *Pharmacol. Rev.* 24:583–655, 1972.

Shagass, C., and Straumanis, J. J. Drugs and human sensory evoked potentials. In *Psychopharmacology: A Generation of Progress*, ed. M. A. Lipton, A. DiMascio, and K. F. Killam. Raven Press, New York, 1978, pp. 699–709.

Snyder, S. H., U'Prichard, D., and Greenberg, D. A. Neurotransmitter receptor binding in the brain. In *Psychopharmacology: A Generation of Progress*, ed. M. A. Lipton, A. DiMascio, and K. F. Killam. Raven Press, New York, 1978, pp. 361–370.

Spencer, P. S. J. Animal models for screening new agents. *Brit. J. Clin. Pharmacol.* (suppl.):5–12, 1976.

Sprague, R. L., and Werry, J. S. Pediatric psychopharmacology. *Psychopharmacol. Bull.* (special issue, *Pharmacotherapy of Children*), 21–23, 1973.

Sudilovsky, A., Gershon, S., and Beer, B., eds. *Predictability in Psychopharmacology: Preclinical and Clinical Correlations.* Raven Press, New York, 1975.

Usdin, E. Classification of psychotropic drugs. In *Principles of Psychopharmacology*, 2nd ed., ed. W. G. Clark and J. Del Guidice. Academic Press, New York, 1978, pp. 193–246.

U.S. Food and Drug Administration. Use of approved drugs for unlabeled indications. *F.D.A. Drug Bull.* 12:4–5, 1982.

Vesell, E. S. Pharmacogenetics. *N. Engl. J. Med.* 287:904–909, 1972.

Weil-Malherbe, H. The biochemistry of the functional psychoses. *Adv. Enzymol.* 29:479–553, 1967.

Wittenborn, J. R., and May, P. R., eds. *Prediction of Response to Pharmacotherapy.* Charles C Thomas, Springfield, Ill., 1966.

Wolf, S. The pharmacology of placebos. *Pharmacol. Rev.* 11:689–704, 1959.

Antipsychotic Chemicals

Alpert, M., Diamond, F., and Laski, E. M. Anticholinergic exacerbation of phenothiazine-induced extrapyramidal syndrome. *Am. J. Psychiatry* 133:1073–1075, 1976.

Alvarez-Mena, S. C., and Frank, M. J. Phenothiazine-induced T-wave abnormalities. *J.A.M.A.* 224:1730–1733, 1973.

American Psychiatric Association Task Force (M. A. Lipton, chairman). *Megavitamin and Orthomolecular Therapy in Psychiatry.* Task Force Report no. 7. American Psychiatric Association, Washington, D.C., 1973.

Anderson, W. H., Kuehnle, J. C., and Catanzano, D. M. Rapid treatment of psychosis. *Am. J. Psychiatry* 133:1076–1078, 1976.

Aubree, J. C., and Lader, M. H. High and very high dosage antipsychotics: A critical review. *J. Clin. Psychiatry* 41:341–350, 1980.

Ayd, F. J. Cardiovascular effects of phenothiazines. *Int. Drug Ther. Newsletter* 5:1–8, 1970.

———Rational pharmacotherapy: Once-a-day drug dosage. *Dis. Nerv. Syst.* 34:371–373, 1973.

Baldessarini, R. J. Antipsychotic drugs. In *The Psychiatric Therapies*, ed. B. Karasu. Washington, D.C., The American Psychiatric Press, 1984, pp. 119–170.

———Clinical and epidemiologic aspects of tardive dyskinesia. *J. Clin. Psychiatry* 46 (4:2):8–13, 1985.

Baldessarini, R. J., Cole, J. O., Davis, J. M., Gardos, G., Simpson, G., and Tarsy, D. *Tardive Dyskinesia*. Task Force Report no. 18. American Psychiatric Association, Washington, D.C., 1980.

Baldessarini, R. J., and Davis, J. M. What *is* the best maintenance dose of neuroleptics in schizophrenia? *Psychiatry Res.* 3:115–122, 1980.

Baldessarini, R. J., Katz, B., and Cotton, P. Dissimilar dosing with high-potency and low-potency neuroleptics. *Am. J. Psychiatry* 141:748–752, 1984.

Baldessarini, R. J., and Tarsy, D. Tardive dyskinesia. In *Psychopharmacology: A Generation of Progress*, ed. M. A. Lipton, A. DiMascio, and K. F. Killam. Raven Press, New York, 1978.

Baldessarini, R. J., and Tarsy, D. Relationship of the actions of neuroleptic drugs to the pathophysiology of tardive dyskinesia. *Int. Rev. Neurobiol.* 21:1–45, 1979.

Ban, T. A. Haloperidol and the butyrophenones. *Psychosomatics* 14:286–297, 1973.

Bannon, M. J., Michaud, R. L., and Roth, R. H. Mesocortical dopamine neurons: Lack of autoreceptors modulating dopamine synthesis. *Mol. Pharmacol.* 19:270–275, 1981.

Beumont, P. J. V., Corker, C. S., Friesen, H. G., et al. The effects of phenothiazines on endocrine function: II. Effect in men and post-menopausal women. *Brit. J. Psychiatry* 124:420–430, 1974.

Beumont, P. J. V., Gelder, M. G., Friesen, H. G., et al. The effects of phenothiazines on endocrine function: I. Patients with inappropriate lactation and amenorrhoea. *Brit. J. Psychiatry* 124:413–419, 1974.

Bowers, M. B., Jr., and Rozitis, A. Regional differences in homovanillic acid concentrations after acute and chronic administration of antipsychotic drugs. *J. Pharm. Pharmacol.* 26:743–745, 1974.

Breunning, S. E., Ferguson, D. G., Davidson, N. A., and Poling, A. D. Effects of thioridazine on the intellectual performance of mentally retarded drug responders and non-responders. *Arch. Gen. Psychiatry* 40:309–313, 1983.

Bunney, B. S., and Aghajanian, G. K. Mesolimbic and mesocortical dopaminergic systems: Physiology and pharmacology. In *Psychopharmacology: A Generation of Progress*, ed. M. A. Lipton, A. DiMascio, and K. F. Killam. Raven Press, New York, 1978, pp. 159–169.

Bunney, B. S., Walters, J. R., Roth, R. H., and Aghajanian, G. K. Dopaminergic neurons: Effect of antipsychotic drugs and amphetamine on single cell activity. *J. Pharmacol. Exp. Ther.* 185:560–571, 1973.

Burgoyne, R. W. Effect of drug ritual change on schizophrenic patients. *Am. J. Psychiatry* 133:284–289, 1976.

Burki, A. R., Ruch, W., and Asper, H. Effects of clozapine, thioridazine, perlapine and haloperidol on the metabolism of the biogenic amines in the brain of the rat. *Psychopharmacologia* 41:27–33, 1975.

Burt, D. R., Enna, S. J., Creese, I., and Snyder, S. H. Dopamine receptor binding in the corpus striatum of mammalian brain. *Proc. Natl. Acad. Sci. USA* 72:4655–4659, 1975.

Caffey, E. M., Diamond, L., Frank, T., et al. Discontinuation or reduction of chemotherapy in chronic schizophrenics. *J. Chronic Dis.* 17:347–358, 1964.

Callahan, E. J., Alevizos, P. N., Teigen, J. R., et al. Behavioral effects of reducing the daily frequency of phenothiazine administration. *Arch. Gen. Psychiatry* 32:1285–1290, 1975.

Campbell, M. Biological interventions in psychoses of childhood. *J. Autism Child. Schizo.* 3:347–373, 1973.

———Psychopharmacology in childhood psychosis. *Int. J. Ment. Health* 4:238–254, 1975.

Campbell, M., Anderson, L. T., Small, A. M., Perry, R., Guen, W. H., and Caplan, R. The effects of haloperidol on learning and behavior in autistic children. *J. Autism Dev. Disord.* 12:167–175, 1982.

Campbell, A., and Baldessarini, R. J. Prolonged pharmacologic activity of neuroleptics. *Arch. Gen. Psychiatry* 42:637, 1985.

Campbell, A., Baldessarini, R. J., and Kula, N. S. Prolonged antidopamine actions of single doses of butyrophenones in the rat. *Psychopharmacology* (in press).

Carlsson, A. Mechanism of action of neuroleptic drugs. In *Psychopharmacology: A Generation of Progress*, ed. M. A. Lipton, A. DiMascio, and K. F. Killam. Raven Press, New York, 1978, pp. 1057–1070.

Carlsson, A., and Lindqvist, M. Effect of chlorpromazine and haloperidol on formation of 3-methoxyltyramine and normetanephrine in mouse brain. *Acta Pharmacol. Toxicol.* (Kbh.) 20:140–144, 1963.

Caroff, S. The neuroleptic malignant syndrome. *J. Clin. Psychiatry* 41:79–83, 1980.

Caroff, S., Rosenberg, H., and Gerber, J. C. Neuroleptic malignant syndrome and malignant hyperthermia. *J. Clin. Psychopharmacol.* 3:120–121, 1983.

Casey, J. F., Lasky, J., Klett, C., and Hollister, L. Treatment of schizophrenic reactions with phenothiazine derivatives: A comparative study. *Am. J. Psychiatry* 117:97–105, 1960.

Chapman, L. J., and Knowles, R. R. The effects of phenothiazine on disordered thought in schizophrenia. *J. Consult. Psychol.* 28:165–169, 1964.

Chase, T. N. Rational approaches to the pharmacotherapy of chorea. In *The Basal Ganglia,* ed. M. D. Yahr. Association for Research in Nervous and Mental Disease Publications, vol. 55. Raven Press, New York, 1976, pp. 337–350.

Chien, C. P., DiMascio, A., and Cole, J. O. Antiparkinson agents and depot phenothiazine. *Am. J. Psychiatry* 131:86–90, 1974.

Chouinard, G., and Jones, B. D. Neuroleptic-induced supersensitivity psychosis: Clinical and pharmacologic characteristics. *Am. J. Psychiatry* 137:16–31, 1980.

Chouinard, G., Pinard, G., Prenoveau, Y., and Tetreault, L. Potentiation of haloperidol by alpha-methyltyrosine in the treatment of schizophrenic patients. *Curr. Ther. Res.* 15:473–483, 1973.

Clark, M. L., Ray, T. S., Paredes, A., Ragland, R. E., Costilee, J. P., Smith, C. W., and Wolf, S. Chlorpromazine in women with chronic schizophrenia: The effects on cholesterol levels and cholesterol-behavioral relationships. *Psychosom. Med.* 29:634–642, 1967.

Clement-Cormier, Y. C., Kebabian, J. W., Petzold, G. L., and Greengard, P. Dopamine-sensitive adenylate cyclase in mammalian brain: A possible site of action of antipsychotic drugs. *Proc. Natl. Acad. Sci. USA* 71:1113–1117, 1974.

Cohen, B. M. The clinical utility of plasma neuroleptic levels. In *Guidelines for the Use of Psychotropic Drugs*, ed. H. Stancer et al. Spectrum Publications, New York, 1984, pp. 245–260.

Cohen, D. J., Detlor, J., and Young, J. G. Clonidine ameliorates Gilles de la Tourette syndrome. *Arch. Gen. Psychiatry* 37:135–137, 1980.

Cohen, M. M., Hirschhorn, K., and Frosch, W. A. Cytogenetic effects of tranquilizing drugs in vivo and in vitro. *J.A.M.A.* 207:2425–2426, 1969.

Cole, J. O. Phenothiazine treatment in acute schizophrenia. *Arch. Gen. Psychiatry* 10:246–261, 1964.

Cole, J. O., ed. Symposium on long-acting phenothiazines in psychiatry. *Dis. Nerv. Syst.* 31 (suppl.):1–71, 1970.

Cole, J. O. Antipsychotic drugs: Is more better? *McLean Hosp. J.* 7:61–87, 1982.

Costall, B., and Naylor, R. J. Mesolimbic involvement with behavioral effects indicating antipsychotic activity. *Eur. J. Pharmacol.* 27:46–58, 1974.

Courvoisier, S., Fournel, J., Ducrot, R., et al. Propriétés pharmacodynamiques du chlorhydrate de chloro-3-(dimethyl-amino-3'-propyl)-10-phenothiazine (4560 RP). *Arch. Int. Pharmacodyn. Ther.* 92:305–361, 1952.

Crane, G. E. A review of clinical literature on haloperidol. *Int. J. Neuropsychiatry* 3 (suppl.):110–123, 1967.

Creese, I., Burt, D. R., and Snyder, S. H. Dopamine receptor binding predicts clinical and pharmacological potencies of antischizophrenic drugs. *Science* 192:481–483, 1976.

Creese, I., Burt, D., and Snyder, S. H. Biochemical actions of neuroleptic drugs: Focus on dopamine receptor. In *Handbook of Psychopharmacology*, vol. 10, ed. L. L. Iversen, S. D. Iversen, and S. H. Snyder. Plenum Press, New York, 1978, pp. 37–89.

Curry, S. H., Marshall, J. H. L., Davis, J. M., and Janowsky, D. S. Chlorpromazine plasma levels and effects. *Arch. Gen. Psychiatry* 22:289–296, 1970.

Davidorf, F. H. Thioridazine pigmentary retinopathy. *Arch. Ophthalmol.* 90:251–255, 1973.

Davis, J. M. Overview: Maintenance therapy in psychiatry: I. Schizophrenia. *Am. J. Psychiatry* 132:1237–1245, 1975.

——Comparative doses and costs of antipsychotic medication. *Arch. Gen. Psychiatry* 33:858–861, 1976.

——Recent developments in the treatment of schizophrenia. *Psychiatr. Annals* 6:71–111, 1976.

——Antipsychotic drugs. In *Comprehensive Textbook of Psychiatry,* 3rd ed., ed. H. L. Kaplan, A. M. Freedman, and B. J. Sadock. Williams and Wilkins, Baltimore, 1980, pp. 2257–2289.

Davis, J. M., and Garver, D. L. Neuroleptics: Clinical use in psychiatry. In *Handbook of Psychopharmacology,* vol. 10, ed. L. L. Iversen, S. D. Iversen, and S. H. Snyder. Plenum Press, New York, 1978, pp. 129–164.

Delay, J., and Deniker, P. Trente-huit cas de psychoses traitées par la cure prolongée et continue de 4560 RP. Le Congres des Al. et Neurol. de Langue Fr. In *Compte rendu du Congres.* Masson et Cie, Paris, 1952.

Delay, J., Deniker, P., and Harl, J. Utilization thérapeutique psychiatrique d'une phénothiazine d'action centrale élective (4560 RP). *Ann. Med. Psychol.* 110:112–117, 1952.

Denber, H., and Bird, E. Chlorpromazine in the treatment of mental illness: IV. Final results with analysis of data on 1,523 patients. *Am. J. Psychiatry* 113:972–978, 1957.

Dimond, R. C., Brammer, S. R., Atkinson, R. L., Jr., et al. Chlorpromazine treatment and growth hormone secretory responses in acromegaly. *J. Clin. Endocrinol. Metab.* 36:1189–1195, 1973.

Dobkin, A. B., Gilbert, R. G. B., and Lamoureu, L. Physiological effects of chlorpromazine. *Anaesthesia* 9:157–174, 1954.

Donaldson, S. R., Gelenberg, A. J., and Baldessarini, R. J. The pharmacological treatment of schizophrenia: A progress report. *Schizophrenia Bull.* 9:504–527, 1983.

——————Current status of medical treatments for schizophrenia. In *American Handbook of Psychiatry,* ed. P. Berger. New York, Academic Press (in press).

Donlon, P. T., and Tupin, J. P. Rapid "digitalization" of decompensated schizophrenic patients with antipsychotic agents. *Am. J. Psychiatry* 131:310–312, 1974.

DuComb, L., and Baldessarini, R. J. Timing and risk of bone marrow depression by psychotropic drugs. *Am. J. Psychiatry* 134:1294–1295, 1977.

Engelhardt, D. M., Polizos, P., Waizer, J., and Hoffman, S. P. A double-blind comparison of fluphenazine and haloperidol. *J. Autism Child. Schizo.* 3:128–137, 1973.

Engelhardt, D. M., Rosen, B., Freedman, N., and Margolis, R. Phenothiazines in prevention of psychiatric hospitalization: A reevaluation. *Arch. Gen. Psychiatry* 16:98–101, 1967.

Ericksen, S. E., Hurt, S. W., and Davis, J. M. Dosage of antipsychotic drugs. *N. Engl. J. Med.* 294:1296–1297, 1976.

Erle, G., Basso, M., Federspil, G., Sicolo, N., and Scandellari, C. Effect of chlorpromazine on blood glucose and plasma insulin in man. *Eur. J. Clin. Pharmacol.* 11:15–18, 1977.

Faretra, G., Dooher, L., and Dowling, J. Comparisons of haloperidol and fluphenazine in disturbed children. *Am. J. Psychiatry* 126:1670–1673, 1970.

Feinberg, A. P., and Snyder, S. H. Phenothiazine drugs: Structure-activity relationships explained by a conformation that mimics dopamine. *Proc. Natl. Acad. Sci. USA* 72:1899–1903, 1975.

Feinsilver, D., and Gunderson, J. Psychotherapy for schizophrenics: Is it indicated? *Schizophr. Bull.* 6:11–23, 1972.

Finnerty, R. J., Goldberg, H. L., Nathan, L., et al. Haloperidol in neurotic outpatients. *Dis. Nerv. Sys.* 37:621–624, 1976.

Fletcher, G. F., and Wenger, N. K. Cardiotoxic effects of Mellaril: Conduction disturbances and supraventricular arrhythmias. *Am. Heart J.* 78:135–138, 1969.

Forrest, I. S., Bolt, A. G., and Serra, M. T. Distribution of chlorpromazine metabolites in selected organs of psychiatric patients chronically dosed up to the time of death. *Biochem. Pharmacol.* 17:2061–2070, 1968.

Forrest, I. S., Carr, C. J., and Usdin, E., eds. *Phenothiazines and Structurally Related Drugs.* Raven Press, New York, 1974.

Forsman, A., and Öhman, R. On the pharmacokinetics of haloperidol. *Nord. Psykiatr. Tidskr.* 28:441–448, 1974.

Frohman, L. A. Clinical neuropharmacology of hypothalamic releasing factors. *N. Engl. J. Med.* 286:1391–1398, 1972.

Galbrecht, C. R., and Klett, C. J. Predicting response to phenothiazines: The right drug for the right patient. *J. Nerv. Ment. Dis.* 147:173–183, 1968.

Gardos, G., and Cole, J. O. The dual action of thiothixene. *Arch. Gen. Psychiatry* 29:222–225, 1973.

——Maintenance antipsychotic therapy: Is the cure worse than the disease? *Am. J. Psychiatry* 133:32–36, 1976.

Garver, D. L., Davis, J. M., Dekirmenjian, H., et al. Pharmacokinetics of red blood cell phenothiazine and clinical effects. *Arch. Gen. Psychiatry* 33:862–866, 1976.

Gelenberg, A. J., and Mandel, M. R. Catatonic reactions to high potency neuroleptic drugs. *Arch. Gen. Psychiatry* 34:947–950, 1977.

Goldberg, S. C., Frosch, W. A., Drossman, A. K., et al. Prediction of response to phenothiazines in schizophrenia: A cross validation study. *Arch. Gen. Psychiatry* 26:367–373, 1972.

Gottschalk, L. A., Biener, R., Noble, E., Birch, H., Wilbert, D., and Heizer, J. Thioridazine plasma levels and clinical response. *Compr. Psychiatry* 16:323–337, 1975.

Grabowski, S. W. Safety and effectiveness of haloperidol for mentally retarded behaviorally disordered and hyperkinetic patients. *Curr. Ther. Res.* 15:856–861, 1973.

Gram, L. F., and Rafaelsen, O. J. Lithium treatment of psychotic children and adolescents: A controlled clinical trial. *Acta Psychiatr. Scand.* 48:252–260, 1972.

Greenblatt, M., Solomon, M. H., Evans, A. S., and Brooks, G. W., eds. *Drug and Social Therapy in Schizophrenia.* Charles C Thomas, Springfield, Ill., 1965.

Grinspoon, L., Ewalt, J. R., and Shader, R. Psychotherapy and pharmacotherapy in chronic schizophrenia. *Am. J. Psychiatry* 124:1645–1652, 1968.

——*Schizophrenia: Pharmacotherapy and Psychotherapy.* Williams and Wilkins, Baltimore, 1972.

Groves, J. E., and Mandel, M. R. The long-acting phenothiazines. *Arch. Gen. Psychiatry* 32:893–900, 1975.

Groves, P. M., and Rebec, G. V. Biochemistry and behavior: Some central actions of amphetamine and antipsychotic drugs. *Ann. Rev. Psychol.* 27:91–127, 1976.

Gualtieri, C. T., Barnhill, J., McGimsey, J., and Schell, D. Tardive dyskinesia and other movement disorders in children treated with psychotropic drugs. *J. Am. Acad. Child Psychiatry* 19:491–510, 1980.

Gunderson, J. G., Frank, A. F., Katz, H. M., Vannicelli, M. L., Frosch, J. P., and Knapp, P. H. Effects of psychotherapy in schizophrenia: II. Comparative outcome of two forms of treatment. *Schizophrenia Bull.* 10:564–598, 1984.

Hanlon, T. E., Michaux, M., Ota, K., et al. The comparative effectiveness of 8 phenothiazines. *Psychopharmacologia* 7:89–106, 1965.

Hirsch, S. R., Gaind, R., Rohde, P. D., Stevens, B. C., and Wing, J. K. Outpatient maintenance of chronic schizophrenic patients with long-acting fluphenazine: Double-blind placebo trial. *Brit. Med. J.* 1:633–637, 1973.

Hogarty, G. E., Goldberg, S. C., and The Collaborative Study Group. Drugs and sociotherapy in the aftercare of schizophrenic patients: One-year relapse rates. *Arch. Gen. Psychiatry* 28:54–62, 1973.

Hogarty, G. E., and Ulrich, R. F. Temporal effects of drug and placebo in delaying relapse in schizophrenic outpatients. *Arch. Gen. Psychiatry* 34:297–301, 1977.

Hollister, L. E., Curry, S. H., Derr, J. E., and Kanter, S. L. Studies of delayed action medication: V. Plasma levels and urinary excretion of chlorpromazine in four different dosage forms given acutely and in steady state conditions. *Clin. Pharmacol. Ther.* 11:49–59, 1970.

Hollister, L. E., Overall, J. E., Kimbell, I., and Pokorny, A. Specific indications for different classes of phenothiazines. *Arch. Gen. Psychiatry* 30:94–99, 1974.

Honigfeld, G., Rosenblum, M. P., Blumenthal, I. J., et al. Behavioral improvement in the older schizophrenic patient: Drug and social therapies. *J. Am. Geriatr. Soc.* 13:57–71, 1965.

Hordern, A. Psychiatry and the tranquilizers. *N. Engl. J. Med.* 265:584–634, 1961.

Iversen, L. L. Dopamine receptors in the brain. *Science* 188:1084–1089, 1975.

Iwahara, S., Iwasaki, T., and Hasegawa, Y. Effects of chlorpromazine and homofenazine on a passive avoidance response in rats. *Psychopharmacologia* 13:320–331, 1968.

Jacobson, G., Baldessarini, R. J., and Manschreck, T. Tardive and withdrawal dyskinesia associated with haloperidol. *Am. J. Psychiatry* 131:910–913, 1974.

Janssen, P. A. J. Chemical and pharmacological classification of neuroleptics. In *Modern Problems in Pharmacopsychiatry: The Neuroleptics,* vol. 5, ed. O. P. Bokon, P. A. J. Janssen, and J. Bokon. S. Karger, Basel, 1970, pp. 34–44.

——— Long-acting neuroleptics and other psychoactive drugs of the future. *Clin. Med.* 79:12–14, 1972.

——— Butyrophenones and diphenylbutylpiperidines. In *Psychopharmacological Agents,* vol. 3, ed. M. Gordon. Academic Press, New York, 1974, pp. 128–158.

Janssen, P. A. J., and Van Bever, W. F. Preclinical psychopharmacology of neuroleptics. In *Principles of Psychopharmacology,* 2nd ed., ed. W. G. Clark and J. Del Guidice. Academic Press, New York, 1978, pp. 279–295.

Jeste, D. V., and Wyatt, R. J. *Understanding and Treating Tardive Dyskinesia.* The Guilford Press, New York, 1982.

Johnson, D. A. W. Further observations on the duration of depot neuroleptic maintenance therapy in schizophrenia. *Brit. J. Psychiatry* 135:524–530, 1979.

Jus, K., Jus, A., Gautier, J., Villeneuve, A., Pires, P., Pineau, R., and Villeneuve, R. Studies of the actions of certain pharmacological agents on tardive dyskinesia and on the rabbit syndrome. *Int. J. Clin. Pharmacol.* 9:138–145, 1974.

Kane, J. M., Rifkin, A., Woerner, M., Reardon, G., Sarantoakos, S., Schiebel, D., and Ramos-Lorenzi, J. Low-dose neuroleptic treatment of outpatient schizophrenics. *Arch. Gen. Psychiatry* 40:896, 1983.

Keepers, G. A., Clappison, V. J., and Casey, D. E. Initial anticholinergic prophylaxis for neuroleptic-induced extrapyramidal syndromes. *Arch. Gen. Psychiatry* 40:113, 1983.

Kiev, A. Double-blind comparison of thiothixene and protriptyline in psychotic depression. *Dis. Nerv. Syst.* 33:811–816, 1973.

Kirven, L. E., and Montero, E. F. Comparison of thioridazine and diazepam on the control of nonpsychiatric symptoms associated with senility: Double-blind study. *J. Am. Geriatr. Soc.* 21:546–551, 1973.

Klawans, H. L., Jr., Bergen, D., and Bruyn, G. W. Prolonged drug-induced parkinsonism. *Confin. Neurol.* 35:368–377, 1973.

Klawans, H. L., Jr., Bergen, D., Bruyn, G. W., and Paulson, G. W. Neuroleptic-induced tardive dyskinesias in nonpsychotic patients. *Arch. Neurol.* 30:338–339, 1974.

Klett, C. J., and Caffey, E. M., Jr. Evaluating the long-term need for antiparkinson drugs by chronic schizophrenics. *Arch. Gen. Psychiatry* 26:374–379, 1972.

Kopelman, A. E., McCullar, F. W., and Heggeness, L. Limb malformations following maternal use of haloperidol. *J.A.M.A.* 231:62–64, 1975.

Korein, J., Fish, B., Shapiro, T., et al. EEG and behavior effects on drug therapy in children: Chlorpromazine and diphenhydramine. *Arch. Gen. Psychiatry* 24:552–563, 1971.

Korpi, E. R., Phelps, B. H., Granger, H., Chang, W-H., Linnoila, M., Meek, J. L., and Wyatt, R. J. Simultaneous determination of haloperidol and its reduced metabolite in serum and plasma by isocratic liquid chromatography with electrochemical detection. *Clin. Chem.* 29:626–628, 1983.

Laborit, H., Huguenard, P., and Alluaume, R. Un nouveau stabilisateur végétatif, le 4560 RP. *Presse Med.* 60:206–208, 1952.

Lasky, J. J., Klett, C. J., Caffey, E. M., Jr., et al. Drug treatment of schizophrenic patients: A comparative evaluation of chlorpromazine, chlorprothixene, fluphenazine, reserpine, thioridazine and triflupromazine. *Dis. Nerv. Syst.* 23:298–306, 1962.

Lee, P. A., Kelly, M. R., and Wallin, J. D. Increased prolactin levels during reserpine treatment of hypertensive patients. *J.A.M.A.* 235:2316–2317, 1976.

Leemsta, J. E., and Koenig, K. L. Sudden death and phenothiazines: A current controversy. *Arch. Gen. Psychiatry* 18:137–148, 1968.

Lehmann, H. F., Ban, T. A., and Suxena, B. M. Nicotinic acid, thioridazine, fluoxymesterone and their combinations in hospitalized geriatric patients. *Am. Psychiatr. Soc. J.* 17:315–320, 1972.

Lehmann, H. E., and Hanrahan, G. E. Chlorpromazine, a new inhibiting agent for psychomotor excitement and manic states. *A.M.A. Arch. Neurol. Psychiatry* 71:227–237, 1954.

Lerner, Y., Lwow, E., Levitan, A., and Belmaker, R. H. Acute high-dose parenteral haloperidol treatment of psychosis. *Am. J. Psychiatry* 136:1061–1064, 1979.

Lipinski, J. F., Zubenko, G., Cohen, B. M., and Barreira, P. Propranolol in the treatment of neuroleptic-induced akathisia. *Am. J. Psychiatry* 141:412–415, 1984.

Loga, S., Curry, S., and Lader, M. Interactions of orphenadrine and phenobarbitone with chlorpromazine: Plasma concentrations and effects in man. *Brit. J. Clin. Pharmacol.* 2:197–208, 1975.

Lord, D. J., and Kidd, C. B. Haloperidol versus diazepam: A double-blind crossover clinical trial. *Med. J. Austr* 1:586–588, 1973.

Man, P. L., and Chen, C. H. Rapid tranquilization of acutely psychotic patients with intramuscular haloperidol and chlorpromazine. *Psychosomatics* 14:59–63, 1973.

Marks, J. Pre-drug behavior as a predictor of response to phenothiazines among schizophrenics. *J. Nerv. Ment. Dis.* 137:597–601, 1963.

Marsden, D. C., Tarsy, D., and Baldessarini, R. J. Spontaneous and drug-induced movement disorders in psychiatric patients. In *Psychiatric Aspects of Neurologic Disease,* ed. D. F. Benson and D. Blumer. Grune and Stratton, New York, 1975, pp. 219–265.

Mason, A. S. Basic principles in the use of antipsychotic agents. *Hosp. Community Psychiatry* 24:825–829, 1973.

Mason, A. S., and Granacher, R. P. *Clinical Handbook of Antipsychotic Drug Therapy.* Brunner/Mazel, New York, 1978.

Matthysse, S. Antipsychotic drug actions: A clue to the neuropathology of schizophrenia? *Fed. Proc.* 32:200–205, 1973.

Matthysse, S., and Sugarman, J. Neurotransmitter theories of schizophrenia. In *Handbook of Psychopharmacology,* vol. 10, ed. L. L. Iversen, S. D. Iversen, and S. H. Snyder. Plenum Press, New York, 1978, pp. 211–242.

May, P. R. A. *Treatment of Schizophrenia: A Comparative Study of Five Treatment Methods.* Science House, New York, 1968.

――――Rational treatment for an irrational disorder: What does the schizophrenic patient need? *Am. J. Psychiatry* 133:1008–1012, 1976.

May, P. R. A., and Van Putten, T. Plasma levels of chlorpromazine in schizophrenia: A critical review of the literature. *Arch. Gen. Psychiatry* 35:1081–1087, 1978.

McAndrew, J. B., Case, Q., and Treffert, D. Effects of prolonged phenothiazine intake on psychotic and other hospitalized children. *J. Autism Child. Schizo.* 2:75–91, 1972.

McClelland, H. A., Blessed, G., Bhate, S., Ali, N., and Clarke, P. A. The abrupt withdrawal of antiparkinsonian drugs in schizophrenic patients. *Brit. J. Psychiatry* 124:151–159, 1974.

McGlashan, T. H. The Chestnut Lodge follow-up study: II. Long-term outcome of schizophrenia and affective disorders. *Arch. Gen. Psychiatry* 41:586–601, 1984.

Meltzer, H. Y., and Stahl, S. M. The dopamine hypothesis of schizophrenia: A review. *Schizophr. Bull.* 2:19–76, 1976.

Messiha, F. S., Knopp, W., Vanecko, S., et al. Haloperidol therapy in Tourette's syndrome: Neurophysiological, biochemical and behavioral correlates. *Life Sci.* 10:449–457, 1971.

Miller, R. J., Horn, A. S., and Iversen, L. L. The action of neuroleptic drugs on dopamine-stimulated adenosine cyclic 3', 5'-monophosphate production in rat neostriatum and limbic forebrain. *Mol. Pharmacol.* 10:759–766, 1974.

Möller Nielsen, I., Pedersen, V., Nymark, M., et al. The comparative pharmacology of flupenthixol and some reference neuroleptics. *Acta Pharmacol. Toxicol.* (Kbh.) 33:353–362, 1973.

Mones, R. J. The use of haloperidol in neurologic patients. In *Butyrophenones in Psychiatry*, ed. A. DiMascio and R. I. Shader. Raven Press, New York, 1972.

Moore, K. E., and Kelly, P. H. Biochemical pharmacology of mesolimbic and mesocortical dopaminergic neurons. In *Psychopharmacology: A Generation of Progress*, ed. M. A. Lipton, A. DiMascio, and K. F. Killam. Raven Press, New York, 1978, pp. 221–234.

Mosher, L. R. Nicotinic acid side-effects and toxicity: A review. *Am. J. Psychiatry* 126:1290–1296, 1970.

Nasrallah, H. A., Donnelly, E. F., Bigelow, L. B., et al. Effects of alpha-methyl-paratyrosine on medicated chronic schizophrenics. *Arch. Gen. Psychiatry* 34:649–655, 1977.

National Institute of Mental Health (NIMH) Psychopharmacology Service Center Collaborative Study Group. Phenothiazine treatment in acute schizophrenia. *Arch. Gen. Psychiatry* 10:246–261, 1964.

National Institute of Mental Health (NIMH) Psychopharmacology Research Branch Collaborative Study Group. Short-term improvement in schizophrenia: The contribution of background factors. *Am. J. Psychiatry* 124:900–909, 1968.

Oldham, A. J., and Bott, M. The management of excitement in a general hospital psychiatric ward by high dosage haloperidol. *Acta Psychiatr. Scand.* 47:369–376, 1971.

Orlov, P., Kasparian, G., DiMascio, A., and Cole, J. O. Withdrawal of antiparkinson drugs. *Arch. Gen. Psychiatry* 25:246–261, 1964.

Overall, J. E. Prior psychiatric treatment and the development of breast cancer. *Arch. Gen. Psychiatry* 35:898–899, 1978.

Overall, J. E., Hollister, L. E., Meyer, F., Kimball, I., and Shelton, J. Imipramine and thioridazine in depressed and schizophrenic patients. *J.A.M.A.* 189:93–96, 1964.

Pisciotta, A. V. Agranulocytosis induced by certain phenothiazine derivatives. *J.A.M.A.* 208:1862–1868, 1969.

Polizos, P., Engelhardt, D. M., Hoffman, S. P., and Waizer, J. Neurological consequences of psychotropic drug withdrawal in schizophrenic children. *J. Autism Child. Schizo.* 3:247–253, 1973.

Post, R. M., and Goodwin, F. K. Time-dependent effects of phenothiazines on dopamine turnover in psychiatric patients. *Science* 190:488–489, 1975.

Prien, R. F., Cole, J. O., and Belkin, N. F. Relapse in chronic schizophrenics: following abrupt withdrawal of tranquilizing medication. *Brit. J. Psychiatry* 115:679–686, 1969.

Prien, R. F., DeLong, S. L., Cole, J. O., and Levine, J. Ocular changes occurring with prolonged high dose chlorpromazine therapy. *Arch. Gen. Psychiatry* 23:464–468, 1970.

Pritchard, M. Prognosis of schizophrenia before and after pharmacotherapy: II. Three-year follow up. *Brit. J. Psychiatry* 113:1353–1359, 1967.

Quitkin, F., Rifkin, A., and Klein, D. F. Very high dosage vs. standard dosage fluphenazine in schizophrenia. *Arch. Gen. Psychiatry* 32:1276–1281, 1975.

Reichlin, S., and Boyd, A. E., III. Neural control of prolactin secretion in man. *Psychoneuroendocrinology* 3:113–130, 1978.

Resnick, M., and Barton, B. T. Droperidol vs. haloperidol in the initial management of acutely agitated patients. *J. Clin. Psychiatry* 45:298–299, 1984.

Rivera-Calimlim, L., Nasrallah, H., Strauss, J., and Lasagna, L. Clinical response and plasma levels: Effect of dose, dosage schedules, and drug interactions on plasma chlorpromazine levels. *Am. J. Psychiatry* 133:646–652, 1976.

Rotrosen, J., Angrist, B. M., Gershon, S., Aronson, M., Gruen, P., Sachar, E., Denning, R. K., Matthysse, S., Stanley, M., and Wilk, S. Thiethylperazine. *Arch. Gen. Psychiatry* 35:1112–1118, 1978.

Sakalis, G., Curry, S. H., Mould, G. P., and Lader, M. H. Physiologic and clinical effects of chlorpromazine and their relationship to plasma level. *Clin. Pharmacol. Ther.* 13:931–946, 1972.

Schooler, N. R., Levine, J., Severe, J. B., Brauzer, B., DiMascio, A., Klerman, G. L., and Tuason, V. B. Prevention of relapse in schizophrenia: An evaluation of fluphenazine decanoate. *Arch. Gen. Psychiatry* 37:16–24, 1980.

Schyve, P. M., Smithline, F., and Meltzer, H. Y. Neuroleptic-induced prolactin level elevation and breast cancer: An emerging issue. *Arch. Gen. Psychiatry* 35:1291–1301, 1978.

Sedvall, G. Receptor feedback and dopamine turnover in CNS. In *Handbook of Psychopharmacology,* vol. 6, ed. L. L. Iversen, S. D. Iversen, and S. H. Snyder. Plenum Press, New York, 1975, pp. 127–177.

Seeman, P. The membrane actions of anesthetics and tranquilizers. *Pharmacol. Rev.* 24:583–655, 1972.

Seeman, P., Chau-Wong, M., Tedesco, J., and Wong, K. Brain receptors for antipsychotic drugs and dopamine: Direct binding assays. *Proc. Natl. Acad. Sci. USA* 72:4376–4380, 1975.

Seeman, P., Lee, T., Chau-Wong, M., and Wong, K. Antipsychotic drug doses and neuroleptic/dopamine receptors. *Nature* 261:717–719, 1976.

Sen, G., and Bose, K. C. *Rauwolfia serpentina,* a new Indian drug for insanity and high blood pressure. *Ind. Med. World* 2:194–201, 1931.

Serrano, A. C., and Forbis, O. L. Haloperidol for psychiatric disorders in children. *Dis. Nerv. Syst.* 34:226–231, 1973.

Shapiro, A. K., Shapiro, E., and Wayne, H. Treatment of Tourette's syndrome. *Arch. Gen. Psychiatry* 28:92–97, 1973.

Shopsin, B., Kim, S. S., and Gershon, S. A controlled study of lithium vs. chlorpromazine in acute schizophrenics. *Brit. J. Psychiatry* 119:435–440, 1971.

Shore, P. A., and Giachetti, A. Reserpine: Basic and clinical pharmacology. In *Handbook of Psychopharmacology,* vol. 10, ed. L. L. Iversen, S. D. Iversen, and S. H. Snyder. Plenum Press, New York, 1978, pp. 197–219.

Siggins, G. R., Hoffer, B. J., Bloom, F. E., and Ungerstedt, U. Cytochemical and electrophysiological studies of dopamine in the caudate nucleus. In *The Basal Ganglia*, ed. M. Yahr, Association for Research in Nervous and Mental Disease Publications, vol. 55. Raven Press, New York, 1976, pp. 227–248.

Simpson, G. M., Cooper, T. B., Bark, N., Sud, I., and Lee, H. J. Effect of antiparkinsonian medication on plasma levels of chlorpromazine. *Arch. Gen. Psychiatry* 37:205–208, 1980.

Simpson, G. M., and Varga, E. Clozapine: A new antipsychotic agent. *Curr. Ther. Res.* 16:679–686, 1974.

Singh, M. M., and Kay, S. R. A comparative study of haloperidol and chlorpromazine in terms of clinical effects and therapeutic reversal with benztropine in schizophrenia. *Psychopharmacologia* 43:103–113, 1975.

Smith, K., Surphlis, W., Gynter, M., and Shimkunas, A. ECT and chlorpromazine compared in the treatment of schizophrenia. *J. Nerv. Ment. Dis.* 144:284–290, 1967.

Snyder, S., Greenberg, D., and Yamamura, H. I. Antischizophrenic drugs and brain cholinergic receptors. *Arch. Gen. Psychiatry* 31:58–61, 1974.

Snyder, S. H., Taylor, K. M., Coyle, J. T., and Meyerhoff, J. L. The role of brain dopamine in behavioral regulation and the actions of psychotropic drugs. *Am. J. Psychiatry* 127:199–207, 1970.

Stawarz, R. J., Hill, H., Robinson, S. E., et al. On the significance of the increase in homovanillic acid (HVA) caused by antipsychotic drugs in corpus striatum and limbic forebrain. *Psychopharmacologia* 43:125–130, 1975.

Sulser, R., and Robinson, S. E. Clinical implications of pharmacological differences among antipsychotic drugs. In *Psychopharmacology: A Generation of Progress*, ed. M. A. Lipton, A. DiMascio, and K. F. Killam. Raven Press, New York, 1978, pp. 943–954.

Swazey, J. P. *Chlorpromazine in Psychiatry: A Study in Therapeutic Innovation.* MIT Press, Cambridge, Mass., 1974.

Tarsy, D., and Baldessarini, R. J. The tardive dyskinesia syndrome. In *Clinical Neuropharmacology*, ed. H. Klawans. Raven Press, New York, 1976, pp. 29–61.

Task Force on Late Neurological Effects of Antipsychotic Drugs (R. J. Baldessarini, chairman). Task Force Report 18: Tardive Dyskinesia. Washington, D.C., American Psychiatric Association, 1980.

Teicher, M. H., and Baldessarini, R. J. Selection of neuroleptic dosage. *Arch. Gen. Psychiatry* 42:636–637, 1985.

Tobias, L. L., and MacDonald, M. L. Withdrawal of maintenance drugs with long-term hospitalized mental patients. *Psychol. Bull.* 81:107–125, 1974.

Tsuang, M. M., Lu, L. M., Stotsky, B. A., and Cole, J. O. Haloperidol vs. thioridazine for hospitalized psychogeriatric patients: Double-blind study. *J. Am. Geriatr. Soc.* 19:593–600, 1971.

Tupin, J. P., and Schuller, A. B. Lithium and haloperidol incompatibility reviewed. *Psychiatr. J. Univ. Ottawa* 3:245–251, 1978.

Van Putten, T. Why do schizophrenic patients refuse to take their drugs? *Arch. Gen. Psychiatry* 31:67–72, 1974.

Van Woert, M. H., Jutkowitz, R., Rosenbaum, D., and Bowers, M. B., Jr. Gilles de la Tourette's syndrome: Biochemical approaches. In *The Basal Ganglia*, ed.

M. D. Yahr. Association for Research in Nervous and Mental Disease Publications, vol. 55. Raven Press, New York, 1976, pp. 459–465.

Waizer, J., Polizos, P., Hoffman, S. P., et al. A single-blind evaluation of thiothixene with out-patient schizophrenic children. *J. Autism Child. Schizo.* 2:378–386, 1972.

Warner, A. M., and Wyman, S. M. Delayed severe extrapyramidal disturbance following frequent depot phenothiazine administration. *Am. J. Psychiatry* 132:743–745, 1975.

Weissman, A. Chemical, pharmacological, and metabolic considerations on thiothixene. In *Thiothixene and the Thioxanthenes*, ed. I. S. Forrest, C. J. Carr, and E. Usdin. Raven Press, New York, 1974, pp. 1–10.

Werry, J. S., Weiss, G., Douglas, V., and Martin, J. Studies on the hyperactive child: III. The effect of chlorpromazine upon behavior and learning ability. *J. Am. Acad. Child. Psychiatry* 5:292–312, 1966.

Wijsenbeek, H., Steiner, M., and Goldberg, S. C. Trifluoperazine: A comparison between regular and high doses. *Psychopharmacologia* 36:147–150, 1974.

Zubenko, G. S., Cohen, B. M., Lipinski, J. F., and Jonas, J. M. The use of clonidine in the treatment of neuroleptic-induced akathisia. *Psychiatry Res.* 13:253–259, 1984.

Lithium Salts

Agulnik, P. L., DiMascio, A., and Moore, P. Acute brain syndrome associated with lithium therapy. *Am. J. Psychiatry* 129:621–623, 1972.

Alexander, P. E., Van Kammen, D. P., and Bunney, W. E., Jr. Antipsychotic effects of lithium in schizophrenia. *Am. J. Psychiatry* 136:283–287, 1979.

Allan, L. D., Desai, G., and Tynan, M. J. Prenatal echocardiographic screening for Ebstein's anomaly for mothers on lithium therapy. *Lancet* 2:875–876, 1982.

Amdisen, A. Monitoring of lithium treatment through determination of lithium concentration. *Danish Med. Bull.* 22:277–291, 1977.

Annell, A. Lithium treatment of children and adolescents. *Acta Psychiat. Scand.* 207 (suppl.):19–30, 1969.

Ayd, F. J., Jr. Lithium and the kidney. *Intl. Drug Ther. Newsletter* 14(7):25–28, 1979.

——— Alternatives for lithium. *Psychiatr. Annals* 14(7):1–4, 1984.

Baastrup, P. C., Hollnagel, P., Sorensen, et al. Adverse reactions in treatment with lithium carbonate and haloperidol. *J.A.M.A.* 236:2645–2646, 1976.

Baastrup, P. C., Paulsen, J. C., Schou, M., and Thomsen, K. Prophylactic lithium: Double-blind discontinuation in manic-depressive and recurrent depressive disorders. *Lancet* 2:326–330, 1970.

Bailey, E., Bond, P. A., Brooks, B. A., et al. The medicinal chemistry of lithium. *Prog. Med. Chem.* 11:193–272, 1975.

Baldessarini, R. J., and Lipinski, J. F. Lithium salts: 1970–1975. *Ann. Intern. Med.* 83:527–533, 1975.

Baldessarini, R. J., and Stephens, J. H. Lithium carbonate for affective disorders: I. Clinical pharmacology and toxicology. *Arch. Gen. Psychiatry* 22:72–77, 1970.

Battle, D. C., Von Riotte, A. B., Gaviria, M., and Grupp, M. Amelioration of polyuria by amiloride in patients receiving long-term lithium therapy. *N. Engl. J. Med.* 312:408–414, 1985.

Berens, S. C., Bernstein, R. S., Robbins, J., and Wolff, J. Antithyroid effects of lithium. *J. Clin. Invest.* 49:1357–1367, 1970.

Biederman, J., Lerner, Y., and Belmaker, R. H. Combination of lithium carbonate and haloperidol in schizoaffective disorder. *Arch. Gen. Psychiatry* 36:327–333, 1979.

Bloom, F. E., Baetge, G., Deyo, S., Ettenberg, A., Koda, L., Magistretti, P. J., Shoemaker, W. J., and Staunton, D. A. Chemical and physiological aspects of the actions of lithium and antidepressant drugs. *Neuropharmacology* 22(3B):359–365, 1983.

Branchey, M. H., Charles, J., and Simpson, G. M. Extrapyramidal side effects of lithium maintenance therapy. *Am. J. Psychiatry* 133:444–445, 1976.

Brenner, R., Cooper, T. B., Yablonski, M. E., Lieberman, J. A., Lesser, M., Siris, S. G., and Rifkin, A. E. Measurement of lithium concentrations in human tears. *Am. J. Psychiatry* 139:678–679, 1982.

Brown, W. A., and Mueller, B. Alleviation of manic symptoms with catecholamine agonists. *Am. J. Psychiatry* 136:230–231, 1979.

Cade, J. F. J. Lithium salts in the treatment of psychotic excitement. *Med. J. Austral.* 2:349–352, 1949.

Campbell, M., Perry, R., and Green, W. H. Use of lithium in children and adolescents. *Psychosomatics* 25:95–106, 1984.

Campbell, M., Small, A. M., Green, W. H., Jennings, S. J., Perry, R., Bennett, W. G., and Anderson, L. Behavioral efficacy of haloperidol and lithium carbonate: A comparison in hospitalized aggressive children with conduct disorder. *Arch. Gen. Psychiatry* 41:650–656, 1984.

Cervi-Skinner, S. J. Lithium-carbonate-induced hypercalcemia. *West. J. Med.* 127:527–528, 1977.

Cho, J. T., Bone, S., Dunner, D. L., et al. The effect of lithium treatment on thyroid function in patients with primary affective disorder. *Am. J. Psychiatry* 136:115–116, 1979.

Christensson, T. A. Lithium, hypercalcaemia, and hyperparathyroidism. *Lancet* 2:144, 1976.

Cohen, B. M., Lipinski, J. F., and Altesman, R. I. Lecithin in the treatment of mania: Double-blind, placebo-controlled trials. *Am. J. Psychiatry* 139:1162–1164, 1982.

Cohen, D. J., Detlor, J., Young, J. G., and Saywitz, B. A. Clonidine ameliorates Gilles de la Tourette's syndrome. *Arch. Gen. Psychiatry* 37:1350–1357, 1980.

Cohen, W. J., and Cohen, N. H. Lithium carbonate, haloperidol and irreversible brain damage. *J.A.M.A.* 230:1283–1287, 1974.

Coppen, A. Mineral metabolism in affective disorders. *Brit. J. Psychiatry* 111:1133–1142, 1965.

Coppen, A., Shaw, D. M., Malleson, A., and Costain, R. Mineral metabolism in mania. *Brit. Med. J.* 1:71–75, 1966.

Cooper, T. B., and Simpson, G. M. The 24-hour lithium level as a prognosticator of dosage requirements: A two-year follow-up study. *Am. J. Psychiatry* 133:440–443, 1976.

——— Kinetics of lithium and clinical response. In *Psychopharmacology: A Generation of Progress*, ed. M. A. Lipton, A. DiMascio, and K. F. Killam. Raven Press, New York, 1978, pp. 923–931.

Cundall, R. L., Brooks, P. W., and Murray, L. G. A controlled evaluation of lithium prophylaxis in affective disorders. *Psychol. Med.* 2:308–311, 1972.

Davis, B. M., Pfefferbaum, A., Krutzik, S., et al. Lithium's effect on parathyroid hormone. *Am. J. Psychiatry* 138:489–492, 1981.

Davis, J. M. Overview: Maintenance therapy in psychiatry. II. Affective disorders. *Am. J. Psychiatry* 133:1–13, 1976.

Davis, J. M., and Fann, W. E. Lithium. *Ann. Rev. Pharmacol.* 11:285–302, 1971.

Davis, K. L., and Berger, P. A. Pharmacological investigations of the cholinergic imbalance hypothesis of movement disorders and psychosis. *Biol. Psychiatry* 13:23–49, 1978.

DeLong, G. R. Lithium carbonate treatment of select behavior disorders in children suggesting manic-depressive illness. *J. Pediatrics* 93:689–694, 1978.

DeLong, G. R., and Nieman, G. W. Lithium-induced behavior changes in children with symptoms suggesting manic-depressive illness. *Psychopharmacol. Bull.* 19:258–265, 1983.

Del Zompo, M., Pitzalis, G. F., Bernardi, F., et al. Antipsychotic effect of apomorphine: A retrospective study. In *Apomorphine and Other Dopaminomimetics, vol. 2: Clinical Pharmacology,* ed. G. U. Corsini and G. L. Gessa. Raven Press, New York, 1981, pp. 65–76.

Demers, R. G., and Heninger, G. R. Electrocardiographic T-wave changes during lithium carbonate treatment. *J.A.M.A.* 218:381–386, 1971.

De Montigny, C., Grunberg, F., Mayer, A., and Deschenes, J.-P. Lithium induces rapid relief of depression in tricyclic antidepressant drug non-responders. *Brit. J. Psychiatry* 138:252–256, 1981.

DePaulo, J. R., Jr., Correa, E. I., and Sapir, D. G. Renal toxicity of lithium and its complications. *Johns Hopkins Med. J.* 149:15–21, 1981.

Dilsaver, S. C. Lithium's effect on muscarinic receptor binding parameters: A relationship to therapeutic efficacy? *Biol. Psychiatry* 19:1551–1565, 1984.

Dunner, D., Patrick, V., and Fieve, R. R. Rapidly cycling manic depressive patients. *Comprehen. Psychiatry* 18:561–566, 1977.

Ekbon, K. Lithium in the treatment of chronic cluster headache. *Headache* 17:39–40, 1977.

Falk, W. E., Mahnke, M. W., and Poskanzer, D. C. Lithium prophylaxis of corticotropin-induced psychosis. *J.A.M.A.* 241:1011–1012, 1979.

Fieve, R. R. Lithium therapy. In *Comprehensive Textbook of Psychiatry,* 3rd ed., ed. H. Kaplan, A. M. Freedman, and B. J. Sadock. Williams and Wilkins, Baltimore, 1980, pp. 2348–2352.

Fieve, R. R., Kumbaraci, T., and Dunner, D. L. Lithium prophylaxis of depression in bipolar I, bipolar II, and unipolar patients. *Am. J. Psychiatry* 133:925–929, 1976.

Fieve, R. R., Platman, S. R., and Plutchick, R. R. The use of lithium in affective disorders: I. Acute endogenous depression. *Am. J. Psychiatry* 125:487–491, 1968.

Forrest, J. J., Jr. Lithium inhibition of cAMP-mediated hormones: A caution. *N. Engl. J. Med.* 292:423–424, 1975.

Franks, R. D., Dabovsky, S. L., Lifshitz, M., Coen, P., Subryan, V., and Walker, S. H. Long-term lithium therapy causes hyperparathyroidism. *Arch. Gen. Psychiatry* 39:1074–1077, 1982.

Freinhar, J. P., and Alvarez, W. H. Use of clonazepam in two cases of acute mania. *J. Clin. Psychiatry* 46:29–30, 1985.

Gattozzi, A. A. *Lithium in the Treatment of Mood Disorders.* U.S. National Clearinghouse for Mental Health Information (NIMH), Publication no. 5033. Government Printing Office, Washington, D.C., 1970.

Gerner, R. H., Post, R. M., Spiegel, A. M., et al. Effects of parathyroid hormone and lithium treatment on calcium and mood in depressed patients. *Biol. Psychiatry* 12:145–151, 1977.

Gerner, R. H., Psarras, J., and Kirschenbaum, M. A. Results of clinical renal function tests in lithium patients. *Am. J. Psychiatry* 137:834–837, 1980.

Gershon, S. Lithium in mania. *Clin. Pharmacol. Ther.* 11:168–187, 1970.

Gershon, S., and Shopsin, B. *Lithium: Its Role in Psychiatric Research and Treatment.* Plenum Press, New York, 1975.

Goldfield, M. D., and Weinstein, M. R. Lithium in pregnancy: A review with recommendations. *Am. J. Psychiatry* 127:888–893, 1971.

————— Lithium carbonate in obstetrics: Guidelines for clinical use. *Am. J. Obstet. Gynecol.* 116:15–22, 1973.

Goodwin, F. K., Murphy, D. L., and Bunney, W. E., Jr. Lithium in depression and mania: A double-blind behavioral and biochemical study. *Arch. Gen. Psychiatry* 21:486–496, 1969.

Grof, P., Lane, J., MacCrimmon, D., et al. Clinical and laboratory correlates of the response to long-term lithium treatment. In *Origin, Intervention, and Treatment of Affective Disorders,* ed. E. Stromgren and M. Schou. Academic Press, New York, 1979, pp. 28–40.

Grof, P., Schou, M., Angst, J., Baastrup, P. C., and Weis, P. Methodological problems of prophylactic trials in recurrent affective disorders. *Brit. J. Psychiatry* 116:599–619, 1970.

Gross, H. A., Ebert, M. H., Faden, V. B., Goldberg, S. C., Nee, L. E., and Kage, W. H. A double-blind trial of lithium carbonate in primary anorexia nervosa. *J. Clin. Psychopharmacol.* 1:376–381, 1981.

Haugaard, E. S., Mickel, R., and Haugaard, N. Actions of lithium ions and insulin on glucose utilization, glycogen synthesis and glycogen synthase in the isolated rat diaphragm. *Biochem. Pharmacol.* 23:1675–1685, 1974.

Hestbach, J., Hansen, H. E., Amdisen, A., et al. Chronic renal lesions following long-term treatment with lithium. *Kidney Int.* 12:205–213, 1977.

Himmelhoch, J. M., Poust, R. I., and Mallinger, A. G. Adjustment of lithium dose during lithium-chlorthiazide therapy. *Clin. Pharmacol. Ther.* 22:225–227, 1977.

Hirschowitz, J., Casper, R., Garver, D. L., et al. Lithium response in good prognosis schizophrenia. *Am. J. Psychiatry* 137:916–920, 1980.

Hwang, S., and Tuason, V. B. Long-term maintenance lithium therapy and possible irreversible renal damage. *J. Clin. Psychiatry* 41:11–19, 1980.

Janowsky, D. S., El-Yousef, M. K., Davis, J. M., et al. Parasympathetic suppression of manic symptoms by physostigmine. *Arch. Gen. Psychiatry* 28:542–547, 1973.

Jefferson, J. W., and Greist, J. H. *Primer of Lithium Therapy.* Williams and Wilkins, Baltimore, 1977.

Jefferson, J. W., Greist, J. H., and Ackerman, D. L. *Lithium Encyclopedia for Clinical Practice.* Lithium Information Center, Department of Psychiatry, University of Wisconsin, Madison, 1983.

Jefferson, J. W., Greist, J. H., Clagnaz, P. J., Eischens, R. R., Marten, W. D., and Eversen, M. A. Effect of strenuous exercise on serum lithium level in man. *Am. J. Psychiatry* 139:1593–1595, 1982.

Johnson, F. N., ed. *Lithium Research and Therapy.* Academic Press, New York, 1975.

————ed. *Handbook of Lithium Therapy.* University Park Press, Baltimore, 1980.

————*The Psychopharmacology of Lithium.* MacMillan Press, London, 1984.

————*The History of Lithium Therapy.* MacMillan Press, London, 1984.

Johnson, F. N., and Johnson, S. *Lithium in Medical Practice.* University Park Press, Baltimore, 1978.

Johnson, G., Gershon, S., Burdock, E. I., et al. Comparative effects of lithium and chlorpromazine in the treatment of acute manic states. *Brit. J. Psychiatry* 119:267–276, 1971.

Jorgensen, F., Larsen, S., Spanager, B., et al. Kidney function and quantitative histological changes in patients on long-term lithium therapy. *Acta Psychiatr. Scand.* 70:455–462, 1984.

Jouvent, R., Lecrubier, Y., Peuch, A. J., et al. Antimanic effect of clonidine. *Am. J. Psychiatry* 137:1275–1276, 1980.

Kane, J., Rifkin, A., Quitkin, F., et al. Extrapyramidal side effects with lithium treatment. *Am. J. Psychiatry* 135:851–853, 1978.

Kudrow, L. Lithium prophylaxis for chronic cluster headache. *Headache* 17:15–18, 1977.

Kukopulos, A., Reginaldi, D., Girardi, P., and Tondo, L. Course of manic-depressive recurrences under lithium. *Compr. Psychiatry* 16:517–524, 1975.

Lewis, J. L., and Winokur, G. The induction of mania: A natural history study with controls. *Arch. Gen. Psychiatry* 39:303–306, 1982.

Lipinski, J. F., Pope, H. G. Possible synergistic action between carbamazepine and lithium carbonate in the treatment of three acutely manic patients. *Am. J. Psychiatry* 139:948–949, 1982.

Lippmann, S. Is lithium bad for the kidneys? *J. Clin. Psychiatry* 43:220–224, 1982.

Livingston, S., Pauli, L., Berman, W. Carbamazepine (Tegretol) in epilepsy: Nine-year follow-up study with special emphasis on untoward reactions. *Dis. Nerv. Syst.* 35:103–107, 1974.

Mandel, M. R., Madsen, J., Miller, A. L., and Baldessarini, R. J. Intoxication associated with lithium and ECT. *Am. J. Psychiatry* 137:1107–1109, 1980.

Mendels, J. Lithium in the treatment of depression. *Am. J. Psychiatry* 133:373–378, 1976.

Merry, J., Reynolds, C. M., Bailey, J., et al. Prophylactic treatment of alcoholism by lithium carbonate: A controlled study. *Lancet* 2:486–488, 1976.

Neil, J. F., Himmelhoch, J. M., and Licata, S. M. Emergence of myasthenia gravis during treatment with lithium carbonate. *Arch. Gen. Psychiatry* 33:1090–1092, 1976.

Nelson, J. C., and Byck, R. Rapid response to lithium in phenelzine non-responders. *Brit. J. Psychiatry* 141:85–86, 1982.

Norman, K. P., Cerrone, K. L., and Reus, V. I. Renal lithium clearance as a rapid and accurate predictor of maintenance dose. *Am. J. Psychiatry* 139:1625–1626, 1982.

Noyes, R., Dempsey, G. M., and Blum, A. Lithium treatment of depression. *Compr. Psychiatry* 15:187–190, 1974.

Pandey, G. N., Dorus, E., Davis, J. M., et al. Lithium transport in human red blood cells. *Arch. Gen. Psychiatry* 36:902–908, 1979.

Perris, C. Morbidity suppression effect of lithium carbonate in cycloid psychosis. *Arch. Gen. Psychiatry* 35:328–331, 1978.

Pert, A., Rosenblatt, J. E., Sivit, C., Pert, C. B., and Bunney, W. E., Jr. Long-term treatment with lithium prevents the development of dopamine receptor supersensitivity. *Science* 201:171–173, 1978.

Pope, H. G., and Lipinski, J. F. Diagnosis in schizophrenia and manic-depressive illness. *Arch. Gen. Psychiatry* 35:811–828, 1978.

Post, R. M., Uhde, T. W., Ballenger, J. C., and Bunney, W. E., Jr. Carbamazepine, temporal lobe epilepsy, and manic depressive illness. *Adv. Biol. Psychiatry* 8:117–156, 1982.

Price, L. H., Yeates, C., and Nelson, J. C. Lithium augmentation of combined neuroleptic-tricyclic treatment in delusional depression. *Am. J. Psychiatry* 140:318–322, 1982.

Prien, R. F., Caffey, E. M., Jr., and Klett, C. J. A comparison of lithium carbonate and chlorpromazine in the treatment of mania. V.A. Cooperative Studies in Psychiatry: Report no. 86, Central Neuropsychiatric Research Lab., Perry Point V.A. Hospital, Maryland, 1971.

———The relationship between serum lithium level and clinical response in acute manics treated with lithium carbonate. *Brit. J. Psychiatry* 120:409–414, 1972.

———Prophylactic efficacy of lithium carbonate in manic-depressive illness. *Arch. Gen. Psychiatry* 28:337–341, 1973.

Prien, R. F., Klett, C. J., and Caffey, E. M., Jr. Lithium carbonate and imipramine in prevention of affective episodes. *Arch. Gen. Psychiatry* 29:420–425, 1973.

Prusoff, B. A., Williams, D. H., Weissman, M. W., et al. Treatment of secondary depression in schizophrenia. *Arch. Gen. Psychiatry* 36:569–575, 1979.

Quitkin, F., Rifkin, A., and Klein, D. F. Prophylaxis of affective disorders. *Arch. Gen. Psychiatry* 33:337–341, 1976.

Quitkin, F., Rifkin, A., Klein, D. F., and Davis, J. M. On prophylaxis in unipolar depressive disorder. *Am. J. Psychiatry* 133:1091–1092, 1976.

Rafaelsen, O. J., Bolwig, T. G., Brun, C., Hetman, O., Ladefoged, J., and Larsen, S. Lithium and the Kidney. Proceedings of the World Psychiatric Association Symposium, Moscow, May 1979.

Ramsey, T. A., Frazer, A., Dyson, W. L., et al. Intracellular lithium and clinical response. *Brit. J. Psychiatry* 128:103–104, 1976.

Ramsey, T. A., and Mendels, J. Lithium as an antidepressant. In *Antidepressants:*

Neurochemical Behavioral and Clinical Perspectives, ed. S. J. Enna, J. B. Malick, and E. Richelson. Raven Press, New York, 1981, pp. 175–182.

Rifkin, A., Kurtin, S. B., Quitkin, F., and Klein, D. F. Lithium-induced folliculitis. *Am. J. Psychiatry* 130:1018–1019, 1973.

Rifkin, A., Quitkin, F., Carrillo, C., et al. Lithium carbonate in emotionally unstable character disorders. *Arch. Gen. Psychiatry* 27:519–523, 1972.

Saton, B. M., and Gaind, R. Lithium. *Clin. Toxicol.* 6:257–269, 1973.

Schou, M. Biology and pharmacology of the lithium ion. *Pharmacol. Rev.* 9:17–58, 1957.

———Lithium in psychiatric therapy and prophylaxis. *J. Psychiatr. Res.* 6:67–95, 1968.

———The biology and pharmacology of lithium: A bibliography. *NIMH Psychopharmacol. Bull.* 5:33–62, 1969.

———Lithium as a prophylactic agent in unipolar affective illness. *Arch. Gen. Psychiatry* 36:849–851, 1979.

Schou, M., Amdisen, A., and Steenstrup, O. R. Lithium and pregnancy: II. Hazards to women given lithium during pregnancy and delivery. *Brit. Med. J.* 2:137–138, 1973.

Schou, M., Amdisen, A., and Trap-Jensen, J. Lithium poisoning. *Am. J. Psychiatry* 125:520–527, 1968.

Selinger, D., Simmons, S., Hailer, A. W., Nurnberger, J. I., Jr., and Gershon, E. S. An effective method for measuring salivary lithium in patients on anticholinergic drugs. *Biol. Psychiatry* 17:1145–1155, 1982.

Shopsin, B., Kim, S. S., and Gershon, S. A controlled study of lithium vs. chlorpromazine in acute schizophrenics. *Brit. J. Psychiatry* 119:435–440, 1971.

Spring, G., and Frankel, M. New data on lithium and haloperidol incompatibility. *Am. J. Psychiatry* 138:818–821, 1981.

Stallone, F., Shelley, E., Mendelwicz, J., and Fieve, R. R. The use of lithium in affective disorders: III. A double-blind study of prophylaxis in bipolar illness. *Am. J. Psychiatry* 130:1006–1010, 1973.

Staunton, D. A., Magistretti, P. J., Shoemaker, W. J., and Bloom, F. E. Effects of chronic lithium treatment on dopamine receptors in the rat corpus striatum: I. Locomotor activity and behavioral supersensitivity. *Brain Research* 232:391–400, 1982.

Staunton, D. A., Magistretti, P. J., Shoemaker, W. J., Devo, S. N., and Bloom, F. E. Effects of chronic lithium treatment on dopamine receptors in the rat corpus striatum: II. No effect on denervation or neuroleptic-induced supersensitivity. *Brain Research* 232:401–412, 1982.

Stokes, P. E., Kocsis, J. H., and Arcuni, O. J. Relationship of lithium chloride dose to treatment response in acute mania. *Arch. Gen. Psychiatry* 33:1080–1084, 1976.

Strayhorn, J. M., and Nash, J. L. Severe neurotoxicity despite "therapeutic" serum levels. *Dis. Nerv. Syst.* 38:107–111, 1977.

Treiser, S. L., Cascio, C. S., O'Donohue, T. L., Thoa, N. B., Jacobwitz, D. M., and Kellar, K. J. Lithium increases serotonin release and decreases serotonin receptors in the hippocampus. *Science* 213:1529–1531, 1981.

Tupin, J. P., and Schuller, A. B. Lithium and haloperidol incompatibility reviewed. *Psychiatr. J. Univ. Ottawa* 3:245–251, 1978.

Van der Velde, C. D. Toxicity of lithium carbonate in elderly patients. *Am. J. Psychiatry* 127:1075–1077, 1971.

Vendsborg, P. B., Bech, P., and Rafaelson, O. J. Lithium treatment and weight gain. *Acta Psychiatr. Scand.* 53:139–147, 1976.

Vestergaard, P., Amdisen, A., Hansen, H. E., and Schou, M. Lithium treatment and kidney function: A survey of 237 patients in long-term treatment. *Acta Psychiatr. Scand.* 60:504–520, 1979.

Vinarova, E., Uhlif, O., Stika, L., and Vinar, O. Side effects of lithium administration. *Act. Nerv. Super.* (Praha) 14:105–107, 1972.

White, M. G., and Fetner, C. D. Treatment of the syndrome of inappropriate secretion of antidiuretic hormone with lithium carbonate. *N. Engl. J. Med.* 292:390–392, 1975.

Williams, D. T., Mehl, R., Yudofsky, S., Adams, D., and Roseman, B. The effect of propranolol on uncontrolled rage outbursts in children and adolescents with organic brain dysfunction. *J. Am. Acad. Child Psychiatry* 21:129–135, 1982.

Wilson, J. H. P., Donker, A. J. M., Van Der Hem., G. K., and Wientjes, J. Peritoneal dialysis for lithium poisoning. *Brit. Med. J.* 2:749–750, 1971.

Winokur, G., Clayton, P. J., and Reich, T. *Manic-Depressive Illness.* C. V. Mosby, St. Louis, 1969.

Woody, J. N., London, W. L., and Wilbands, G. D., Jr. Lithium toxicity in a newborn. *Pediatrics* 47:94–96, 1971.

Youngerman, J., and Canino, I. A. Lithium carbonate use in children and adolescents. *Arch. Gen. Psychiatry* 35:216–224, 1978.

Antidepressant Agents

Alexanderson, B., and Sjoqvist, F. Individual differences in the pharmacokinetics of monomethylated tricyclic antidepressants: Role of genetic and environmental factors and clinical importance. *Ann. N.Y. Acad Sci.* 179:739–751, 1971.

Alino, J. J., Gutierrez, J. L., and Iglesias, M. J. 5-Hydroxytryptophan (5-HTP) and an MAOI (nialamide) in the treatment of depressions: A double-blind controlled study. *Int. Pharmacopsychiatry* 11:8–15, 1976.

American Psychiatric Association Task Force on the Use of Laboratory Tests in Psychiatry (A. H. Glassman, chairman). Tricyclic antidepressants: Blood level measurements and clinical outcome. *Am. J. Psychiatry* 142:155–162, 1985.

Amsterdam, J., Brunswick, D., and Mendels, J. The clinical application of tricyclic antidepressant pharmacokinetics and plasma levels. *Am. J. Psychiatry* 137:653–662, 1980.

Andén, N-E, Dahlstrom, A., Fuxe, K., et al. Ascending neurons to the telencephalon and diencephalon. *Acta Physiol. Scand.* 67:313–326, 1966.

Angst, J., Woggon, B., and Schoepf, J. The treatment of depressions with L-5-hydroxytryptophan versus imipramine. *Arch. Psychiatr. Nervenkr.* 24:175–186, 1977.

Annell, A. Amitriptyline in childhood depressions. *Acta Psychiatr. Scand.* 207 (suppl.):19–30, 1969.

Appel, P., Eckel, K., and Harrer, G. Veranderungen des Blasen- und Blasensphinktertonus durch Thymoleptika: Zystomanometrische Untersuchungen beim Menschen. *Int. Pharmacopsychiatry* 6:15–16, 1971.

Asakura, M., Tsukamoto, T., and Hasegawa, K. Modulation of rat brain alpha$_2$ and beta-adrenergic receptor sensitivity following long-term treatment with antidepressants. *Brain Res.* 235:192–197, 1982.

Åsberg, M. Plasma nortriptyline levels: Relationship to clinical effects. *Clin. Pharmacol. Ther.* 16:215–229, 1974.

———Treatment of depression with tricyclic drugs, pharmacokinetic and pharmacodynamic aspects. *Pharmakopsychiatrie* 9:18–26, 1976.

Asnis, G. M., Asnis, D., Dunnes, D. L., et al. Cogwheel rigidity during chronic lithium therapy. *Am. J. Psychiatry* 136:1225–1226, 1979.

Avery, D., and Winokur, G. The efficacy of electroconvulsive therapy and antidepressants in depression. *Biol. Psychiatry* 12:507–523, 1977.

Axelrod, J., Whitby, L. G., and Hertting, G. Effect of psychotropic drugs on the uptake of H^3-norepinephrine by tissues. *Science* 133:383–384, 1961.

Ayuso-Gutierrez, J. L., and Lopez-Ibor, A. J. Tryptophan and an MAOI (nialamide) in the treatment of depression. *Int. Pharmacopsychiatry* 6:92–97, 1971.

Baldessarini, R. J. Biogenic amine hypotheses in affective disorders. In *The Nature and Treatment of Depression*, ed. F. F. Flach and S. Draghi. Plenum Press, New York, 1975, pp. 347–385.

———The basis for amine hypotheses in affective disorders: A critical evaluation. *Arch. Gen. Psychiatry* 32:1087–1093, 1975.

———Mood drugs. *Disease-a-Month* 11:1–65, 1977.

———Status of psychotropic drug blood level assays and other biochemical measurements in clinical practice. *Am. J. Psychiatry* 136:1177–1180, 1979.

———A summary of biomedical aspects of mood disorders. *McLean Hosp. J.* 6:1–24, 1981.

———Recent advances in antidepressant pharmacology and pharmacotherapy. *Directions in Psychiatry* 1(2):1–8, 1981.

———Overview of recent advances in antidepressant pharmacology. *McLean Hosp. J.* 7:1–27, 1982.

———How do antidepressants work? In *Issues in Psychiatry: Affective Disorders,* ed. S. Frazier. Washington, D.C., APA Press, 1983, pp. 243–260.

———Treatment of depression by altering monoamine metabolism: Precursors and metabolic inhibitors. *Psychopharmacol. Bull.* 20:224–239, 1984.

Baldessarini, R. J., and Karobath, M. Biochemical physiology of central synapses. *Ann. Rev. Physiol.* 35:273–304, 1973.

Ban, T. A. Amoxapine and viloxazine: Review of literature with special reference to clinical studies. *Psychopharmacology Bull.* 15:22–25, 1979.

Beckman, H., and Goodwin, F. K. Antidepressant response to tricyclics and urinary MHPG in unipolar patients. *Arch. Gen. Psychiatry* 32:17–21, 1975.

Berger, F. M. Depression and antidepressant drugs. *Clin. Pharmacol. Ther.* 18:241–248, 1975.

Bialos, D., Giller, E., and Jatlow, P. Recurrence of depression after the discontinuation of long-term amitriptyline treatment. *Am. J. Psychiatry* 139:325–329, 1982.

Bickel, M. H., and Weder, H. J. The total fate of a drug: Kinetics of distribution, excretion, and formation of 14 metabolites in rats treated with imipramine. *Arch. Int. Pharmacodyn. Ther.* 173:433–440, 1968.

Biederman, J., Herzog, D. B., Rivinus, T. M., Harper, G. P., Ferber, R. A., Rosenbaum, J. F., Harmatz, J. S., Tondorf, R., Orsulak, P. J., and Schildkraut, J. J. Amitriptyline in the treatment of anorexia nervosa: A double-blind, placebo-controlled study. *J. Clin. Psychopharmacology* 5:10–16, 1985.

Bielski, R. J., and Friedel, R. O. Prediction of tricyclic antidepressant response. *Arch. Gen. Psychiatry* 33:1479–1489, 1976.

Biggs, J. T., Spiker, D. C., Petit, J. M., et al. Tricyclic antidepressant overdose: Incidence of symptoms. *J.A.M.A.* 238:135–138, 1977.

Biggs, J. T., and Ziegler, V. E. Protriptyline plasma levels and antidepressant response. *Clin. Pharmacol. Ther.* 22:269–273, 1977.

Blackwell, B., Stefopoulos, A., and Enders, P. Anticholinergic activity of two tricyclic antidepressants. *Am. J. Psychiatry* 135:722–724, 1978.

Bloomingdale, L. M., and Bressler, B. Rapid intramuscular administration of tricyclic antidepressants. *Am. J. Psychiatry* 136:1092–1093, 1979.

Bojanovsky, J., and Tolle, R. Dihydroergotamin gegen die Kreislaufwirkungen der Thymoleptika. *Dtsch. Med. Wochenschr.* 99:1064–1065, 1974.

Bopp, B., and Biel, J. H. Antidepressant drugs. *Life Sci.* 14:415–423, 1974.

Boston Collaborative Drug Surveillance Program. Adverse reactions to the tricyclic-antidepressant drugs. *Lancet* 1:529–531, 1972.

Brackenridge, R. G. Cardiotoxicity of amitriptyline. *Lancet* 2:929–930, 1972.

Bradley, C. The behavior of children receiving benzedrine. *Am. J. Orthopsychiatry* 94:577–585, 1937.

Braithwaite, R., Goulding, R., Theano, G., et al. Amitriptyline plasma levels and therapeutic response. *Clin. Pharmacol. Ther.* 19:795–801, 1976.

Brogdon, R., Heel, R. C., Speight, T. M., et al. Nomifensine: A review of its pharmacologic properties and therapeutic efficacy in depressive illness. *Drugs* 18:1–24, 1979.

Brown, D., Winsberg, B. G., Bialer, I., and Press, M. Imipramine therapy and seizures: Three children treated for hyperactive behavior disorders. *Am. J. Psychiatry* 130:210–212, 1973.

Brunswick, D. J., Amsterdam, J. D., Mendels, J., and Stern, S. L. Prediction of steady-state imipramine and desmethylimipramine plasma concentrations from single-dose data. *Clin. Pharmacol. Ther.* 25:605–610, 1979.

Brunswick, D. J., and Mendels, J. Reduced levels of tricyclic antidepressants in plasma from Vacutainers. *Commun. Psychopharmacol.* 1:131–134, 1977.

Bunney, W. E., Jr., Murphy, D. L., and Goodwin, F. K. The "switch process" in manic-depressive illness. *Arch. Gen. Psychiatry* 27:295–302, 1972.

Burgess, C. D., and Turner, P. Cardiotoxicity of antidepressant drugs. *Neuropharmacology* 19:1195–1199, 1980.

Burrows, C. D., and Davis, B. Antidepressants and barbiturates. *Brit. Med. J.* 3:331–334, 1971.

Burrows, G., Scoggins, B. A., Turecek, L. R., et al. Plasma nortriptyline and clinical response. *Clin. Pharmacol. Ther.* 16:639–644, 1974.

Burrows, G. D., Vohra, J., Hunt, D., Sloman, J. G., Soggins, B. A., and Davies, B. Cardiac effects of different tricyclic antidepressant drugs. *Brit. J. Psychiatry* 129:335–341, 1976.

Carlson, G. A., and Cantwell, D. P. Unmasking masked depression in children and adolescents. *Am. J. Psychiatry* 137:445–449, 1980.

Carroll, B. J. Monoamine precursors in the treatment of depression. *Clin. Pharmacol. Ther.* 12:743–761, 1972.

Cassem, N. Cardiovascular effects of antidepressants. *J. Clin. Psychiatry* 43(11:2):22–28, 1982.

Charney, D. S., Menkes, D. B., and Henninger, G. R. Receptor sensitivity and the mechanism of action of antidepressant treatment. *Arch. Gen. Psychiatry* 38:1160–1180, 1981.

Clements-Jewery, S., Robson, P. A., and Chidley, L. J. Biochemical investigations into the mode of action of trazodone. *Neuropharmacology* 19:1165–1173, 1980.

Cloney, P. E. Tricyclic antidepressants in the treatment of peptic ulcer disease. *Hosp. Pharm.* 17:620–621, 1982.

Cobbin, D. M., Requin-Blow, B., Williams, L. R., and Williams, W. D. Urinary MHPG levels and tricyclic antidepressant drug selection. *Arch. Gen. Psychiatry* 36:1111–1115, 1979.

Cohen, B. J., Harris, P. Q., Altesman, R. I., and Cole, J. O. Amoxapine: A neuroleptic as well as an antidepressant? *Am. J. Psychiatry* 139:1165–1167, 1982.

Cole, J. O., Branconnier, R., Salomen, M., et al. Tricyclic use in the cognitively impaired elderly. *J. Clin. Psychiatry* 44:14–19, 1983.

Cole, J. O., Hartmann, E., and Brigham, P. L-tryptophan: Clinical studies. *McLean Hosp. J.* 5:37–71, 1980.

Cooper, A. J. Tryptophan antidepressant: Physiological sedative, fact or fancy? *Psychopharmacology* (Berlin) 61:97–102, 1979.

Cooper, T. B., and Simpson, G. M. Prediction of individual dosage of nortriptyline. *Am. J. Psychiatry* 135:333–335, 1978.

Cooper, T. B., Simpson, G. M., and Lee, T. H. Thymoleptic and neuroleptic drug plasma levels in psychiatry: Current status. *Int. Rev. Neurobiol.* 19:269–309, 1976.

Coppen, A., Ghose, K., Montgomery, S., et al. Continuation therapy with amitriptyline in depression. *Brit. J. Psychiatry* 133:28–33, 1978.

Coppen, A., Whybrow, P. C., Noguera, R., et al. The comparative antidepressant value of L-tryptophan and imipramine with and without attempted potentiation by liothyronine. *Arch. Gen. Psychiatry* 26:234–241, 1972.

Couch, J. R., Ziegler, D. K., and Hassanein, R. Amitriptyline in the prophylaxis of migraine. *Neurology* 26:121–127, 1976.

Couper-Smartt, J. D., and Rodham, R. A technique for surveying side-effects of tricyclic drugs with reference to reported sexual effects. *J. Int. Med. Res.* 1:473–476, 1973.

Coupet, J., Rauh, C. E., Szues-Myers, V. A., and Yunger, L. M. Amoxapine, an antidepressant with antipsychotic properties: A possible role for 7-hydroxy-amoxapine. *Biochem. Pharmacol.* 28:2514–2515, 1979.

Crews, F. T., Paul, S. M., and Goodwin, F. K. Acceleration of beta-receptor desensitization in combined administration of antidepressants and phenoxybenzamine. *Nature* 290:787–789, 1981.

Crews, F. T., and Smith, C. B. Presynaptic alpha-receptor subsensitivity after long-term antidepressant treatment. *Science* 202:322–324, 1978.

Crombie, D. L., Pinsent, R. J., and Fleming, D. Imipramine in pregnancy. *Brit. Med. J.* 1:745–746, 1972.

Crome, P., Dawling, S., and Braithwaite, R. A. Effect of activated charcoal on absorption of nortriptyline. *Lancet* 2:1203–1205, 1977.

Cytryn, L., McKnew, D. H., and Bunny, W. E., Jr. Diagnosis of depression in children: A reassessment. *Am. J. Psychiatry* 135:22–25, 1980.

Davies, R. K., Tucker, G. J., Harrow, M., and Detre, T. P. Confusional episodes and antidepressant medication. *Am. J. Psychiatry* 128:95–99, 1971.

Davis, J. M. Antidepressant drugs. In *Comprehensive Textbook of Psychiatry*, 3rd ed., ed. H. I. Kaplan, A. M. Freedman, and B. J. Sadock. Williams and Wilkins, Baltimore, 1980, pp. 2290–2315.

Davis, J. M., and Vogel, C. Efficacy of trazodone: Data from European and United States studies. *J. Clin. Psychopharmacol.* 1:27S–34S, 1981.

DeMontigny, C., and Aghajanian, G. K. Tricyclic antidepressants: Long-term treatment increases responsivity of rat forebrain neurons to serotonin. *Science* 202:1303–1305, 1978.

Dilsaver, S. C., Feinber, M., and Greden, J. F. Antidepressant withdrawal symptoms treated with anticholinergic agents. *Am. J. Psychiatry* 140:249–251, 1983.

DiMascio, A., Heninger, G., and Klerman, G. L. Psychopharmacology of imipramine and desipramine: A comparative study of their effects in normal males. *Psychopharmacologia* 5:361–371, 1964.

Dinsmore, P. R., and Ryback, R. Lithium in schizoaffective disorders. *Dis. Nerv. Sys.* 33:771–776, 1972.

Dunner, D. L., and Fieve, R. R. Affective disorders: Studies with amine precursors. *Am. J. Psychiatry* 132:180–183, 1975.

Eggermont, E., Raveschot, J., Deneve, V., and Casteels-Van Daele, M. The adverse influence of imipramine on the adaption of the newborn infant to extrauterine life. *Acta Paediat. Belg.* 26:197–204, 1972.

Enna, S. J., Malick, J. B., and Richelson, E. *Antidepressants: Neurochemical, Behavioral, and Clinical Perspectives.* Raven Press, New York, 1981.

Everett, G. M., and Tolman, J. E. P. Mode of action of rauwolfia alkaloids and motor activity. In *Biological Psychiatry,* ed. J. Masserman. Grune and Stratton, New York, 1959, pp. 75–81.

Everett, H. C. The use of bethanechol chloride with tricyclic antidepressants. *Am. J. Psychiatry* 132:1202–1204, 1975.

Fawcett, J., Maas, J. W., and Dekirmenjian, H. Depression and MHPG excretion: Response to dextroamphetamine and tricyclic antidepressants. *Arch. Gen. Psychiatry* 26:246–251, 1972.

Feighner, J. P. Pharmacology: New antidepressants. *Psychiat. Ann.* 10:388–395, 1980.

Feighner, J. P., King, L. F., Schuckit, M. A., et al. Hormonal potentiation of imipramine and ECT in primary depression. *Am. J. Psychiatry* 128:1230–1238, 1972.

Fibiger, H. C., and Phillips, A. G. Increased intracranial self-stimulation in rats after long-term administration of desipramine. *Science* 214:683–685, 1981.

Fink, M. *Convulsive Therapy: Theory and Practice.* Raven Press, New York, 1979.

Fischbach, R. Die vegetativen Effekte der Antidepressiva im Bereich des Gastro-Intestinaltraktes. *Wien. Med. Wochenschr.* 123 (suppl. 5):3–26, 1973.

Flemenbaum, A. Pavor nocturnus: A complication of single daily tricyclic or neuroleptic dosage. *Am. J. Psychiatry* 133:570–572, 1976.

Folks, D. G., King, L. D., Dowdy, S. B., et al. Carbamazepine treatment of selected affectively disordered inpatients. *Am. J. Psychiatry* 139:115–117, 1982.

Freeman, C. P., Basson, J. V., and Crighton, A. Double-blind controlled trial of electroconvulsive therapy (ECT) and simulated ECT in depressive illness. *Lancet* 1:738–740, 1978.

Freeman, J. W., Mundy, G. R., Beattie, R. R., and Ryan, C. Cardiac abnormalities in poisoning with tricyclic antidepressants. *Brit. Med. J.* 2:610–611, 1969.

Frommer, E. A. Treatment in childhood depression with antidepressant drugs. *Brit. Med. J.* 1:729–732, 1967.

Fujiwara, J., and Otsuki, S. Subtype of affective psychoses classified by response on amine precursors and monoamine metabolism. *Folia Psychiatr. Neurol. Japon.* 28:93–100, 1974.

Garfinkel, B. D., Wender, P. H., Sloman, L., and O'Neil, I. Tricyclic antidepressant and methylpheindate treatment of attention deficit disorder in children. *J. Am. Acad. Child Psychiatry* 22:343–348, 1983.

Garver, D. L., and Davis, J. M. Biogenic amine hypotheses of affective disorders. *Life Sciences* 24:383–394, 1979.

Gastfriend, D. R., Biederman, J., and Jellinek, M. S. Desipramine in the treatment of adolescents with attention deficit disorders. *Am. J. Psychiatry* 141:906–908, 1984.

Gelenberg, A. J., Gibson, C. J., and Wojcik, J. D. Neurotransmitter precursors for the treatment of depression. *Psychopharmacol. Bull.* 18:7–18, 1982.

Geller, B., Perel, J. M., Knitter, E. F., Lycaki, H., and Farook, Z. Q. Nortriptyline in major depressive disorder in children: Response steady-state plasma levels, predictive kinetics and pharmacokinetics. *Psychopharmacol. Bull.* 19:62–65, 1983.

Gershon, S., Mann, J., Newton, R., et al. Evaluation of trazodone in the treatment of endogenous depression: Results of a multi-center double-blind study. *J. Clin. Psychopharmacol.* 1:395–445, 1981.

Ghose, K., Gifford, L. A., Turner, P., and Leighton, M. Studies of the interaction of desmethylimipramine with tyramine in man after a single oral dose, and its correlation with plasma concentration. *Brit. J. Pharmacol.* 3:334–337, 1976.

Gillen, J. C., Wyatt, R. J., Fram, D., et al. The relationship between changes in REM sleep and clinical improvement in depressed patients treated with amitriptyline. *Psychopharmacology* 59:267–272, 1978.

Gittelman-Klein, R., and Klein, D. F. Controlled imipramine treatment of school phobia. *Arch. Gen. Psychiatry* 25:204–207, 1971.

———School phobia: Diagnostic considerations in the light of imipramine effects. *J. Nerv. Ment. Dis.* 156:199–215, 1973.

Glassman, A. H., and Bigger, J. T., Jr. Cardiovascular effects of therapeutic doses of tricyclic antidepressants. *Arch. Gen. Psychiatry* 38:815–820, 1981.

Glassman, A. H., Bigger, J. T., Jr., Giardina, E. V., et al. Clinical characteristics of imipramine-induced orthostatic hypotension. *Lancet* L:468–472, 1979.

Glassman, A. H., Giardina, E. V., Perel, J. M., Bigger, J. T., Kantor, S. J., and Davies, M. Clinical characteristics of imipramine-induced orthostatic hypotension. *Lancet* 1:468–470, 1979.

Glassman, A. H., and Perel, J. M. The clinical pharmacology of imipramine. *Arch. Gen. Psychiatry* 28:649–653, 1973.

Glassman, A. H., Perel, J. M., Shostak, M., et al. Clinical implications of imipramine plasma levels for depressive illness. *Arch. Gen. Psychiatry* 34:197–204, 1977.

Glowinski, J., and Baldessarini, R. J. Metabolism of norepinephrine in the central nervous system. *Pharmacol. Rev.* 18:1201–1238, 1966.

Goodwin, F. K. The impact of tricyclic antidepressants and lithium on the time course of recurrent affective disorders. *McLean Hosp. J.* 8:1–16, 1983.

Goodwin, F. K., Cowdry, R. W., and Webster, M. H. Predictors of drug response in the affective disorders: Toward an integrated approach. In *Psychopharmacology: A Generation of Progress*, ed. M. A. Lipton, A. DiMascio, and K. F. Killam. Raven Press, New York, 1978.

Goodwin, F. K., Prange, A. J., Post, R. M., Muscettola, G., and Lipton, M. A. Potentiation of antidepressant effects by L-triiodothyronine in tricyclic nonresponders. *Am. J. Psychiatry* 139:34–38, 1982.

Gram, L. F., Christiansen, J., and Overo, K. F. Pharmacokinetic interaction between tricyclic antidepressants and other psychopharmaca. *Acta Psychiatr. Scand.* (suppl.)243:52–53, 1973.

Granacher, R. P., and Baldessarini, R. J. Physostigmine: Its use in acute anticholinergic syndrome with antidepressant and antiparkinson drugs. *Arch. Gen. Psychiatry* 32:375–380, 1975.

Greenblatt, M., Grosser, G. H., and Wechsler, H. A comparative study of selected antidepressant medications and EST. *Am. J. Psychiatry* 119:144–153, 1962.

Grof, P., and Vinar, O. Maintenance and prophylactic imipramine doses in recurrent depressions. *Activ./Nerv. Sup.* (Praha) 8:383–385, 1966.

Grunthal, E. Utersuchungen uber die besondere psychologische Wirkung des Thymolepticums TOFRANIL. *Psychiatr. Neurol. Wochenschr.* 136:402–408, 1958.

Gruvstad, M. Plasma levels of antidepressants and clinical response. *Lancet* 1:95–96, 1973.

Gualtieri, C. T., Golden, R., Evans, R. W., and Hicks, R. E. Blood level measurement of psychoactive drugs in pediatric psychiatry. *Therap. Drug Monitoring* 6:127–141, 1984.

Halen, K. A., Eckert, E., and Falk, J. R. Cyproheptadine, an antidepressant and weight-inducing drug for anorexia nervosa. *Psychopharmacol. Bull.* 19:103–105, 1982.

Hayes, T. A., Panitch, M. L., and Barker, E. Imipramine dosage in children: A comment on "imipramine and electrocardiographic abnormalities in hyperactive children." *Am. J. Psychiatry* 132:546–547, 1975.

Heal, D. J. Phenylephrine-induced activity in mice as a model of central α_1-adrenoreceptor function: Effects of acute and repeated administration of antidepressant drugs and electroconvulsive shock. *Neuropharmacology* 23:1241–1251, 1984.

Herrington, R. N., Bruce, A., Johnstone, E. C., and Lader, M. H. Comparative trial of L-tryptophan and amitriptyline in depressive illness. *Psychol. Med.* 6:673–678, 1976.

Hill, D. Amphetamine in psychopathic states. *Brit. J. Addiction* 44:50–54, 1947.

Hoehn, R., Gross, M., and Lasagna, L. A double-blind comparison of placebo and imipramine in the treatment of depressed patients in a state hospital. *J. Psychiatr. Res.* 1:76–91, 1961.

Hoenig, J., and Vistram, S. Amitriptyline vs. imipramine in depressive psychoses. *Brit. J. Psychiatry* 110:840–845, 1964.

Holinger, P. C., and Klawans, H. L. Reversal of tricyclic-overdosage-induced central anticholinergic syndrome by physostigmine. *Am. J. Psychiatry* 133:1018–1023, 1976.

Hollister, L. E. Doxepin hydrochloride. *Ann. Intern. Med.* 81:360–363, 1974.

——— Tricyclic antidepressants. *N. Engl. J. Med.* 299:1106–1109, 1168–1172, 1978.

Hollister, L. E., Davis, K. L., and Berger, P. A. Subtypes of depression based on excretion of MHPG and response to nortriptyline. *Arch. Gen. Psychiatry* 37:1107–1110, 1980.

Hollister, L., Overall, J., Shelton, J., et al. Drug therapy of depression: Amitriptyline, perphenazine, and their combination in different syndromes. *Arch. Gen. Psychiatry* 17:486–493, 1967.

Huessy, H. R., and Wright, A. L. The use of imipramine in children's behavior disorders. *Acta Paedopsychiatr.* (Basel) 37:194–199, 1970.

Idanpaan-Heikkila, J., and Saxen, L. Possible teratogenicity of imipramine and chlorimipramine. *Lancet* 2:282–284, 1973.

Jacobsen, E. The theoretical basis of the chemotherapy of depression. In *Depression: Proceedings of a Symposium at Cambridge, September 1959,* ed. E. B. Davies. Cambridge University Press, New York, 1964, p. 208.

Janowski, D. S., El-Yousef, M. K., and Davis, J. M. Acetylcholine and depression. *Psychosom. Med.* 36:248–257, 1974.

Jefferson, J. W. A review of the cardiovascular effects and toxicity of tricyclic antidepressants. *Psychosom. Med.* 37:160–179, 1975.

Jones, R. S. G. Enhancement of 5-hydroxytryptamine-induced behavioral effects following chronic administration of antidepressant drugs. *Psychopharmacology* 69:307–311, 1980.

Kaiser, G., and Zirkle, C. L. Antidepressant drugs. In *Medicinal Chemistry*, 2nd ed., ed. A. Burger. John Wiley, New York, 1970, pp. 1470–1497.

Kane, J. M., and Lieberman, J. The efficacy of amoxapine, maprotiline and trazodone in comparison to imipramine and amitriptyline: A review of the literature. *Psychopharmacol. Bull.* 20:240–260, 1984.

Kanof, P. D., and Greengard, P. Brain histamine receptors as targets for antidepressant drugs. *Nature* 272:329–333, 1978.

Kantor, S. J., Bigger, J. T., Jr., Glassman, A. H., et al. Imipramine-induced heart block. *J.A.M.A.* 231:1364–1366, 1975.

Keller, M. B., Klerman, G. L., Lavori, P. W., Coryell, W., Endicott, J., and

Taylor, J. Long-term outcome of episodes of major depression: Clinical and public health significance. *J.A.M.A.* 252:788–792, 1984.

Keller, M. B., Klerman, G. L., Lavori, P. W., Fawcett, J. A., Coryell, W., and Endicott, J. Treatment received by depressed patients. *J.A.M.A.* 248:1848–1855, 1982.

Keller, M. B., Lavori, P. N., Endicott, J., Coryell, W., and Klerman, G. L. "Double depression": Two-year follow-up. *Am. J. Psychiatry* 140:689–694, 1983.

Kinnier, W. J., Chuang, D.-M., Gwynn, G., and Costa, E. Characteristics and regulation of high-affinity [^{3}H]imipramine binding to rat hippocampal membranes. *Neuropharmacology* 20:411–419, 1981.

Klein, D. F., and Fink, M. Psychiatric reaction patterns to imipramine. *Am. J. Psychiatry* 119:432–438, 1962.

Klerman, G. F., and Cole, J. O. Clinical pharmacology of imipramine and related antidepressant compounds. *Pharmacol. Rev.* 17:101–141, 1965.

Klerman, G. L. Drug therapy of clinical depressions. *J. Psychiatr. Res.* 9:253–270, 1972.

Kline, N. S. Antidepressant medications. *J.A.M.A.* 227:1158–1160, 1974.

Kline, N. S., Pare, M., Hallstrom, C., and Cooper, T. B. Amitriptyline protects patients on MAOIs from tyramine reactions. *J. Clin. Psychopharmacol.* 2:434–435, 1982.

Kline, N. S., Sacks, W., and Simpson, G. M. Further studies on one day treatment of depression with 5-HTP. *Am. J. Psychiatry* 121:379–381, 1964.

Kragh-Sorenson, P., Åsberg, M., and Eggert-Hansen, C. Plasma nortriptyline levels in endogenous depression. *Lancet* 1:113–115, 1973.

Kragh-Sorenson, P., Hansen, C. E., Baastrup, P. C., et al. Self-inhibiting action of nortriptyline's antidepressant effects at high plasma levels. *Psychopharmacologia* 45:305–312, 1976.

Krenzelok, E. P., North, D. S., and Elkins, B. R. Physostigmine's use questioned for amoxapine overdose. *Am. J. Hosp. Pharm.* 38:1882–1889, 1981.

Kuenssberg, E. V., and Knox, J. D. E. Imipramine in pregnancy. *Brit. Med. J.* 2:292–293, 1972.

Kuhn, R. The treatment of depressive states with G22355 (imipramine hydrochloride). *Am. J. Psychiatry* 115:459–464, 1958.

Kupfer, D. J., Coble, P., Kane, J., et al. Imipramine and EEG sleep in children with depressive symptoms. *Psychopharmacology* 60:117–123, 1979.

Kupfer, D. J., Foster, F. G., Reich, L., et al. EEG sleep changes as predictors in depression. *Am. J. Psychiatry* 133:622–626, 1976.

Kupfer, D. J., Spiker, D. G., Coble, P. A., et al. Sleep and treatment prediction in endogenous depression. *Am. J. Psychiatry* 138:429–434, 1981.

Kvinesdal, B., Molin, J., Fröland, A., and Gram, L. F. Imipramine treatment of painful diabetic neuropathy. *J.A.M.A.* 251:1727–1730, 1984.

Lambert, P. A. Les effets indésirables des antidépresseurs tricycliques. *Thérapie* (Paris) 28:269–305, 1973.

Larochelle, P., Hamet, P., and Enjalbert, M. Responses to tyramine and norepinephrine after imipramine and trazodone. *Clin. Pharmacol. Ther.* 26:24–30, 1979.

Law, W., III, Petti, T. A., and Kazdin, A. E. Withdrawal symptoms after graduated cessation of imipramine in children. *Am. J. Psychiatry* 138:647–651, 1981.

Lee, C.-M., and Snyder, S. H. Norepinephrine neuronal uptake binding sites in rat brain membranes labeled with [³H]desipramine. *Proc. Natl. Acad. Sci. USA* 78:5250–5254, 1981.

Lehmann, H. E., Cohn, C. H., and De Verteuil, R. L. The treatment of depressive conditions with imipramine (G22355). *Canad. Psychiatr. Assoc. J.* 3:155–160, 1958.

Linnoila, M., George, L., and Guthrie, S. Interaction between antidepressants and perphenazine in psychiatric patients. *Am. J. Psychiatry* 139:1329–1331, 1982.

Linnoila, M., George, L., Guthrie, S., and Leventhal, B. Effect of alcohol consumption and cigarette smoking on antidepressant levels of depressed patients. *Am. J. Psychiatry* 138:841–842, 1981.

Lipper, S., Murphy, D. L., Slater, S., and Bucksbaum, M. S. Comparative behavioral effects of clorgyline and pargyline in man: A preliminary evaluation. *Psychopharmacology* (Berlin) 62:123–128, 1979.

Loo, H., and Bousser, M. G. Incidents et accidents des chimiothérapies par les antidépresseurs. *Cah. Med.* (Paris) 13:777–794, 1972.

Lowe, M. C., Horita, A., Gelenberg, A. J., and Klerman, G. L. Preclinical pharmacology of antidepressants. In *Principles of Psychopharmacology*, 2nd ed., ed. W. G. Clark and J. Del Guidice. Academic Press, New York, 1978, pp. 311–323.

Lucas, A. R., Lockett, H. J., and Grimm, F. Amitriptyline in childhood depression. *Dis. Nerv. Syst.* 26:105–110, 1965.

Lydiard, R. B., and Gelenberg, A. J. Amoxapine: An antidepressant with neuroleptic properties? *Pharmacotherapy* 1:163–178, 1981.

Maas, J. W. Clinical implications of pharmacological differences among antidepressants. In *Psychopharmacology: A Generation of Progress,* ed. M. A. Lipton, A. DiMascio, and K. F. Killam. Raven Press, New York, 1978, pp. 955–960.

Maas, J. W., Fawcett, J. A., and Dekirmenjian, H. Catecholamine metabolism, depressive illness and drug response. *Arch. Gen. Psychiatry* 26:252–262, 1972.

Maj, J., Mogilnicka, E., and Klimek, V. The effect of repeated administration of antidepressant drugs on the responsiveness of rats to catecholamine agonists. *J. Neural. Transmission* 44:221–235, 1979.

Malitz, S., and Kanzler, M. Are antidepressants better than placebo? *Am. J. Psychiatry* 127:1605–1611, 1971.

McBride, N. G., and Morrow, A. W. Limb deformities associated with iminodibenzyl hydrochloride. *Med. J. Austral.* 1:492 and 831, 1972.

McCauley, R. B. Monoamine oxidases and the pharmacology of monoamine oxidase inhibitors. In *Neuropharmacology of Central Nervous System and Behavioral Disorders,* ed. G. C. Palmer. Academic Press, New York, 1981, pp. 93–109.

McGuire, P. S., and Seiden, L. S. The effects of tricyclic antidepressants on performance under a differential-reinforcement-of-low-rates schedule in rats. *J. Pharmacol. Exp. Ther.* 214:635–641, 1980.

McMillen, B. A., Warnack, W., German, D. C., and Shore, P. A. Effects of chronic desipramine treatment on rat brain noradrenergic responses to beta-adrenergic drugs. *Eur. J. Pharmacol.* 61:239–246, 1980.

Mendels, J., Stinnert, J. L., Burns, D., and Frazer, A. Amine precursors and depression. *Arch. Gen. Psychiatry*, 32:22–30, 1975.

Menkes, D. B., Aghajanian, G. K., and Gallagher, D. W. Chronic antidepressant treatment enhances agonist affinity of brain alpha$_1$-adrenoreceptors. *Eur. J. Pharmacol.* 87:35–41, 1983.

Moir, D. C. Tricyclic antidepressants and cardiac disease. *Am. Heart J.* 84:841–842, 1973.

Moir, D. C., Dingwall-Fordyce, I., and Weir, R. D. Medicines evaluation and monitoring group: A follow-up study of cardiac patients receiving amitriptyline. *Eur. J. Clin. Pharmacol.* 6:98–101, 1973.

Möller-Nielsen, I. Tricyclic antidepressants: General pharmacology. In *Psychotropic Agents: Antipsychotics and Antidepressants,* vol. 55, part I, *Handbook of Experimental Pharmacology,* ed. F. Hoffmeister and G. Stille. Springer-Verlag, Berlin, 1980, pp. 399–410.

Montgomery, S. A. Review of antidepressant efficacy in inpatients. *Neuropharmacology* 19:1185–1190, 1980.

Moody, J., Tait, A., and Todrick, A. Plasma levels of imipramine and desmethylimipramine during therapy. *Brit. J. Psychiatry* 113:183–193, 1967.

Morgan, M. H., and Read, A. E. Antidepressants and liver disease. *Gut* 13:697–701, 1972.

Morris, J. B., and Beck, A. T. The efficacy of antidepressant drugs. *Arch. Gen. Psychiatry* 30:667–674, 1974.

Murphy, D. L., Campbell, I., and Costa, J. L. Current status of the indoleamine hypothesis of the affective disorders. In *Psychopharmacology: A Generation of Progress,* ed. M. A. Lipton, A. DiMascio, and K. F. Killam. Raven Press, New York, 1978, pp. 1235–1248.

Nagy, A., and Johansson, R. Plasma levels of imipramine and desipramine in man after different routes of administration. *Naunyn Schmiedeberg's Arch. Pharmacol.* 209:145–160, 1975.

Nelson, J. C., and Bowers, M. B., Jr. Delusional unipolar depression: Description and drug response. *Arch. Gen. Psychiatry* 35:1321–1328, 1978.

Nelson, J. C., Jatlow, P., Quinlan, D. M., and Bowers, M. B., Jr. Desipramine plasma concentration and antidepressant response. *Arch. Gen. Psychiatry* 39:1419–1422, 1982.

Nicotra, M. B., Rivera, M., Pool, J. L., and Noall, M. W. Tricyclic antidepressant overdose: Clinical and pharmacological observations. *Clin. Toxicol.* 18:599–613, 1981.

Nies, A., Robinson, D. S., Friedman, M. J., Green, R., Cooper, T. B., Ravaris, C. L., and Ives, J. O. Relationship between age and tricyclic antidepressant plasma levels. *Am. J. Psychiatry* 134:790–793, 1977.

Noble, J., and Matthew, H. Acute poisoning by tricyclic antidepressants: Clinical features and management of 100 patients. *Clin. Toxicol.* 2:403–421, 1969.

Nouri, A., and Cuendet, J. F. Ateintes oculaires au cours des traitements aux thymoleptiques. *Schweiz. Med. Wochenschr.* 101:1178–1180, 1971.

Nurnberg, H. G., and Coccaro, E. F. Response of panic disorder and resistance of depression to imipramine. *Am. J. Psychiatry* 139:1060–1062, 1982.

Olphe, H. R., and Schellenberg, A. Reduced sensitivity of neurons to noradrenaline after chronic treatment with antidepressant drugs. *Eur. J. Pharmacol.* 63:7–13, 1980.

Ostroff, R. B., and Docherty, J. P. Tricyclics, bioequivalence, and clinical response. *Am. J. Psychiatry* 135:1560–1561, 1979.

Paul, S. M., Rehavi, M., Pice, K., et al. Does high-affinity [³H] imipramine binding label serotonin reuptake sites in brain and platelet? *Life Sciences* 28:2253–2260, 1981.

Paykel, E. S. Management of acute depression. In *Psychopharmacology of Affective Disorders,* ed. E. S. Paykel and A. Coppen. Oxford University Press, New York, 1979, pp. 235–247.

Peroutka, S. J., and Snyder, S. H. Long-term antidepressant treatment decreases spiroperidol-labeled serotonin receptor binding. *Science* 210:88–90, 1980.

———Interactions of antidepressants with neurotransmitter receptor sites. In *Antidepressants: Neurochemical, Behavioral, and Clinical Perspectives,* ed. S. J. Enna, J. B. Malick, and E. Richelson. Raven Press, New York, 1981, pp. 75–90.

Petersen, K. E., Andersen, O. O., and Hansen, T. Mode of action and relative value of imipramine and similar drugs in the treatment of nocturnal enuresis. *Eur. J. Clin. Pharmacol.* 7:187–194, 1974.

Pinder, R. M. Antidepressants. *Ann. Reports Med. Chem.* 15:1–11, 1980.

Pinder, R. M., Brogden, R. N., Speight, T. M., and Avery, G. S. Maprotiline: A review of its pharmacologic properties and therapeutic efficacy in mental depressive states. *Drugs* 13:321–352, 1977.

Pohl, R., Berchou, R., and Rainey, J. M. Tricyclic antidepressants and monoamine oxidase inhibitors in the treatment of agoraphobia. *J. Clin. Psychopharmacol.* 2:399–407, 1983.

Poldinger, W., and Gammel, G. Differences in effect between nomifensine and nortriptyline. *Int. Pharmacopsychiatry* 13:58–62, 1978.

Pond, S. M., Graham, G. G., Birkett, D. J., and Wade, D. N. Effects of tricyclic antidepressants on drug metabolism. *Clin. Pharmacol. Ther.* 18:191–199, 1975.

Pope, H. G., Jr., Hudson, J. I., and Jonas, J. M. Antidepressant treatment of bulimia: Preliminary experience and practical recommendations. *J. Clin. Psychopharmacology* 3:264–279, 1983.

Pope, H. G., Jr., Hudson, J. I., Jonas, J. M., and Yurgelun-Todd, D. Bulimia treated with imipramine: A placebo-controlled double-blind study. *Am. J. Psychiatry* 140:554–558, 1983.

Praag, H. M. van. Amine hypotheses of affective disorders. In *Handbook of Psychopharmacology,* vol. 13, ed. L. L. Iversen, S. D. Iversen, and S. H. Snyder. Plenum Press, New York, 1978, pp. 187–297.

Preskorn, S. H., and Othmer, S. C. Evaluation of bupropion hydrochloride: The first of a new class of atypical antidepressants. *Pharmacotherapy* 4:20–34, 1984.

Prien, R. F. Long-term maintenance therapy in affective disorders. In *Schizophrenia and Affective Disorders: Biology and Drug Treatment,* ed. A. Rifkin. Wright-PSG, Boston, 1983, pp. 95–115.

Prien, R. F., Kupfer, D. J., Mansky, P. A., Small, J. G., Tuason, V. B., Voss, C. B., and Johnson, W. E. Drug therapy in the prevention of recurrences of unipolar and bipolar affective disorders. *Arch. Gen. Psychiatry* 41:1096–1104, 1984.

Puig-Antich, J., Blau, S., Marx, N., Greenhill, L. L., and Chambers, W. Prepubertal major depressive disorder. *J. Am. Acad. Child Psychiatry* 17:695–707, 1978.

Quitkin, F., Rifkin, A., and Klein, D. F. Prophylaxis of affective disorders: Current status of knowledge. *Arch. Gen. Psychiatry* 33:337–341, 1976.

Raisfeld, I. H. Cardiovascular complications of antidepressant therapy: Interactions at the adrenergic neuron. *Am. Heart J.* 83:129–133, 1972.

Randrup, A., and Braestrup, C. Uptake inhibition of biogenic amines by newer antidepressant drugs: Relevance to the dopamine hypothesis of depression. *Psychopharmacology* 53:309–314, 1977.

Rasmussen, J. Poisoning with amitriptyline, imipramine and nortriptyline. *Dan. Med. Bull.* 16:201–203, 1966.

Rausch, J. L., Pavlinac, D. M., and Newman, P. E. Complete heart block following a single dose of trazodone. *Am. J. Psychiatry* 141:1472–1473, 1984.

Ravaris, C. L., Robinson, D. S., Ives, J. O., et al. Phenelzine and amitriptyline in the treatment of depression. *Arch. Gen. Psychiatry* 37:1075–1080, 1980.

Rehavi, M., Ramot, O., Yavetz, B., and Sokolovsky, M. Amitryptyline: Long-term treatment elevates alpha-adrenergic and muscarinic receptor binding in mouse brain. *Brain Res.* 194:443–453, 1980.

Reynolds, C. F., Marin, R. S., and Spiker, D. Clinical considerations in prescribing antidepressants for geriatric patients. *Geriat. Med. Today* 2:45–55, 1983.

Riblet, L. A., and Taylor, D. P. Pharmacology and neurochemistry of trazodone. *J. Clin. Psychopharmacol.* 1:117S–22S, 1981.

Richels, K., Chung, H. R., Csanalosi, I., et al. Iprindole and imipramine in nonpsychotic depressed out-patients. *Brit. J. Psychiatry* 123:329–339, 1973.

Richelson, E. Tricyclic antidepressants and H_1 receptors. *Mayo Clinic Proc.* 54:669–674, 1979.

——— Tricyclic antidepressants: Interactions with histamine and muscarinic acetylcholine receptor. In *Antidepressants: Neurochemical, Behavioral, and Clinical Perspectives,* ed. S. J. Enna, J. B. Malick, and E. Richelson. Raven Press, New York, 1981, pp. 53–73.

——— Antimuscarinic and other receptor-blocking properties of antidepressants. *Mayo Clinic Proc.* 58:40–46, 1983.

Richelson, E., and Diventz-Romero, S. Blockade by psychotropic drugs on muscarinic acetylcholine receptor in cultured nerve cells. *Biol. Psychiatry* 12:771–785, 1977.

Rickels, K., Chung, H. R., Feldman, H. S., et al. Amitriptyline, diazepam and phenobarbital sodium in depressed outpatients. *J. Nerv. Ment. Dis.* 157:442–451, 1973.

Rickels, K., Ward, C., and Schut, L. Different populations, different drug responses: A comparative study of two antidepressants, each used in two different patient groups. *Am. J. Med. Sci.* 247:328–335, 1964.

Risch, S. C., Janowsky, D. S., and Huey, L. Y. Plasma levels of tricyclic antidepressants and clinical efficacy. In *Antidepressants: Neurochemical, Behavioral, and Clinical Perspectives,* ed. S. J. Enna, J. B. Malick, and E. Richelson. Raven Press, New York, 1981, pp. 183–217.

Rogers, S. C., and Clay, P. M. A statistical review of controlled studies of imipramine and placebo in the treatment of depressive illnesses. *Brit. J. Psychiatry* 127:599–603, 1975.

Rotblatt, M. D. Antidepressants and seizures. *Drug Intell. Clin. Pharmacol.* 16:749–750, 1982.

Sano, I. L-5-Hydroxytryptophan (L-5-HTP) therapie. *Folia Psychiatr. Neurol. Japon.* 26:7–17, 1972.

Saraf, K., and Klein, D. F. The safety of a single daily dose schedule for imipramine. *Am. J. Psychiatry* 128:483–484, 1971.

Sathananthan, G. L., and Gershon, S. Imipramine withdrawal: An akathisia-like syndrome. *Am. J. Psychiatry* 130:1286–1287, 1973.

Sathananthan, G. L., Gershon, S., Almeida, M., et al. Correlation between plasma and cerebrospinal fluid levels of imipramine. *Arch. Gen. Psychiatry* 33:1109–1110, 1976.

Schatzberg, A. F., Orsulak, P. J., Rosenbaum, A. H., et al. Toward a biochemical classification of depressive disorders: V. Heterogeneity of unipolar depressions. *Am. J. Psychiatry* 139:471–475, 1982.

Schatzberg, A. F., and Rosenbaum, A. H. Studies on MHPG levels as predictors of antidepressant response. *McLean Hosp. J.* 6:138–157, 1981.

Schatzberg, A. F., Rosenbaum, A. H., Orsulak, P. J., et al. Toward a biochemical classification of depressive disorders: III. Pretreatment urinary MHPG levels as predictors of response to treatment with maprotiline. *Psychopharmacology* 75:34–38, 1981.

Schildkraut, J. J. *Neuropsychopharmacology and the Affective Disorders.* Little, Brown, Boston, 1970.

——— Norepinephrine metabolites as biochemical criteria for classifying depressive disorders and predicting responses to treatment: Preliminary findings. *Am. J. Psychiatry* 130:695–699, 1973.

Schildkraut, J. J., Roffman, M., Orsulak, P. J., et al. Effects of short- and long-term administration of tricyclic antidepressants and lithium on norepinephrine turnover in brain. *Pharmacopsychiatry* 9:193–202, 1976.

Schilgen, B., and Tolle, R. Partial sleep deprivation as therapy for depression. *Arch. Gen. Psychiatry* 37:267–271, 1980.

Sellinger-Barnette, M. M., Mendels, J., and Frazer, A. The effect of psychoactive drugs on beta-adrenergic receptor binding sites in rat brain. *Neuropharmacology* 19:447–454, 1980.

Selvini, A., Ross, C., Belli, C., et al. Antidepressant treatment with maprotiline in the management of emotional disturbances in patients with acute myocardial infarction: A controlled study. *J. Int. Med. Res.* 4:42–46, 1976.

Settle, E. C., and Ayd, F. J. Trimipramine: Twenty years' worldwide clinical experience. *J. Clin. Psychiatry* 41:266–274, 1980.

Shatan, C. Withdrawal symptoms after abrupt termination of imipramine. *Can. Psychiatr. Assoc. J.* 2:150–157, 1966.

Shopsin, B. Second-generation antidepressants. *J. Clin. Psychiatry* 41 (12, sec. 2):45–46, 1980.

Shopsin, B., Cassano, G. B., and Conti, L. An overview of new "second-generation" antidepressant compounds: Research and treatment implications. In *Antidepressants: Neurochemical, Behavioral, and Clinical Perspectives,* ed. S. J. Enna, J. B. Malick, and E. Richelson. Raven Press, New York, 1981, pp. 219–251.

Siggins, G. R., and Schultz, J. E. Chronic treatment with lithium or desipramine alters discharge frequency and norepinephrine responsiveness of cerebellar Purkinje cells. *Proc. Natl. Acad. Sci. USA* 76:5987–5991, 1979.

Simpson, G. M., Amin, M., Angus, J. W. S., et al. Role of antidepressants and neuroleptics in the treatment of depression. *Arch. Gen. Psychiatry* 27:337–345, 1972.

Simpson, G. M., Lee, J. H., Cuculic, Z., and Kellner, R. Two dosages of imipramine in hospitalized endogenous and neurotic depressives. *Arch. Gen. Psychiatry* 33:1093–1102, 1976.

Simpson, G. M., White, K. L., Boyd, J. L., et al. Relationships between plasma antidepressant levels and clinical outcome for inpatients receiving imipramine. *Am. J. Psychiatry* 139:358–360, 1982.

Siris, S. G., Cooper, T. B., Rifkin, A. E., Brenner, R., and Lieberman, J. A. Plasma imipramine concentrations in patients receiving concomitant fluphenazine decanoate. *Am. J. Psychiatry* 139:104–105, 1982.

Smith, R. C., Chojnacki, M., Hu R., and Mann, E. Cardiovascular effects of therapeutic doses of tricyclic antidepressants: Importance of blood level monitoring. *J. Clin. Psychiatry* 41 (12, sec. 2):57–63, 1980.

Snyder, S. H., and Yamamura, H. Antidepressants and the muscarinic acetylcholine receptor. *Arch. Gen. Psychiatry* 34:236–239, 1977.

Spiker, D. G., and Biggs, J. T. Tricyclic antidepressants: Prolonged plasma levels after overdose. *J.A.M.A.* 236:1711–1712, 1976.

Spiker, D. G., Edwards, D., Hanin, I., et al. Urinary MHPG and clinical response to amitriptyline in depressed patients. *Am. J. Psychiatry* 137:1183–1187, 1980.

Sulser, F. Pharmacology: Current antidepressants. *Psychiatr. Ann.* 10:381–387, 1980.

Sulser, F., and Mobley, P. L. Biochemical effects of antidepressants in animals. In *Psychotropic Agents: Antipsychotics and Antidepressants,* vol. 55, part I, *Handbook of Experimental Pharmacology,* ed. F. Hoffmeister and G. Stille. Springer-Verlag, Berlin, 1980, pp. 471–490.

Sulser, F., Vetulani, J., and Mobley, P. I. Mode of action of antidepressant drugs. *Biochem. Pharmacol.* 27:257–261, 1978.

Svenssen, T. H., and Usdin, T. Feedback inhibition of brain noradrenaline neurons by tricyclic antidepressants: Alpha-receptor mediation. *Science* 202:1089–1091, 1978.

U'Prichard, D. C., Greenberg, D. A., Sheehan, P. P., and Snyder, S. H. Tricyclic antidepressants: Therapeutic properties and affinity for alpha-noradrenergic receptor binding sites in the brain. *Science* 199:197–198, 1978.

Van Hiele, L. J. L-5-hydroxytryptophan in depression: The first substitution therapy in psychiatry? *Neuropsychobiology* 6:230–240, 1980.

Van Kammen, D. P., and Murphy, D. L. Prediction of imipramine antidepressant response by a one-day d-amphetamine trial. *Am. J. Psychiatry* 135:1179–1184, 1978.

Van Praag, H. M. Amine hypotheses of affective disorders. In *Handbook of Psy-*

chopharmacology, vol. 13, ed. L. L. Iversen, S. D. Iversen, and S. H. Snyder. Plenum Press, New York, 1978, pp. 187–297.

——In search of the mode of action of antidepressants. 5-HTP/tyrosine mixtures in depressions. *Neuropharmacology* 22(3B):433–440, 1983.

Van Scheyen, J. D., and Van Kammen, D. P. Clomipramine-induced mania in unipolar depression. *Arch. Gen. Psychiatry* 36:560–565, 1979.

Veith, R. C., Raskind, M. A., and Caldwell, J. H. Cardiovascular effects of tricyclic antidepressants in depressed patients with chronic heart disease. *N. Engl. J. Med.* 306:954–959, 1982.

Vetulani, J., Stawarz, R. J., Dingell, J. V., et al. A possible common mechanism of action of antidepressant treatments. *Naunyn-Schmiedeberg's Arch. Pharmacol.* 239:109–114, 1976.

Vogel, G. W., Vogel, F., McAbee, R. S., et al. Improvement of depression by REM sleep deprivation. *Arch. Gen. Psychiatry* 37:247–253, 1980.

Vohra, J., and Burrows, G. D. Cardiovascular complications of tricyclic antidepressant overdose. *Drugs* 8:432–437, 1974.

Waal, H. J. Propranolol-induced depression. *Brit. Med. J.* 2:50, 1967.

Waizer, J., Hoffman, S. P., Polizos, P., and Engelhardt, D. M. Outpatient treatment of hyperactive school children with imipramine. *Am. J. Psychiatry* 131:587–591, 1974.

Walter, C. J. S. Clinical significance of plasma imipramine levels. *Proc. Roy. Soc. Med.* 64:282–285, 1971.

Wang, R. Y., and Aghajanian, G. K. Enhanced sensitivity of amygdaloid neurons to serotonin and norepinephrine after chronic antidepressant treatment. *Comm. Psychopharmacol.* 4:83–90, 1980.

Wehr, T. A., Wirz-Justice, A., Duncan, W., et al. Phase advance of the circadian sleep-waking cycle as an antidepressant. *Science* 206:710–713, 1979.

Weil-Malherbe, H. The biochemistry of the functional psychoses. *Adv. Enzymol.* 29:479–553, 1967.

Weissman, M. M. The psychological treatment of depression. *Arch. Gen. Psychiatry* 36:1261–1269, 1979.

Weller, E. B., Preskorn, S. H., Weller, R. A., and Croskell, M. Childhood depression: Imipramine levels and response. *Psychopharmacol. Bull.* 19:59–62, 1983.

Wells, B. G., and Gelenberg, A. J. Evaluation of maprotiline hydrochloride. *Pharmacotherapy* 1:121–139, 1981.

Williams, R. B., and Sherter, C. Cardiac complications of tricyclic antidepressant therapy. *Ann. Intern. Med.* 74:395–398, 1971.

Wilson, I. C., Prange, A. J., McClane, T. K., et al. Thyroid hormone enhancement of imipramine in non-retarded depressions. *N. Engl. J. Med.* 282:1063–1067, 1970.

Winokur, G., Clayton, P., and Reich, T. *Manic-Depressive Disease.* Mosby, St. Louis, 1970.

Winsberg, B. G., Goldstein, S., Yepes, L. E., and Perel, J. M. Imipramine and electrocardiographic abnormalities in hyperactive children. *Am. J. Psychiatry* 132:542–545, 1975.

Wittenborn, J., Plante, M., Burgess, F., and Maurer, H. Comparison of imipramine, ECT, and placebo in the treatment of depression. *J. Nerv. Ment. Dis.* 135:131–137, 1962.

Wright, G., Galloway, L., Kim, J., Dalton, M., Miller, L., and Stern, W. Bupropion in the long-term treatment of cyclic mood disorders: Mood stabilizing effects. *J. Clin. Psychiatry* 46:22–25, 1985.

Ziegler, V. E., Biggs, J. T., and Wylie, L. T. Doxepin kinetics. *Clin. Pharmacol. Ther.* 23:573–579, 1978.

Zis, A. P., and Goodwin, F. K. Novel antidepressants and the biogenic amine hypothesis of depression. *Arch. Gen. Psychiatry* 36:1097–1107, 1979.

Zis, A., Grof, P., Webster, M., et al. Prediction of relapse in recurrent affective disorders. *Psychopharmacol. Bull.* 16:47–49, 1980.

Zitrin, C. M., Klein, D. F., Woener, M. G., et al. Treatment of phobias: I. Comparison of imipramine hydrochloride and placebo. *Arch. Gen. Psychiatry* 40:125–138, 1983.

Zung, W. Effect of antidepressant drugs on sleeping and dreaming. Proceedings of the Fourth World Congress of Psychiatry, Madrid. In *Excerpta Medica, International Congress Series* 150:1804–1826, 1966.

MAO Inhibitors and Stimulants

Atkinson, R. M., and Ditman, K. S. Tranylcypromine: A review. *Clin. Pharmacol. Ther.* 6:631–655, 1965.

Ayd, F., ed. Combined tricyclic-MAO antidepressant therapy. *Int. Drug Ther. Newsletter* 10:5–7, 1975.

Baldessarini, R. J. Pharmacology of amphetamines. *Pediatrics* 49:694–701, 1972.

——— Treatment of depression by altering monoamine metabolism: Precursors and metabolic inhibitors. *Psychopharmacol. Bull.* 20:224–239, 1984.

Barsa, J., and Sanders, J. C. A comparative study of tranylcypromine and pargyline. *Psychopharmacologia* 6:295–298, 1964.

Bender, L., and Cottington, F. The use of amphetamine sulfate (Benzedrine) in child psychiatry. *Am. J. Psychiatry* 99:116–121, 1942.

Blackwell, B., Marley, E., Price, J., and Taylor, D. Hypertensive interactions between monoamine-oxidase inhibitors. *Brit. J. Psychiatry* 113:349–365, 1967.

Bloch, R., Dooneieff, A., Buchberg, A., and Spellman, S. The clinical effects of isoniazid and iproniazid in the treatment of pulmonary tuberculosis. *Ann. Intern. Med.* 40:881–900, 1954.

Bradley, C. The behavior of children receiving Benzedrine. *Am. J. Psychiatry* 94:577–585, 1937.

Bradley, C., and Bowen, M. Amphetamine (Benzedrine) therapy of children's behavior disorders. *Am. J. Orthopsychiatry* 11:92–103, 1941.

Brumback, R. A., and Weinberg, W. A. Relationship of hyperactivity and depression in children. *Percept. Motor Skills* 45:247–251, 1977.

Conners, C. K. Psychological effects of stimulant drugs in children with minimal brain dysfunction. *Pediatrics* 49:702–708, 1972.

Conners, C. K., Rothschild, G., Eisenberg, L., et al. Dextroamphetamine sulfate in children with learning disorders. *Arch. Gen. Psychiatry* 21:182–190, 1969.

Conners, C. K., Taylor, E., Meo, G., et al. Magnesium pemoline and dextroamphetamine: A controlled study in children with minimal brain dysfunction. *Psychopharmacologia* 26:321–336, 1972.

Crane, G. E. Iproniazid (Marsilid) phosphate: A therapeutic agent for mental disorders and debilitating disease. *Psychiatr. Res. Rep.* 8:142–152, 1957.

Davies, B. E. A pilot study of nialamide at Cambridge. *J. Soc. Genet. Med.* 123:163–172, 1959.

De La Cruz, F. F., Fox, B. H., and Roberts, R. H., eds. Minimal brain dysfunction. *Ann. N.Y. Acad. Sci.* 205:1–396, 1973.

Denckla, M. B., Bemporad, J. R., and MacKay, M. C. Tics following methylphenidate administration: A report of 20 cases. *J.A.M.A.* 235:1349–1351, 1976.

Elsworth, J. D., Glover, V., Reynolds, G. P., et al. Deprenyl administration in man: A selective monoamine oxidase B inhibitor without the "cheese effect." *Psychopharmacology* (Berlin) 57:33–38, 1978.

Evans, D., Davison, K., and Pratt, R. The influence of acetylator phenotype on the effect of treating depression with phenelzine. *Clin. Pharmacol. Ther.* 6:430–435, 1965.

Finberg, J. P. M., and Youdim, M. B. H. Selective MAO A and B inhibitors: Their mechanism of action and pharmacology. *Neuropharmacology* 22(3B):441–446, 1983.

Folks, D. G. Monoamine oxidase inhibitors: Reappraisal of dietary considerations. *J. Clin. Psychopharmacol.* 3:249–252, 1983.

Freeman, R. D. Drug effects on learning in children: A selective review of the past thirty years. *J. Special Ed.* 1:17–44, 1966.

Geller, E., Ritvo, E. R., Freeman, B. J., and Yuwiler, A. Preliminary observations on the effect of fenfluramine on blood serotonin and symptoms in three autistic boys. *N. Engl. J. Med.* 307:165–169, 1982.

Gilbert, J., Donnelly, K. J., Zimmer, L. E., and Kubis, J. F. Effect of magnesium pemoline and methylphenidate on memory improvement and mood in normal aging subjects. *Aging Hum. Devel.* 4:35–51, 1973.

Guilleminault, C., Wilson, R. A., and Dement, W. C. A study on cataplexy. *Arch. Neurol.* 31:225–261, 1974.

Johnstone, E. C., and Marsh, W. Acetylator status and response to phenelzine in depressed patients. *Lancet* 1:567–570, 1973.

Katon, W., Raskind, M. Treatment of depression in the medically ill elderly with methylphenidate. *Am. J. Psychiatry* 137:963–965, 1980.

Kelly, D., Guirguis, W., Frommer, E., et al. Treatment of phobic states with antidepressants. *Brit. J. Psychiatry* 116:387–398, 1970.

Kline, N. S. Clinical experience with iproniazid (Marsilid). *J. Clin. Exp. Psychopathol.* 19 (suppl.):72–78, 1958.

Knoll, J. Analysis of the pharmacological effects of selective monoamine oxidase inhibitors. In *Monoamine Oxidase and Its Inhibition,* ed. G. E. W. Wolstenholme and J. Knight. Elsevier Press, Amsterdam, 1976, pp. 135–161.

Levine, R. J., and Sjoerdsma, A. Estimation of monoamine oxidase activity in man: Techniques and applications. *Ann. N.Y. Acad. Sci.* 107:966–974, 1963.

Levy, B. F. Treatment of hypertension with pargyline hydrochloride. *Curr. Ther. Res.* 8:343–346, 1966.

Liebowitz, M. R., Quitkin, F. M., Stewart, J. W., McGrath, P. J., Harrison, W., Rabkin, J., Tricamo, E., Markowitz, J. S., and Klein, D. F. Phenelzine vs. imipramine in atypical depression. *Arch. Gen. Psychiatry* 41:669–677, 1984.

Lopez-Ibor, A. J., Ayuso-Gutierrez, J. L., and Iglesias, M. L. 5-Hydroxytryptophan (5-HTP) and a MAOI (nialamide) in the treatment of depression: A double-blind controlled study. *Int. Pharmacopsychiatry* 11:8–15, 1976.

Lowe, T. L., Cohen, D. J., Detlor, J., Kremenitzer, M. W., and Shaywitz, B. A. Stimulant medications precipitate Tourette's syndrome. *J.A.M.A.* 247:1729–1731, 1982.

Mann, J. J., Frances, A., Kaplan, R. D., et al. The relative efficacy of L-deprenyl, a selective monoamine oxidase type B inhibitor, in endogenous and non-endogenous depression. *Clin. Psychopharmacol.* 2:54–57, 1982.

Mattes, J. A., and Gittleman, R. Growth of hyperactive children on a maintenance regimen of methylphenidate. *Arch. Gen. Psychiatry* 40:317–321, 1983.

Maxwell, R. A., and White, H. L. Tricyclic and monoamine oxidase inhibitor antidepressants: Structure-activity relationships. In *Handbook of Psychopharmacology,* vol. 14, ed. L. L. Iversen, S. D. Iversen, and S. H. Snyder. Plenum Press, New York, 1978, pp. 83–155.

Mendelwicz, J., and Youdim, M. B. H. Antidepressant potentiation of 5-hydroxytryptophan by L-deprenil in affective illness. *J. Affect. Disord.* 2:137–146, 1980.

———— L-deprenil, a selective monoamine oxidase type B inhibitor in the treatment of depression: A double-blind evaluation. *Brit. J. Psychiatry* 142:509–511, 1983.

Mendis, N., Pare, C. M. B., Sandler, M., et al. Is the failure of (−)deprenyl, a selective monoamine oxidase B inhibitor, to alleviate depression related to freedom from the cheese effect? *Psychopharmacology* 73:87–90, 1981.

Murphy, D. L., Lipper, S., Campbell, I. C., et al. Comparative studies of MAO-B inhibitors in man. In *Monoamine Oxidase: Structure, Function, and Altered Functions,* ed. T. P. Singer, R. W. VonKorff, and D. L. Murphy. Academic Press, New York, 1979, pp. 457–475.

Nelson, J. C., and Byck, R. Rapid response to lithium in phenelzine nonresponders. *Brit. J. Psychiatry* 141:85–86, 1982.

O'Malley, J. E., and Eisenberg, L. The hyperkinetic syndrome. *Semin. Psychiatry* 5:95–103, 1973.

Overall, J. E., Hollister, L. E., Shelton, J., et al. Tranylcypromine compared with dextroamphetamine in hospitalized depressed patients. *Dis. Nerv. Syst.* 27:653–658, 1966.

Page, J. G., Bernstein, J. E., Janicki, R. S., and Michelli, F. A. A multi-clinic trial of pemoline in childhood hyperkinesis. In *Clinical Use of Stimulant Drugs in Children,* ed. C. K. Connors. Excerpta Medica, The Hague, Netherlands, 1974.

Pickar, D., Murphy, D. L., Cohen, R. M., et al. Selective and nonselective monoamine oxidase inhibitors. *Arch. Gen. Psychiatry* 39:535–540, 1982.

Pohl, R., Berchou, R., and Rainey, J. M. Tricyclic antidepressants and monoamine oxidase inhibitors in the treatment of agoraphobia. *J. Clin. Psychopharmacol.* 2:399–407, 1982.

Pollitt, J., and Young, J. Anxiety state or masked depression? A study based on the action of monoamine oxidase inhibitors. *Brit. J. Psychiatry* 119:143–149, 1971.

Post, R. M., Kotin, J., and Goodwin, F. K. The effects of cocaine on depressed patients. *Am. J. Psychiatry* 131:511–517, 1974.

Potter, W. Z., Murphy, D. L., Wehr, T. A., et al. Clorgyline: A new treatment for patients with refractory rapid-cycling disorder. *Arch. Gen. Psychiatry* 39:505–510, 1982.

Quitkin, F., Rifkin, A., and Klein, D. F. Monoamine oxidase inhibitors. *Arch. Gen. Psychiatry* 36:749–759, 1979.

Rabkin, J. G., Quitkin, E. M., McGrath, P., Harrison, W., and Tricamo, E. Adverse reactions to monoamine oxidase inhibitors. *J. Clin. Psychopharmacol.* 5:2–9, 1985.

Rao, D. B., and Norris, J. R. A double-blind investigation of Hydergine in the treatment of cerebrovascular insufficiency in the elderly. *Johns Hopkins Med. J.* 130:317–324, 1972.

Rapoport, J. L., Buchsbaum, M. S., Zahn, T. P., Weingartner, H., Ludlow, C., and Mikkelsen, E. J. Dextroamphetamine: Cognitive and behavioral effects in normal prepubertal boys. *Science* 199:560–563, 1978.

Rapoport, J. L., Quinn, P. O., Bradbard, G., et al. Imipramine and methylphenidate treatments of hyperactive boys. *Arch. Gen. Psychiatry* 30:789–793, 1974.

Raskin, A. Adverse reactions to phenelzine: Results of a nine-hospital depression study. *J. Clin. Pharmacol.* 12:22–25, 1972.

Robinson, D. S., Nies, A., Ravaris, C. L., Ives, J. O., and Bartlett, D. Clinical pharmacology of phenelzine. *Arch. Gen. Psychiatry* 35:629–635, 1978.

Safer, D. J., and Allen, R. P. Factors influencing the suppressant effects of two stimulant drugs on the growth of hyperactive children. *Pediatrics* 51:660–667, 1973.

Satterfield, J. H., Cantwell, D., Saul, R. E., et al. Response to stimulant drug treatment in hyperactive children: Prediction from EEG and neurological findings. *J. Autism Child. Schizo.* 3:36–48, 1973.

Savage, D. D., Mendels, J., and Frazer, A. Monoamine oxidase inhibitors and serotonin uptake inhibitors: Differential effects of [^{3}H]serotonin binding sites in rat brain. *J. Pharmacol. Exp. Ther.* 212:259–263, 1980.

Sethna, E. R. A study of refractory cases of depressive illness and their response to combined antidepressant therapy. *Brit. J. Psychiatry* 124:265–272, 1974.

Singer, T. P., Von Korff, D. W., and Murphy, D. L., eds. *Monoamine Oxidase: Structure, Function and Altered Functions.* Academic Press, New York, 1979.

Sjoqvist, F. Interaction between monoamine oxidase (MAO) inhibitors and other substances. *Proc. R. Soc. Med.* 58:967–978, 1965.

Sleator, E. K., Von Neumann, A., and Sprague, R. L. Hyperactive children: A continuous long-term placebo-controlled follow-up. *J.A.M.A.* 229:316–317, 1974.

Solyon, L., Heseltine, G. F. D., McClure, D. J., et al. Behavior therapy vs. drug therapy in the treatment of phobic neurosis. *Canad. Psychiatr. Assoc. J.* 18:25–31, 1973.

Spiker, D. G., and Pugh, D. D. Combining tricyclic and monoamine oxidase inhibitor antidepressants. *Arch. Gen. Psychiatry* 33:828–830, 1976.

Sprague, R. L., and Sleator, E. K. Effects of psychopharmacologic agents on learning disorders. *Pediatr. Clin. North Am.* 20:719–735, 1973.

——— Methylphenidate in hyperkinetic children: Differences in dose effects on learning and social behavior. *Science* 198:1274–1276, 1977.

Stockley, I. H. Monoamine oxidase inhibitors: I. Interactions with sympathomimetic amines. *Pharmacol. J.* 210:590–594, 1973.

Stotsky, B. A., Cole, J. O., Lu, L. M., and Smiflin, C. A controlled study of the efficacy of pentylenetetrazole in hard-core hospitalized psychogeriatric patients. *Am. J. Psychiatry* 129:387–391, 1972.

Tyrer, P., Candy, J., and Kelly, D. Phenelzine in phobic anxiety: A controlled trial. *Psychol. Med.* 3:120–124, 1973.

——— A study of the clinical effects of phenelzine and placebo in the treatment of phobic anxiety. *Psychopharmacologia* 32:237–254, 1973.

Walsh, B. T., Stewart, J. W., Wright, L., Harrison, W., Roose, S. P., and Glassman, A. H. Treatment of bulimia with monoamine oxidase inhibitors. *Am. J. Psychiatry* 139:1629–1630, 1982.

Wender, P. H. *Minimal Brain Dysfunction in Children.* Wiley-Interscience, New York, 1971.

Wender, P. H., Reimherr, F. W., and Wood, D. R. Attention deficit disorders ("minimal brain dysfunction") in adults: A replication study of diagnosis and drug treatment. *Arch. Gen. Psychiatry* 38:449–456, 1981.

Wharton, R. N., Perel, J. M., Dayton, P. G., and Malitz, S. A potential clinical use for methylphenidate with tricyclic antidepressants. *Am. J. Psychiatry* 127:1619–1625, 1971.

White, K., and Simpson, G. Combined MAOI-tricyclic antidepressant treatment: A reevaluation. *J. Clin. Psychopharmacol.* 1:264–282, 1981.

Winsberg, B. G., Bialer, I., Kupietz, S., and Tobias, J. Effects of imipramine and dextroamphetamine on behavior of neuropsychiatrically impaired children. *Am. J. Psychiatry* 128:1425–1431, 1972.

Wyatt, R. J., Fram, D. H., Buchbinder, R., and Snyder, F. Treatment of intractable narcolepsy with a monoamine oxidase inhibitor. *N. Engl. J. Med.* 285:987–991, 1971.

Antianxiety Agents

Allquander, C. Dependence on sedative and hypnotic drugs. *Acta Psychiatr. Scand.* (suppl.) 270:1–120, 1978.

American Medical Association Committee on Alcoholism and Drug Dependence. Barbiturates and barbiturate-like drugs: Considerations in their medical use. *J.A.M.A.* 230:1440–1441, 1974.

Avant, G. R., Speeg, K. V., Jr., Freemon, F. R., Schenker, S., and Berman, M. L. Physostigmine reversal of diazepam-induced hypnosis. *Ann. Intern. Med.* 91:53–55, 1979.

Balter, M. B., Levine, J., and Manheimer, D. I. Cross-national study of the extent of antianxiety/sedative drug use. *N. Engl. J. Med.* 290:769–774, 1974.

Berger, F. The relation between the pharmacological properties of meprobamate and the clinical usefulness of the drug. In *Psychopharmacology: A Review of*

Progress, 1957–1967, ed. D. H. Efron. U.S. Public Health Service Publication no. 1836, Government Printing Office, Washington, D.C., 1969, pp. 139–152.

Berger, F. M. The pharmacological properties of 2-methyl-2-n-propyl-1,3 propanediol dicarbamate (MILTOWN), a new interneuronal blocking agent. *J. Pharmacol. Exp. Ther.* 112:413–423, 1954.

Blackwell, B. The role of diazepam in medical practice. *J.A.M.A.* 225:1637–1641, 1973.

Braestrup, C., and Squires, R. Specific benzodiazepine receptors in the rat brain characterized by high-affinity ^{3}H-diazepam binding. *Proc. Natl. Acad. Sci. USA* 74:3905–3809, 1977.

Busto, U., Kaplan, H. L., and Sellers, E. M. Benzodiazepine-associated emergencies in Toronto. *Am. J. Psychiatry* 137:226–227, 1980.

Chouinard, G., Annable, L., Fontaine, R., and Solyom, L. Alprazolam in the treatment of generalized anxiety and panic disorders. *Psychopharmacology* 77:229–233, 1982.

Cohen, I. M. The benzodiazepines. In *Discoveries in Biological Psychiatry,* ed. F. J. Ayd and B. Blackwell. J. B. Lippincott, Philadelphia, 1970.

Cole, J. O., Haskell, D. S., and Orzack, M. H. Problems with benzodiazepines: An assessment of the available evidence. *McLean Hosp. J.* 6:46–74, 1981.

Cole, J. O., Orzack, M. H., Beake, B., et al. Assessment of the abuse liability of buspirone in recreational sedative users. *J. Clin. Psychiatry* 43:69–74, 1982.

Covi, L., Lipman, R. S., Pattison, J. H., et al. Length of treatment with anxiolytic sedatives and response to their sudden withdrawal. *Acta Psychiatr. Scand.* 49:51–64, 1973.

Davis, J. M. Minor tranquilizers, sedatives, and hypnotics. In *Comprehensive Textbook of Psychiatry,* ed. H. Kaplan, A. M. Freedman, and B. J. Sadock. Williams and Wilkins, Baltimore, 1980, pp. 2316–2332.

DiMascio, A., Shader, R. I., and Harmatz, J. Psychotropic drugs and induced hostility. *Psychosomatics* 10:46–47, 1969.

Dundee, J. W., McGowan, W. A. W., Lilburn, J. K., et al. Comparison of the actions of diazepam and lorazepam. *Brit. J. Anaesth.* 51:439–446, 1979.

Edwards, J. G. Adverse effects of antianxiety drugs. *Drugs* 22:495–514, 1981.

Essig, C. F. Addiction to non-barbiturate sedative and tranquilizing drugs. *Clin. Pharmacol. Ther.* 5:334–343, 1964.

Fabre, L. F., and McLendon, D. M. A double-blind study comparing the efficacy and safety of alprazolam with diazepam and placebo in anxious outpatients. *Curr. Ther. Res.* 19:661–668, 1976.

Fabre, L. F., McLendon, D. M., and Stephens, A. G. Comparison of the therapeutic effect, tolerance and safety of benzodiazepines administered for several months to outpatients with chronic anxiety neurosis. *J. Int. Med. Res.* 246:1568–1570, 1981.

Finkle, B. S., McCloskey, K. L., and Goodman, L. S. Diazepam and drug-associated deaths: A survey in the United States and Canada. *J.A.M.A.* 242:429–434, 1979.

Garattini, S., Mussini, E., and Randall, L. O., eds. *The Benzodiazepines.* Raven Press, New York, 1973.

Goldberg, H. L., and Finnerty, R. J. A double-blind study of prochlorperazine, chlordiazepoxide and placebo in psychoneurotic outpatients with dominant symptoms of anxiety. *Int. Pharmacopsychiatry* 14:264–277, 1979.

——Comparative efficacy of buspirone and diazepam in the treatment of anxiety. *Am. J. Psychiatry* 136:1184–1187, 1979.

Goldstein, B. J., and Brauzer, B. Pharmacological considerations in the treatment of anxiety and depression in medical practice. *Med. Clin. North Am.* 55:485–494, 1971.

Gottschalk, L. A. Pharmacokinetics of the minor tranquilizers and clinical response. In *Psychopharmacology: A Generation of Progress,* ed. M. A. Lipton, A. DiMascio, and D. F. Killam. Raven Press, New York, 1978, pp. 975–985.

Greenblatt, D. J., and Shader, R. I. Meprobamate: A study of irrational drug use. *Am. J. Psychiatry* 127:1297–1304, 1971.

——*Benzodiazepines in Clinical Practice.* Raven Press, New York, 1974.

——Pharmacotherapy of anxiety with benzodiazepines and beta-adrenergic blockers. In *Psychopharmacology: A Generation of Progress,* ed. M. A. Lipton, A. DiMascio, and K. F. Killam. Raven Press, New York, 1978.

Greenblatt, D. J., Shader, R. I., and Abernethy, D. R. Current status of benzodiazepines. *N. Engl. J. Med.* 309:354–358, 1983.

Hall, R. C. W., and Disook, S. Paradoxical reactions to benzodiazepines. *Brit. J. Clin. Pharmacol.* 11 (suppl 1):99S–104S, 1981.

Hoehn-Saric, R. Neurotransmitters in anxiety. *Arch. Gen. Psychiatry* 39:735–742, 1982.

Hollister, L. E., Conley, F. K., Britt, R. H., and Shuer, L. Long-term use of diazepam. *J.A.M.A.* 246:1568–1570, 1981.

Hollister, L. E., Greenblatt, D. J., Rickels, K., Aud, F. J., and Greiner, G. E. Benzodiazepines: Current update. *Psychosomatics* 21 (suppl. 1):1–32, 1980.

Hunkeler, W., Mohler, H., Pieri, L., Polc, P., Bonetti, E. P., Cumin, R., Schaffner, R., and Haefeley, W. Selective antagonists of benzodiazepines. *Nature* 290:514–516, 1981.

Kalant, H., LeBlanc, A. E., and Gibbons, R. J. Tolerance to and dependence on some nonopiate psychotropic drugs. *Pharmacol. Rev.* 23:135–191, 1971.

Kales, A., Allen, C., Scharf, M. B., and Kales, J. D. Hypnotic drugs and their effectiveness: All night EEG studies of insomniac patients. *Arch. Gen. Psychiatry* 23:226–232, 1970.

Kanto, J. Plasma concentrations of diazepam and its metabolites after peroral, intramuscular, and rectal administration. *Int. J. Clin. Pharmacol.* 12:427–432, 1975.

Kathol, R. G., Noyes, R., Jr., Sylmen, D. J., Crowe, R. R., Clancy, J., and Kerber, R. E. Propranolol in chronic anxiety disorders. *Arch. Gen. Psychiatry* 37:1361–1365, 1980.

Kelly, D., Brown, C. C., and Shafter, J. W. A controlled physiological, clinical and psychological evaluation of chlordiazepoxide. *Brit. J. Psychiatry* 115:1387–1392, 1969.

Lader, M. Minor tranquilizers. In *The Psychiatric Therapies,* part 1: *The Somatic Therapies,* ed. B. Karasu. American Psychiatric Association, Washington, D.C., 1984, pp. 53–84.

Lasagna, L. The role of benzodiazepines in non-psychiatric medical practice. *Am. J. Psychiatry* 134:656–658, 1977.

Linnoila, M., Otterstrom, S., and Antilla, M. Serum chlordiazepoxide, diazepam, and thioridazine concentrations after the simultaneous ingestion of alcohol or placebo drink. *Ann. Clin. Res.* 6:4–6, 1974.

Mandelli, M., Tognoni, G., and Garattini, S. Clinical pharmacokinetics of diazepam. *Clin. Pharmacokinet.* 3:72–91, 1978.

Matthew, H., ed. *Acute Barbiturate Poisoning.* Excerpta Medica, Amsterdam, 1971.

McDonall, A., Owen, S., and Robin, A. A. A controlled comparison of diazepam and amylobarbitone in anxiety states. *Brit. J. Psychiatry* 112:629–631, 1966.

McNair, D. M. Antianxiety drugs and human performance. *Arch. Gen. Psychiatry* 29:609–617, 1973.

Mellinger, G. D., and Balter, M. B. Prevalence and patterns of use of psychotherapeutic drugs: Results of a 1979 national survey of American adults. In *Proceedings of the International Seminar on the Epidemiological Impact of Psychotropic Drugs,* ed. G. Tognoni, C. Bellantuono, and M. Lader. Elsevier/North Holland Press, Amsterdam, 1981, pp. 117–135.

Mennini, T., and Garattini, S. Benzodiazepine receptors: Correlation with pharmacological responses in living animals. *Life Sciences* 31:2025–2035, 1982.

Mishara, B. L., and Kastenbaum, R. Wine in the treatment of long-term geriatric patients in mental institutions. *J. Am. Geriatr. Soc.* 22:88–94, 1974.

Paul, S., Skolnick, J., Tallman, J., and Usdin, E., eds. *Pharmacology of Benzodiazepines.* Macmillan, New York, 1983.

Petersen, R. C., and Ghoneim, M. M. Diazepam and human memory: Influence on acquisition, retrieval, and state-dependent learning. *Prog. Neuropsychopharmacol.* 4:81–89, 1980.

Petursson, H., and Lader, M. H. Withdrawal from long-term benzodiazepine treatment. *Brit. Med. J.* 283:643–645, 1981.

Rickels, K. Benzodiazepines in the treatment of anxiety: North American experiences. In *The Benzodiazepines: From Molecular Biology to Clinical Practice,* ed. E. Costa. Raven Press, New York, 1983, pp. 295–310.

Rickels, K., Downing, R. W., and Winokur, A. Antianxiety drugs: Clinical use in psychiatry. In *Handbook of Psychopharmacology,* vol. 13, ed. L. L. Iversen, S. D. Iversen, and S. H. Snyder. Plenum Press, New York, 1978, pp. 395–430.

Rickels, K., Weisman, K., Norstad, D. O., et al. Buspirone and diazepam in anxiety: A controlled study. *J. Clin. Psychiatry* 43:81–86, 1982.

Rosenbaum, J. F. The drug treatment of anxiety. *N. Engl. J. Med.* 306:401–404, 1982.

Safra, M. J., and Oakley, G. P., Jr. Association between cleft lip with or without cleft palate and prenatal exposure to diazepam. *Lancet* 2:478–480, 1975.

Sepinwall, J., and Cook, L. Behavioral pharmacology of antianxiety drugs. In *Handbook of Psychopharmacology,* vol. 13, ed. L. L. Iversen, S. D. Iversen, and S. H. Snyder. Plenum Press, New York, 1978, pp. 345–393.

Shader, R. I., Goodman, M., and Gever, J. Panic disorders: Current perspectives. *J. Clin. Psychopharmacol.* 2 (suppl.):2–10, 1982.

Shader, R. I., and Greenblatt, D. J. Clinical implications of benzodiazepine pharmacokinetics. *Am. J. Psychiatry* 134:652–656, 1977.

Sheehan, D. V. Panic attacks and phobias. *N. Engl. J. Med.* 307:156–158, 1980.

Sheehan, D. V., Ballenger, J., and Jacobsen, G. Treatment of endogenous anxiety with phobic, hysterical and hypochondriacal symptoms. *Arch. Gen. Psychiatry* 36:51–59, 1980.

Skolnick, P., and Paul, S. M. Benzodiazepine receptors in the central nervous system. *Intl. Rev. Neurobiol.* 23:103–140, 1982.

Solomon, K., and Hart, R. Pitfalls and prospects in clinical research on anti-anxiety drugs: Benzodiazepines and placebo—A research review. *J. Clin. Psychiatry* 39:823–831, 1978.

Spier, S. A., Tesar, G. E., Rosenbaum, J. F., and Woods, S. W. Clonazepam in the treatment of panic disorder and agoraphobia. *J. Clin. Psychiatry* (in press).

Sternbach, L. H. Chemistry of 1,5-benzodiazepines and some aspects of the structure-activity relationship. In *The Benzodiazepines*, ed. S. Garattini, E. Mussini, and L. O. Randall. Raven Press, New York, 1973, pp. 1–26.

Study, R. E., and Barker, J. L. Cellular mechanisms of benzodiazepine action. *J.A.M.A.* 247:2147–2151, 1982.

Tallman, J. F., Paul, S. M., Skolnick, P., and Gallager, D. W. Receptors for the age of anxiety: Pharmacology of the benzodiazepines. *Science* 207:274–281, 1980.

Taylor, R. L., Maurer, J. E., and Tinklenberg, J. R. Management of "bad trips" in an evolving drug scene. *J.A.M.A.* 213:422–425, 1970.

Tyrer, P. J. Use of beta-blocking drugs in psychiatry and neurology. *Drugs* 20:300–308, 1980.

Winstead, D. K., Anderson, A., Eilers, M. K., et al. Diazepam on demand: Drug-seeking behavior in psychiatric inpatients. *Arch. Gen. Psychiatry* 30:349–351, 1974.

Yamamura, H. I., ed. The mechanism of action of the benzodiazepines. *Fed. Proc.* 39:3016–3055, 1980.

Drug Interactions and Toxicology

Alexander, C. S., and Nino, A. Cardiovascular complications in young patients taking psychotropic drugs. *Am. Heart J.* 78:757–769, 1969.

American Pharmaceutical Association. *Evaluations of Drug Interactions,* 2nd ed. American Pharmaceutical Association, Washington, D.C., 1976.

Ban, T. A. Drug interactions with psychoactive drugs. *Dis. Nerv. Syst.* 36:164–166, 1975.

Boston Collaborative Drug Surveillance Program: Reserpine and breast cancer. *Lancet* 2:669–671, 1974.

Bourne, P. G., ed. *A Treatment Manual for Acute Drug Abuse Emergencies.* National Clearinghouse for Drug Abuse Information, Rockville, Md., 1974.

Breckenridge, A., and Orme, M. Clinical implications of enzyme induction. *Ann. N.Y. Acad. Sci.* 179:421–431, 1971.

Briant, R. H., Reid, J. L., and Dollery, C. T. Interaction between clonidine and desipramine in man. *Brit. Med. J.* 1:522–523, 1973.

Caranasos, G. J., Stewart, R. B., and Cluff, L. E. Drug-induced illness leading to hospitalization. *J.A.M.A.* 228:713–717, 1974.

Cohen, S. N., and Armstrong, M. F. *Drug Interactions: A Handbook for Clinical Use.* Williams and Wilkins, Baltimore, 1974.

Conney, A. H. Pharmacological implications of microsomal enzyme induction. *Pharmacol. Rev.* 19:317–366, 1967.

Davis, J. M., Bartlett, E., and Termini, B. Overdosage of psychotropic drugs: A review. *Dis. Nerv. Syst.* 29:157–164, 246–256, 1968.

Davis, J. M., Sekerke, J., and Janowsky, D. S. Drug interactions involving the drugs of abuse. *Drug Intel. Clin. Pharm.* 8:120–142, 1974.

El-Yousef, M. K., Janowsky, D. S., Davis, J. M., and Sekerke, H. J. Reversal of antiparkinsonian drug toxicity by physostigmine: A controlled study. *Am. J. Psychiatry* 130:141–145, 1973.

Fann, W. E. Some clinically important interactions of psychotropic drugs. *South. Med. J.* 66:661–665, 1973.

Formiller, M., and Cohon, M. S. Coumarin and indanedione anticoagulants: Potentiators and antagonists. *Am. J. Hosp. Pharm.* 26:574–582, 1969.

Garg, S. *Clinical Guide to Undesirable Drug Interactions and Interferences.* Springer, New York, 1973.

Glasscote, R., Sussex, J. N., Jaffe, J. H., et al. *The Treatment of Drug Abuse.* American Psychiatric Association, Washington, D.C., 1972.

Gram, L. F., and Overo, K. F. Drug interaction: Inhibitory effect of neuroleptics on metabolism of tricyclic antidepressants in man. *Brit. Med. J.* 1:463–465, 1972.

Granacher, R. P., and Baldessarini, R. J. The usefulness of physostigmine in neurology and psychiatry. In *Clinical Neuropharmacology,* vol. 1, ed. H. L. Klawans. Raven Press, New York, 1976, pp. 63–79.

Greenblatt, D. J., and Shader, R. I. Drug abuse and the emergency room physician. *Am. J. Psychiatry* 131:559–562, 1974.

Griffen, J. P., and D'Arcy, P. F. *A Manual of Adverse Drug Interactions.* J. Wright and Sons, Bristol, 1975.

Hansten, P. D. *Drug Interactions,* 3rd ed. Lea & Febiger, Philadelphia, 1975.

Hollister, L. E. Adverse reactions to psychotherapeutic drugs. In *Drug Treatment of Mental Disorders,* ed. L. L. Simpson. Raven Press, New York, 1976, pp. 267–288.

Hurwitz, N. Predisposing factors in adverse reactions to drugs. *Brit. Med. J.* 1:536–539, 1969.

Janowsky, D. S., El-Yousef, M. K., Davis, J. M., and Fann, W. E. Guanethidine antagonism by antipsychotic drugs. *J. Tenn. Med. Assoc.* 65:620–622, 1972.

Jick, H. Drugs—remarkably non-toxic. *N. Engl. J. Med.* 291:824–828, 1974.

Kaufmann, J. S. Drug interactions involving psychotherapeutic agents. In *Drug Treatment of Mental Disorders,* ed. L. L. Simpson. Raven Press, New York, 1976, pp. 289–309.

Kline, N. S., Alexander, S. F., and Chamberlain, A. *Psychotropic Drugs: A Manual for Emergency Management of Overdosage.* Medical Economics, Oradell, N.J., 1974.

Kuntzman, R. Drugs and enzyme induction. *Ann. Rev. Pharmacol.* 9:21–36, 1969.

Lemberger, L. Clinically important antihypertensive drug interactions. *Drug Therapy* 49–55, December 1974.

Lennard, H. L., Epstein, L. J., Bernstein, A., and Ransom, D. C. Hazards implicit in prescribing psychoactive drugs. *Science* 169:438–441, 1970.

Lilienfeld, A. M., Chang, L., Thomas, C. B., and Levin, M. L. Rauwolfia derivatives and breast cancer. *Johns Hopkins Med. J.* 139:41–50, 1975.

Linnoila, M., Mattila, M. J., and Kitchell, B. S. Drug interactions with alcohol. *Drugs* 18:299–311, 1979.

Lubran, M. The effects of drugs on laboratory values. *Med. Clin. North Am.* 53:211–222, 1969.

Mack, T. M., Henderson, B. E., Gerkins, V. R., et al. Reserpine and breast cancer in a retirement community. *N. Engl. J. Med.* 292:1366–1371, 1975.

Marsden, C. D., Tarsy, D., and Baldessarini, R. J. Spontaneous and drug-induced movement disorders in psychiatric patients. In *Psychiatric Aspects of Neurologic Disease,* ed. D. F. Benson and D. Blumer. Grune and Stratton, New York, 1975, pp. 219–265.

Martin, E. W. *Hazards of Medication.* Lippincott, Philadelphia, 1971.

Miller, R. R. Hospital admissions due to adverse drug reactions: A report from the Boston Collaborative Drug Surveillance Program. *Arch. Intern. Med.* 134:219–223, 1974.

Morselli, P. L., Cohen, S. N., and Garattini, S., eds. *Drug Interactions.* Raven Press, New York, 1974.

Nies, A. S. Drug interactions. *Med. Clin. North Am.* 58:965–975, 1974.

Raisfeld, I. H. Clinical pharmacology of drug interactions. *Ann. Rev. Med.* 24:385–418, 1973.

Raskind, M. A. Psychosis, polydipsia and water intoxication. *Arch. Gen. Psychiatry* 30:112–114, 1974.

Sayers, A. C., and Burki, H. R. Antiacetylcholine activities of psychoactive drugs: A comparison of the [^{3}H]quinuclidinylbenzilate binding assay with conventional methods. *J. Pharm. Pharmacol.* 28:252–253, 1976.

Scientific Review Subpanel on Psychotherapeutic Agents. *Evaluation of Drug Interactions.* American Pharmaceutical Association, Washington, D.C., 1973.

Seidl, L. G., Thornton, F., Smith, J. W., and Cluff, L. E. Studies on the epidemiology of adverse drug reactions: III. Reactions in patients on a general medical service. *Bull. Johns Hopkins Hosp.* 119:229–315, 1966.

Seppala, T., Linnoila, M., Elonen, E., Mattita, M. J., and Maki, M. Effect of tricyclic antidepressants and alcohol on psychomotor skills related to driving. *Clin. Pharmacol. Ther.* 17:515–522, 1975.

Shader, R. I., ed. *Psychiatric Complications of Medical Drugs.* Raven Press, New York, 1972.

Shader, R. I., and DiMascio, A., eds. *Psychotropic Drug Side Effects: Clinical and Theoretical Perspectives.* Williams and Wilkins, Baltimore, 1970.

Sher, S. P. Drug enzyme induction and drug interactions: Literature tabulation. *Toxicol. Appl. Pharmacol.* 18:780–834, 1973.

Sigg, E. B. Autonomic side-effects induced by psychotherapeutic agents. In *Psychopharmacology: A Review of Progress, 1957–1967,* ed. D. H. Efron, J. O. Cole, J. Levine, and J. R. Wittenborn. Government Printing Office, Washington, D.C., 1968, pp. 581–588.

Swidler, G. *Handbook of Drug Interactions.* Wiley-Interscience, New York, 1971.

Wilkinson, G. R. Treatment of drug intoxication: A review of some scientific principles. *Clin. Toxicol.* 3:249–265, 1970.

Index

"Tricyclics." *See* Antidepressants; Antipsychotics
Tryptophan, 223–226
TSH. *See* Thyroid-stimulating hormone
Tybamate, 235
Tyramine, 210, 214

Ulcer. *See* Peptic ulcer
Uptake. *See* Amines

Valium. *See* Diazepam
Valproic acid, 127

Vasodilators, 271–275
Vasopressin, 273
Verapamil, 91, 129

Wellbutrin. *See* Bupropion
Withdrawal, 257
Withdrawal-emergent dyskinesias, 79
Withholding treatment, 293

Xanax. *See* Alprazolam; Benzodiazepines

Zimelidine, 227